Control of Hospital Infection

Fourth edition

Control of Hospital Infection

Infection

A practical handbook

Fourth edition

Edited by

Graham A J Ayliffe MD FRCPath

Emeritus Professor of Medical Microbiology, University of Birmingham; Honorary Consultant and former Director, Hospital Infection Research Laboratory, City Hospital NHS Trust, Birmingham

Adam P Fraise MB BS FRCPath

Consultant Medical Microbiologist and Director, Hospital Infection Research Laboratory, City Hospital NHS Trust, Birmingham

Alasdair M Geddes CBE, FRCP (Ed and Lond), FRCPath, FFPHM

Professor of Infection, University of Birmingham; Consultant Physician, University Hospital NHS Trust, Birmingham and former Consultant Adviser in Infectious Diseases, Department of Health, London

The late Kathy Mitchell RGN

Clinical Nurse Specialist in Infection Control, City Hospital NHS Trust, Birmingham

A member of the Hodder Headline Group
LONDON
Co-published in the USA by Oxford University Press Inc., New York

First published in Great Britain in 2000 by
Arnold, a member of the Hodder Headline Group,
338 Euston Road, London NW1 3BH

http://www.arnoldpublishers.com

Co-published in the USA by
Oxford University Press Inc.,
198 Madison Avenue, New York, NY10016
Oxford is a registered trademark of Oxford University Press

British Library Cataloguing in Publication Data
A catalogue record for this book is available from the British Library

Library of Congress Cataloging-in-Publication Data
A catalog record for this book is available from the Libary of Congress

ISBN 0 340 75911 9

1 2 3 4 5 6 7 8 9 10

Commissioning Editor: Georgina Bentliff
Production Editor: James Rabson
Production Controller: Iain McWilliams
Cover designer: Terry Griffiths

Typeset in 10/13pt Sabon by Saxon Graphics Ltd, Derby.
Printed and bound in Great Britain by MPG Books Ltd, Bodmin.

CONTENTS

LIST OF CONTRIBUTORS

Graham A J Ayliffe Emeritus Professor of Medical Microbiology, University of Birmingham; Honorary Consultant and former Director, Hospital Infection Research Laboratory, City Hospital NHS Trust, Birmingham

John Babb Laboratory Manager, Hospital Infection Research Laboratory, City Hospital NHS Trust, Birmingham

Iain Blair Consultant in Communicable Disease Control, Sandwell Health Authority

Christina Bradley Senior Biomedical Scientist, Hospital Infection Research Laboratory, City Hospital NHS Trust, Birmingham

Nigel Cripps Principal Engineer, Estates Business Agency, Coventry

Rebecca Evans Clinical Nurse Specialist – Infection Control, City Hospital NHS Trust, Birmingham

Adam P Fraise Consultant Medical Microbiologist and Director, Hospital Infection Research Laboratory, City Hospital NHS Trust, Birmingham

Alasdair M Geddes Professor of Infection, University of Birmingham, Consultant Physician, University Hospital NHS Trust, Birmingham and former Consultant Adviser in Infectious Diseases, Department of Health, London

Richard H George Consultant Microbiologist, Children's Hospital, Birmingham

The late Kathy Mitchell Clinical Nurse Specialist in Infection Control, City Hospital NHS Trust, Birmingham

Deenan Pillay Consultant Medical Virologist, Birmingham Public Health Laboratory and University of Birmingham Medical School

PREFACE TO FOURTH EDITION

This handbook was first produced as infection control guidance for the West Midlands Region of the UK in the early 1970s. The first edition, published in 1975, was widely used throughout the UK and many other countries. The original contributors were mainly microbiologists, surgeons and physicians from the Midlands, and the original editors, Edward Lowbury, Graham Ayliffe, Alasdair Geddes and David Williams continued to edit and contribute to the recommendations in the second and third editions. For this fourth edition, Professors Lowbury and Williams decided to retire and were replaced by Adam Fraise and Kathy Mitchell. Kathy who was a Clinical Nurse Specialist in Infection Control, was highly enthusiastic about her involvement in a new edition with more nursing input. Sadly, she died suddenly last year and was unable to complete the task. Her final contribution was greatly missed. We are grateful to Rebecca Evans for her comments on the nursing aspects.

The basic techniques and problems of prevention of infection are mainly similar to those described in previous editions, but clinical techniques have progressed and some 'new' and 'old' infections have emerged or re-emerged as major problems.

The increased use of heat-labile equipment, particularly flexible fibre-optic endoscopes, has highlighted the necessity for effective decontamination methods. New disinfectants and sterilizing technologies have emerged and are being assessed to replace glutaraldehyde, which has continued to cause irritant reactions and hypersensitivity in staff, unless adequate ventilation equipment and safe working practices are in place. The importance of cleaning medical and other equipment continues to be stressed, and automated washing machines have provided improved standards of cleaning and staff safety.

The problems of bloodborne viruses (hepatitis B and C and HIV) continue to influence hospital practice, and guidance on preventing transmission to and from health-care workers has been published by government agencies in most countries. 'Universal' precautions or 'body substance isolation' techniques are accepted as important by most infection control staff. However, they are expensive and the efficacy of using gloves as a substitute for handwashing has not been substantiated. Nevertheless, contaminated needles and sharp instrument injuries are a potential hazard to staff, and the implementation of good handling and disposal techniques is essential.

One of the major problems world-wide is the increase in antibiotic-resistant strains of bacteria, mainly in hospitals, but also in the community and in animal husbandry. Epidemic strains of methicillin-resistant *Staphylococcus aureus* (MRSA) have spread in hospitals in most countries, and have proved difficult to control without considerable resources and expenditure. The reports of vancomycin-resistant strains are particularly worrying. Strains of glycopeptide-resistant enterococci (GRE) (often referred to as vancomycin-resistant enterococci or VRE), which produce β-lactamase and are resistant to high levels of aminoglycosides, are particularly difficult to treat. These are also starting to spread more widely in hospitals. Highly resistant strains of Gram-negative bacilli also continue to spread in hospitals, and outbreaks of *Clostridium difficile* remain common in elderly care units. Highly resistant strains of *Mycobacterium tuberculosis* are causing therapy problems in many parts of the world, particularly in developing countries, and isolation facilities for patients with resistant organisms are often inadequate.

The possibility of reducing resistance by controlling the use of antibiotics is a logical approach, but so far the implementation of effective policies has proved difficult in most situations. Clinicians are loath to restrict the use of any effective antibiotic in the treatment of individual patients. Infection control techniques can have a greater initial influence on the spread of resistant organisms in hospitals, and are easier to implement. However, a combined approach of antibiotic restriction, effective surveillance and good infection control practices is essential if antibiotic resistance is to be overcome.

The costs of hospital care have increased considerably, and the use of evidence-based guidelines and the elimination of rituals applies as much to infection control as to other aspects of care. Claims for negligence in many countries are now very high and they redirect urgently needed funds away from patient care. Improvements in quality control, the use of audits and risk assessment are therefore being encouraged by most governments. The effect of these methods on patient outcome (e.g. infection rates) is an obvious criterion for administrators wishing to demonstrate the quality of their services. Surveillance of infection alone can reduce infection but, depending on the method chosen, it can also provide useful information on infection rates. However, the use of rates to compare the incidence of infection in different hospitals is still rarely possible due to the problem of correcting for risk factors and the early discharge of patients from hospital. Patient care in hospitals and the community is becoming more closely integrated, and the community section in this book has been expanded in order to address administrative structure, outbreaks of infection and the particular problems of infection control in the community.

In recent years, Directives and many Standards have emerged from the European Union, as well as guidelines from government agencies and professional organizations. European legislation and standards represent a consensus of opinion from many countries, often with different infection control philosophies, and they may not be appropriate throughout Europe or elsewhere. Many of these regulations and guidelines have been referenced in this book, but these recommendations are not necessarily endorsed where they are considered to be inappropriate. It is hoped that the book will continue to be of interest and useful to infection control workers in all countries. Infection control staff should make their own assessments based, where possible, on scientific evidence or on knowledge of the behaviour of micro-organisms in the patient and in the environment. The safety of patients and staff is the main consideration, and all hospitals should have an infection control manual based (where relevant) on national guidelines.

This book is intended as a practical guide and is not a comprehensive textbook. All of the chapters have been revised and updated where necessary. Only a limited number of references have been included in each chapter, but a more general bibliography has been provided at the end of the book. For more information, the reader is referred to specialist journals on hospital infection, such as the *Journal of Hospital Infection, Infection Control* and *Hospital Epidemiology,* and the *American Journal of Infection Control*, and to larger textbooks and books on policies and guidelines.

This handbook has been prepared as a guide for use mainly by hospital staff. It is intended for infection control staff, other doctors and nurses, physiotherapists, radiographers and others involved in the treatment and care of patients. It will also be useful in part for administrators, architects, engineers, pharmacists, sterile services staff, domestic and catering managers and others whose work may influence the risk of infection among patients and staff.

ACKNOWLEDGEMENTS

We should like to thank Norman Hicks, Sterile Services Manager, and Andrew Barnes, formerly Quality Control Pharmacist, from the City Hospital NHS Trust, Birmingham, for their helpful comments.

We should also like to thank John Gowar, Consultant Surgeon, Plastic Surgery and Burns Unit and Alasdair Robertson, Consultant Physician, Occupational Health Department, both from the University Hospital Birmingham NHS Trust, Birmingham, as well as Neil Rowe, Solicitor, for comments on the legal section, and the members of the original working party who are listed in the first and second editions of the book. We would also particularly like to thank Marie Baxter for typing the manuscript.

chapter 1

INTRODUCTION

DEFINITIONS

The term *infection* is generally used to refer to the deposition and multiplication of bacteria and other micro-organisms in tissues or on surfaces of the body with an associated tissue reaction. If the response of the host is slight or absent, it is usually termed *colonization*. A carriage site is a normal area of skin or mucous membrane (e.g. nose) in which organisms are multiplying, but without any host response. *Sepsis* is the presence of inflammation, pus formation and other signs of illness in wounds colonized by micro-organisms, and in tissues to which such infection has spread. Other types of infective illness are described by terms which refer to the site of infection (e.g. tonsillitis, peritonitis, gastroenteritis, pneumonia), or to the specific disease when this is distinctive (e.g. tuberculosis, measles, tetanus). The term *contamination* refers to the soiling of inanimate objects or living material with harmful, potentially infectious or unwanted matter.

Hospital (or *'nosocomial'*) *infection* is infection acquired either by patients while they are in hospital, or by members of hospital staff. The term *hospital-acquired infection* (HAI) is sometimes used, and this may be associated with sepsis or other forms of infective illness, either in hospital or after the patient has returned home. *Cross- or exogenous infection* means infection acquired in hospital from other people, either patients or staff. *Self- (or endogenous) infection* refers to infection caused by microbes which the patient carries on normal or septic areas of his or her own body (normal bacterial flora), including organisms which these areas have acquired in hospital (e.g. self-infection supervening on cross-infection or on infection from the environment).

For obvious reasons, all infections of operation wounds are hospital infections. However, in other sites, it is often impossible to say whether an infection was acquired by the patient in hospital or before he or she came into hospital. The term *hospital-associated infection* has been used to cover such infections, as well as those acquired in hospital.

A *source* of hospital infection may be defined as a place where *pathogenic* (i.e. potentially disease-producing) micro-organisms are growing or have grown, and from which they are transmitted to patients (e.g. an infected wound, the nose or faeces of a carrier, contaminated food, contaminated solutions). A *reservoir* is a place where pathogens can survive or sometimes grow outside the body and from which they could be transferred – directly or indirectly – to patients (e.g. static equipment, furniture, floors). Although the term is sometimes used inter-changeably with the term *source*, it is usually accepted that the source is the part of the reservoir which provides organisms that infect or colonize one or more patients. A *vehicle* is a mobile object which can carry pathogenic organisms to a patient (e.g. dust particles, bedpans, blankets, toys, etc.). The word *vector* is commonly used interchangeably with vehicle, but it is sometimes used in the specialized sense of an insect which carries pathogenic micro-organisms (i.e. an *insect vector*), and should probably be restricted to this usage. These categories overlap. For example, a fluid in which bacteria multiply may be a vehicle as well as a source of infection, and will have acquired the organism from some antecedent source (e.g. a patient with pseudomonas infection).

THE IMPORTANCE OF HOSPITAL INFECTION

Prevalence surveys of hospital infection in many countries have shown that about 1 in 10 patients in hospital have acquired an infection, and a similar number of infections are acquired in the community (e.g. Meers *et al.*, 1981; Maryon-White *et al.*, 1988, Emmerson *et al.*, 1996). The main acquired infections are those of the urinary tract, surgical wounds, lower respiratory tract and skin. The frequency and severity vary with the age of the patient, the type of operation in surgical cases, the duration of catheterization (urinary and vascular), immunosuppressive treatment and other factors. It is necessary to take these 'risk' factors into account when comparing the incidence or prevalence of infection in different hospitals, and in the prediction of expected infection in individual patients or wards in hospitals (Emmerson and Ayliffe, 1996).

The *prevalence* rate is the proportion of a defined group that has an infection at any one point in time. The *incidence* rate is the proportion of a defined group that develops an infection within a stated period, and is lower than the prevalence rate. The incidence of hospital-acquired infection is about 5%. This continuous and apparently universal, although variable incidence is described as *endemic* infection. However, there is sometimes a large increase in the commonly occurring types of infection (e.g. post-operative wound sepsis) or the appearance of infection of a type that is not normally present in the hospital (e.g. salmonella infections in babies, or pseudomonas infections after eye surgery); this is called *epidemic* infection. Typing by serological, bacteriophage, bacteriocine or the newer molecular methods shows that epidemic infection is usually due to a single type, which can often be traced to a source (e.g. a carrier of a virulent strain of *Staphylococcus aureus,* or a solution contaminated with *Pseudomonas aeruginosa).* If aseptic and hygienic infection control measures in a hospital break down, the frequency of infection caused by multiple types of bacteria (i.e. *endemic* infection as defined above) may be increased to epidemic proportions.

The importance of hospital infection can be considered in terms of both the patient's illness and the prolonged occupancy of hospital beds. Illness due to hospital infection is now rarely a cause of death, although this may occur in patients with poor resistance (e.g. those with extensive burns or multi-system failure) or from highly pathogenic organisms (e.g. some strains of hepatitis B virus). The cost of a prolonged stay is a convenient measure of the cost of infection, as it equates to a reduction in the number of beds available to fulfil contracts and reduce waiting-lists (Daschner, 1989).

Additional costs may include consumables such as wound-care dressings and antibiotics. Estimates of the mean number of extra in-patient days in hospital range from 2 to 24, with costs per patient ranging from £250 to £3000 (Coello *et al.*, 1993; Department of Health, 1995). The overall reduction in length of stay means that many patients who would previously have been treated for an infection in hospital will now be treated in the community. This will increase the costs of medical and nursing care in the community. Other more personal 'costs' include the emotional and psychological trauma to the patient and their family, loss of income and the cost of financial support.

FACTORS INVOLVED IN HOSPITAL INFECTION

The occurrence and effects of hospital infection depend largely on the following factors:
1 the micro-organisms;
2 the host (patients and staff);
3 the environment;
4 treatment.

THE MICRO-ORGANISMS

Although virtually any infection may be acquired by patients or staff in hospital, there are certain pathogenic organisms which are particularly likely to be associated with hospital infection, and some which rarely cause infection in other environments. Their role as a cause of hospital infection depends both on their *pathogenicity* or *virulence* (the ability of the species or strain to cause disease) and on their numbers. It also depends on the patient's defences, and as many patients in hospital have lowered resistance because of their disease or treatment, organisms which are relatively harmless to healthy people may cause disease in hospital. Such 'opportunistic' organisms (e.g. *Pseudomonas aeruginosa)* are usually resistant to many antibiotics and able to flourish under conditions in which most disease-producing organisms cannot multiply. In surgical wound infection, Gram-negative bacilli, particularly *Escherichia coli*, play a predominant role, but *Staphylococcus aureus* is still of major importance in clean surgery. *Staphylococcus epidermidis* infections have been increasing, particularly in cases of prosthetic implant surgery, vascular catheterisation and leukaemia, and in premature neonates. Haemolytic streptococci of Group A (*Streptococcus pyogenes*), which were formerly a much feared cause of invasive and rapidly fatal wound infection, are now a relatively infrequent cause of wound or burn infection and have remained fully sensitive to penicillin. However, despite its apparently diminished invasiveness, *Streptococcus pyogenes* is more likely to cause the complete failure of skin grafts than other bacteria if it gains access to full-skin-thickness burns, and it is still an occasional cause of septicaemia and death. Over the last few years streptococcal necrotizing fasciitis has received considerable publicity, although it is doubtful whether the number of cases has increased.

Tetanus and gas gangrene are dangerous infections, but they are very rare, despite the fact that the bacteria which cause them are commonly found in dust and human faeces. Their anaerobic growth requirements make it difficult or impossible for these organisms to colonize tissues that have a good blood supply or are exposed to the air. A group of anaerobes that are more commonly responsible for clinical infection in hospital consists of the family of non-sporing anaerobic bacilli, including *Bacteroides* species. These organisms are normal inhabitants of the large intestine, where they greatly outnumber *E. coli* and other aerobes. In lower intestinal operations, *Bacteroides fragilis* has recently been recognized as a major pathogen, often causing peritonitis and wound infection together with aerobic organisms. Concurrent growth of aerobic organisms in the wound may increase the risks of anaerobic infection by reducing the oxygen content of the tissues. In highly susceptible patients, such as those who have had transplants, those infected with the human immunodeficiency virus (HIV) and those requiring prolonged immunosuppressive treatment, certain atypical mycobacteria (e.g. *Mycobacterium avium-intracellulare*), fungi (e.g. *Candida albicans,* aspergilli and *Cryptococcus neoformans*), viruses (e.g. herpes simplex and cytomegalovirus) and protozoa (e.g. *Pneumocystis carinii*) are a cause of severe and often fatal infections. Cryptosporidia are a cause of severe diarrhoea in patients with HIV infection. Arthropod parasites (e.g. itch mites, scabies and lice) may also be transmitted in hospital.

Other organisms that are occasionally responsible for hospital infection include bloodborne viruses, e.g. hepatitis B (HBV), hepatitis C (HCV) and human immunodeficiency virus (HIV). Prions (agents that cause Creutzfeld-Jacob disease and human BSE) are a potential but very rare blood borne hazard. Ebola, Lassa and other haemorrhagic viral infections have spread in hospitals, but as yet are not a major problem outside sub-Saharan Africa. Outbreaks of infection (epidemic infection) may be caused by the agents of specific infectious diseases, usually due to the admission of an infected patient or the presence of a carrier in the ward. These may be viral infections (e.g. varicella, respiratory syncytical virus and rotavirus) usually in paediatric wards. Food-poisoning outbreaks, especially those due to *Salmonella*, have been responsible for large outbreaks in hospitals (Department of Health and Social Security, 1986a), but are usually less of a problem than such outbreaks in the community. Verotoxin-producing strains of *E. coli* (*E. coli* 0157-H7) have caused an increasing number of outbreaks, mainly in the community, and have been associated with severe infections, especially in the elderly. However, outbreaks of hospital infection are often caused by transmissible strains of antibiotic-resistant organisms (e.g. methicillin-resistant *Staphylococcus aureus* (MRSA), vancomycin-resistant enterococci (VRE) and highly resistant Gram-negative bacilli such as *Enterobacter* and *Klebsiella* species). They may also occur as a result of exceptional errors in asepsis or sterile supply (e.g. infection by Gram-negative bacilli due to contamination of eyedrops or infusion fluids).

THE HOST (PATIENT OR MEMBER OF STAFF)

The susceptibility of the host and the virulence of the micro-organisms are independent variables which have the same relevance to infection as do the qualities of soil and seed in agriculture.

A patient may have poor general resistance (e.g. in infancy, before antibodies have been formed and when the tissues that produce antibodies are imperfectly developed), or poor resistance may be associated with disease (e.g. uncontrolled diabetes, leukaemia or severe burns), with poor nutrition or with certain forms of treatment (e.g. the use of immunosuppressive drugs given to prevent the rejection of transplanted organs or in the chemotherapy of cancer). General resistance may also be reduced by infection, the extreme example of this being HIV infection.

The patient may also have poor local resistance because of an imperfect blood supply to the tissues, or because of the presence of dead tissue or blood clot in which bacteria can grow without interference from the natural defences. Foreign bodies, including sutures and prostheses, also increase the susceptibility of the tissues to local sepsis. Surgical operations and instrumentation (e.g. catheterization) allow access of bacteria to tissues which are normally protected against contamination. Some of these, particularly the chambers of the eye, the meninges, the joints, the endocardium and the urinary tract, have very low resistance to bacterial invasion and are therefore peculiarly susceptible to infection with organisms of low virulence.

Not only the patients but also the staff (including laboratory staff) are exposed to special hazards of infection with virulent organisms. The risk of infection among members of staff through contamination with blood and exudates of patients with HBV, HCV or HIV has received much attention in recent years. The risk in most hospitals, especially with regard to HIV, is extremely low, but fear of AIDS has not surprisingly been associated with an excessive response in terms of preventative measures.

THE ENVIRONMENT

The place where the patient is treated has an important influence on the likelihood of his or her acquiring infection and on the nature of such infection. A wide variety of micro-organisms, including virulent strains, is likely to be found in hospitals where many people, including some with infection, are in close proximity to one another. These organisms are likely to include a large proportion of antibiotic-resistant bacteria (e.g. MRSA, which can flourish where antibiotic usage has led to the suppression of sensitive bacteria).

Different areas of the hospital are associated with different infection hazards. In the operating-theatre there is a special hazard of wound infection because of the exposure – often for several hours – of susceptible tissues, and the presence of a number of potential human and inanimate sources. In wards, the patients may be exposed for many weeks to contaminants from which open surgical wounds will usually be protected by some form of cover, although this is imperfect in many patients, especially those with wound drains. Special hazards exist in neonatal wards through possible contamination of feeds, suction and resuscitation equipment, etc., and because of the frequent handling of infants, and similar problems exist in intensive-care units and burns wards. In Infectious Diseases Hospitals there is a special hazard of infection with the agents of acute communicable diseases. There is a risk of Legionnaire's disease through airborne contamination of aerosols containing *Legionella pneumophila* from cooling towers, humidifiers or water-supply systems colonized by the organism (Department of Health and Social Security, 1986b). *Aspergillus* spores in the environment may cause infection in immunocompromised patients, particularly after liver or bone-marrow transplants.

One objective in control of hospital infection is to expose patients to an environment at least as free from microbial hazard as that which they would encounter outside hospital.

TREATMENT

The clinical results of microbial contamination are influenced by details of treatment – favourably by correct surgical or medical procedures and antimicrobial chemotherapy, and adversely (as mentioned above) by treatment with immunosuppressive drugs or steroids. Antibiotic treatment may often select strains of organisms which are resistant to several antibodies in addition to the single agent used for therapy.

SOURCES AND ROUTES OF INFECTION (Figure 1.1)

Self-infection (endogenous infection) of an operation wound may be due to bacteria transferred from an area where they are causing infection (e.g. boils), or by the normal bacterial flora carried by the patient without symptoms on the skin or the nose (mostly staphylococci), but occasionally in the mouth (especially streptococci), the intestines (especially coliform bacilli and *Bacteroides* species). Endogenous infection with *Bacteroides* species and coliform bacilli is especially important in the lower intestinal tract, but the upper intestine and stomach may be heavily colonized by these bacteria in patients with gastric carcinoma or other pathological states, and during treatment with H_2-receptor blockers.

Cross-infection (exogenous infection) with some of these organisms may occur from other patients or members of staff either by contact or by airborne routes. Infection may be transferred on the hands or clothing of staff, visitors or ambulant patients, on unsterile objects or in fluids used in treatment, food, etc. Members of staff (e.g. nurses, physiotherapists, doctors) who attend to many patients are likely to transfer infective organisms from one patient to another. Visitors who only attend one patient present a smaller hazard, although they may transfer their own micro-organisms. A fetus may be infected by the mother (e.g. with cytomegalovirus) *in utero* or on delivery (e.g. with *Neisseria gonorrheae*). Airborne transfer may occur through the dispersal of skin scales that are shed continuously from the surface of the body and often carry staphylococci, or on droplet nuclei dispersed from the potential source of airborne infection, especially from a patient with respiratory tract infection. Droplet nuclei are small particles less than 5 μ in diameter which dry, leaving a small nucleus which may contain viable bacteria or viruses. The droplet nuclei are carried by convection currents of air and rarely fall to the floor. However, larger droplets fall rapidly to the floor, usually within several feet, and are not usually regarded as airborne spread. Epidemic infections arise through the presence of a case of an infectious disease or of a carrier of the causal organism in the ward, theatre or other place in the hospital where a number of patients may be exposed to contamination. The route or routes of transfer vary, depending on the survival of the organisms outside the body as well as other factors. Infection may also occur through contamination with organisms acquired from inanimate sources, such as Gram-negative bacilli on inadequately decontaminated equipment. Insect vectors (e.g. cockroaches, ants, flies) may convey infective organisms either to patients or to sterilized equipment. Legionnaire's disease appears to be acquired from the inanimate environment only and, although rare, it is potentially dangerous. Hepatitis B and C and HIV infections have the potential for spread in hospitals from the blood of infected patients or carriers, usually from a needlestick or other injury or – in the past – from transfused blood or blood products.

Although the relative importance of different sources and routes can rarely be stated with any precision, there are certain patterns which are relevant to the choice of methods for controlling hospital infection. Of the sources, those in which bacteria are multiplying (e.g. patients with infectious disease and septic wounds, but also healthy surfaces of the body and contaminated solutions) are, in general, more important than dry objects or surfaces on which organisms may survive but cannot multiply. Infected patients and septic wounds are more likely to be a dangerous source than healthy surfaces of the body, because the bacteria in the former can be assumed to be virulent, while those on healthy intact surfaces may often be avirulent. Vehicles which can convey the pathogenic organisms directly to the patient's susceptible sites (e.g. fluids used for aseptic procedures, surgical instruments, food, the hands of nurses handling newborn babies) are more likely to cause infection than sources or reservoirs which do not come into contact with such sites or with the patient. Some of the latter (e.g. floors, walls, furniture) are of very little importance unless incorrect procedures (e.g. sweeping with a brush) are used. The larger the number of stages of contact transfer from a source or reservoir, the smaller the numbers of bacteria that will reach the patients. Contact transfer is more important than airborne transfer, particularly for organisms that do not survive well under dry conditions outside the body. Gram-negative bacilli (e.g. typhoid and dysentery bacilli and *Pseudomonas aeruginosa*), which have this characteristic because they are highly sensitive to drying, are more capable than Gram-positive cocci of survival in water, and are therefore more likely to be transferred in a fluid vector. However, a sufficient number may survive the effects of drying for them to be transmissible on the hands of nurses, doctors and other human contacts.

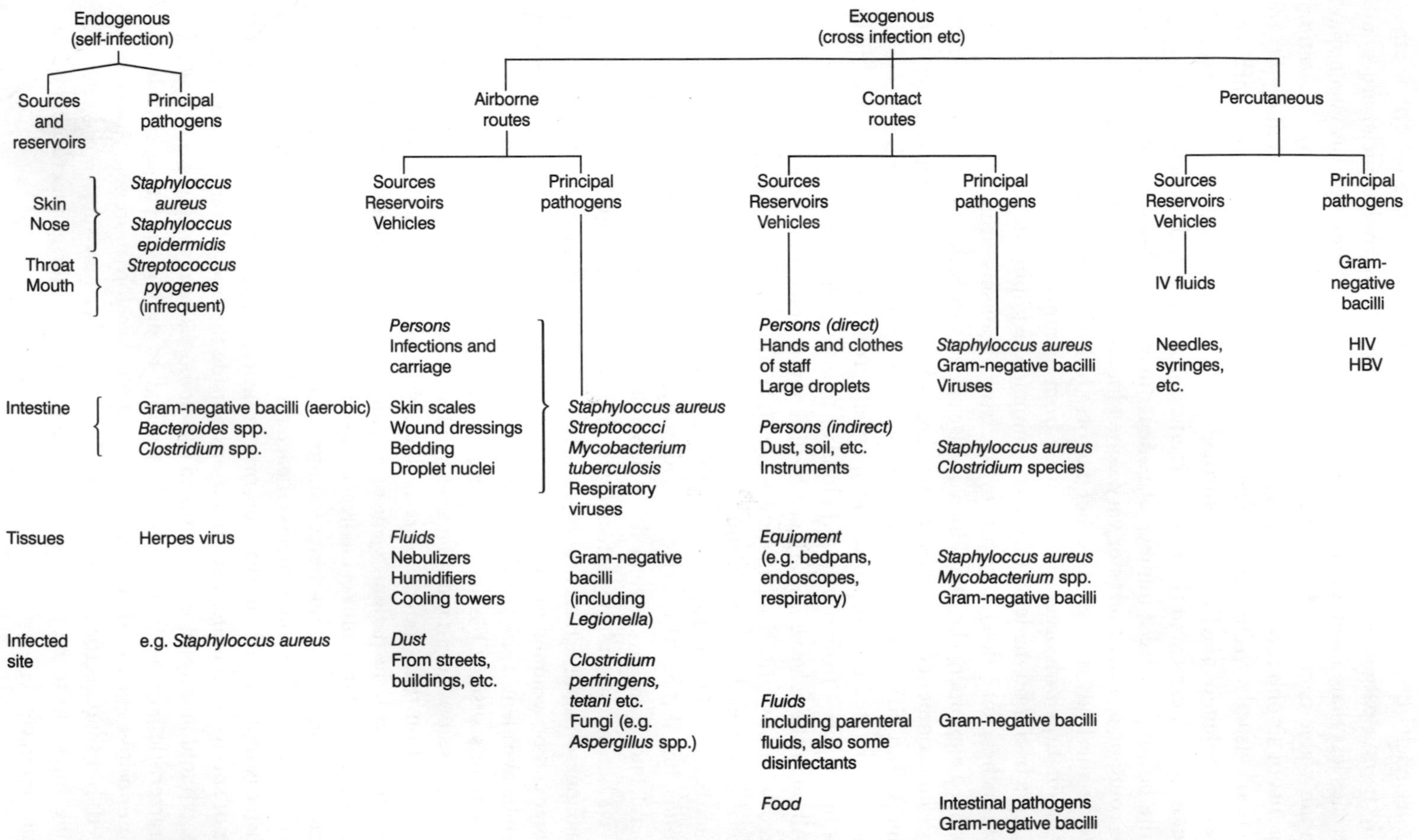

Figure 1.1 Sources of routes of infection

Endogenous (self-infection)

Sources and reservoirs	Principal pathogens
Skin / Nose / Throat / Mouth	*Staphylococcus aureus* / *Staphylococcus epidermidis* / *Streptococcus pyogenes* (infrequent)
Intestine	Gram-negative bacilli (aerobic) / *Bacteroides* spp. / *Clostridium* spp.
Tissues	Herpes virus
Infected site	e.g. *Staphylococcus aureus*

Exogenous (cross infection etc)

Airborne routes

Sources Reservoirs Vehicles	Principal pathogens
Persons — Infections and carriage; Skin scales, Wound dressings, Bedding, Droplet nuclei	*Staphylococcus aureus* / *Streptococci* / *Mycobacterium tuberculosis* / Respiratory viruses
Fluids — Nebulizers, Humidifiers, Cooling towers	Gram-negative bacilli (including *Legionella*)
Dust — From streets, buildings, etc.	*Clostridium perfringens, tetani* etc. / Fungi (e.g. *Aspergillus* spp.)

Contact routes

Sources Reservoirs Vehicles	Principal pathogens
Persons (direct) — Hands and clothes of staff, Large droplets	*Staphyloccus aureus* / Gram-negative bacilli / Viruses
Persons (indirect) — Dust, soil, etc. Instruments	*Staphyloccus aureus* / *Clostridium* species
Equipment (e.g. bedpans, endoscopes, respiratory)	*Staphyloccus aureus* / *Mycobacterium* spp. / Gram-negative bacilli
Fluids including parenteral fluids, also some disinfectants	Gram-negative bacilli
Food	Intestinal pathogens / Gram-negative bacilli

Percutaneous

Sources Reservoirs Vehicles	Principal pathogens
IV fluids	Gram-negative bacilli
Needles, syringes, etc.	HIV / HBV

PRINCIPLES OF CONTROL OF INFECTION

Patients are protected against infection in hospital by a whole system of methods, including surgical asepsis and hospital hygiene, the purpose of which can be summarised as follows:

1 to remove the sources or potential sources of infection (or, more usually, to remove disease-producing microbes from potential sources of infection) – this includes treatment of infected patients as well as sterilizing, disinfection and cleaning of contaminated materials and surfaces;
2 to block the routes of transfer of bacteria from those potential sources and reservoirs to uninfected patients, which include isolation of infected or susceptible patients, aseptic operations, 'no-touch' dressing techniques and particularly the wearing of gloves and handwashing;
3 to enhance the patient's resistance to infection (e.g. during operations by careful handling of tissues and removal of slough and foreign bodies, and also by enhancing the general defences, reinforcement of immunity to tetanus, and the use of antibiotic prophylaxis if and when this is indicated).

Methods advocated for the control of infection can be classified under the following four headings (Medical Research Council, 1968):

1 established methods, for which good evidence is available;
2 provisionally established methods, for which there is some evidence;
3 rational methods, which are consistent with our knowledge of bacteria but which cannot be evaluated by experiments (e.g. avoidance of 'clutter' in operating-rooms);
4 'rituals' – methods which have been shown by experiment or observation to have no value, or even to be harmful.

Other methods of classification (e.g. Garner, 1996) are discussed in Chapter 2.

From a large amount of research conducted in recent years we know that much infection can be prevented and some lives can be saved by applying certain methods of controlling infection. At the same time, in many hospitals there is a continuing incidence of endemic infection at levels which are similar to those reported many years ago. This may be due, in part, to more adventurous surgery and medicine, and to the presence of more patients who are highly susceptible to infection, but there is also evidence of erratic and unstandardized aseptic and hygienic methods which are probably largely responsible for the incidence of cross-infection.

One of the major problems world-wide is the increase in highly antibiotic-resistant organisms. Many of these are associated with hospital infections where antibiotic usage is high and there are frequent opportunities for spread from one patient to another in the same ward. Control of outbreaks can be very costly. Methicillin-resistant *Staphylococcus aureus* (MRSA) is a typical example. It is present in the hospitals of most countries, and new epidemic strains appeared in the UK in the 1980s which have since spread widely throughout the country. Control methods which were previously successful have often failed and some strains are only sensitive to vancomycin or teicoplanin (Combined Working Party of the British Society for Antimicrobial Chemotherapy, Hospital Infection Society and Infection Control Nurses Association, 1998). The increased presence of MRSA in the community and greater movement of patients and staff both between and within hospitals has increased the difficulties in control of infection.

More recently, the emergence of vancomycin-resistant enterococci in intensive-care and other high-risk units has been causing anxiety. These strains are increasingly being reported in non-specialised wards, especially in the USA, and some severe infections are untreatable with antibiotics available for routine use. Outbreaks of *Clostridium difficile* in wards for the elderly have also been causing many problems in some hospitals.

Highly antibiotic-resistant strains of *Mycobacterium* tuberculosis have recently been responsible for small outbreaks of hospital infection, especially in immunocompromised patients. Prevention of spread to staff by the use of particulate respirators has received much attention, particularly in the USA. *Pseudomonas aeruginosa* is still a common cause of death in patients with severe burns in developing countries. Outbreaks of infection with other antibiotic-resistant Gram-negative bacilli (e.g. *Klebsiella* species, *Enterobacter* species, *Serratia marcescens* and *Acinetobacter* species) are commonly reported, particularly in intensive-care units, liver-transplant units and urological wards. These infections are usually controllable by good aseptic techniques and avoidance of excessive use of antibiotics.

The risk of spread of hepatitis B and C viruses and HIV in hospitals, although low, has demonstrated the importance of care in handling blood, the safe disposal of needles and the effective decontamination of medical equipment. Glutaraldehyde has been used for many years for the disinfection of heat-labile medical equipment, but recently problems have arisen with regard to irritancy and allergy involving the skin and respiratory tract of staff. Alternative disinfectants, such as peracetic acid, chlorine dioxide and peroxygen compounds, are being investigated. Difficulties in cleaning and possible infection risks have led to a large increase in the use of single-use items. However, the cost of some of these items can be very high, and reprocessing is often considered, although it has legal implications and requires high standards.

These bloodborne diseases have also been responsible for the introduction of universal precautions or body substance isolation in many countries (Garner, 1996). Universal precautions involve the wearing of gloves as well as other precautions in the handling of blood and body fluids of all patients, and body substance isolation extends these to all secretions, wound discharges and excretions. These universal precautions can be expensive, and data supporting them remain limited.

The Study on the Efficacy of Nosomial Infection Control (SENIC) conducted in the USA from 1975–1980 still provides the best evidence of the value of an infection control team and of efficient control and surveillance of infection (Haley *et al.*, 1985). In the UK there have been many changes in the health service administration and guidance on the administration of infection control has been updated

(Department of Health, 1995). The key role in infection control in hospitals remains that of the infection control team, consisting of the infection control doctor (officer) and the infection control nurse (ICN). The main changes in the administration of control of infection have been in the setting up of the role of the Consultant in Communicable Disease Control (CCDC), and in the increased emphasis on surveillance associated with the wider use of computers in hospitals (Emmerson and Ayliffe, 1996).

Surgical procedures have been changing, and many techniques, (e.g. cholecystectomy) can now be carried out by endoscopic techniques. This minimal-access surgery has enabled patients to go home on the day of surgery or after only 1 or 2 days. This considerably reduces hotel costs and probably infection rates as well, although limited data is available as many more post-operative infections are now first manifesting themselves in the community. The change towards more community care has demonstrated a need for more infection control nurses in the community, and has increased the responsibilities of the CCDC.

MOLECULAR METHODS IN INFECTION CONTROL

Molecular methods have become established as useful and powerful tools in many branches of medicine. The main role for molecular methods in infection control is in the field of typing organisms for epidemiological purposes – so-called 'molecular epidemiology'.

Molecular typing methods involve extracting DNA from organisms and identifying differences in the DNA sequence of those organisms. By comparing organisms which are thought to be involved in an outbreak, cross-infection can be identified.

One fundamental point about typing which needs to be recognized is that these techniques can only differentiate between strains, and they cannot prove that two strains are the same. For this reason, strains which appear identical when typed are said to be *indistinguishable*.

PULSED-FIELD GEL ELECTROPHORESIS (PFGE)

PFGE is a technique which allows large fragments of DNA to be separated on an agarose gel. When used as a typing method, the DNA extracted from the organism is cut with enzymes known as restriction enzymes. Restriction enzymes identify specific sequences within the organism's DNA and cut the DNA at that point. The enzymes used in PFGE typing are chosen to recognize infrequent sequences, and they therefore break the DNA into a small number of relatively large fragments. When cut DNA is run on a gel, stained and visualized under ultraviolet (UV) light, a series of bands can be seen. The positions of the DNA fragments of distinguishable organisms have different banding patterns. By convention, two organisms which have more than three bands in different positions are said to be distinguishable.

RANDOM AMPLIFICATION OF POLYMORPHIC DNA (RAPD)

This technique utilizes the occurrence of repetitive DNA sequences which are found in many bacteria. These sequences are often found as multiple copies distributed throughout the organism's genome. Genetic changes alter the position of these sequences and can thus be used to differentiate between strains.

Oligonucleotide primers which are complementary to parts of these sequences are incorporated into a polymerase chain reaction (PCR) with the organism's DNA. This yields a PCR product which, when run on an agarose gel, will demonstrate a banding pattern that can be used to distinguish strains, although reproducibility is often a problem with this technique.

RIBOTYPING

This technique is similar to RAPD in that it relies on the presence of multiple copies of a known sequence. In this case, the sequence is the ribosomal RNA gene (*rrn*) and an oligonucleotide probe is manufactured to bind to the *rrn* genes. This probe is labelled with either a radioactive molecule or (more commonly) with a visible label such as digoxigenin.

The strain's DNA is extracted and run on an agarose gel. Following transfer to a nylon membrane, the preparation is exposed to the probe and bands can be visualized. This technique is well established, but it is technically difficult and thus time-consuming and expensive.

THE FUTURE OF INFECTION CONTROL

The Directives and Standards produced by the European Union are having an increasing influence on infection control in the UK, particularly with regard to the disinfection and sterilization of medical devices. Extension of legislation into other aspects of infection control could increase the problems as countries in Europe often have different infection-control philosophies.

Nevertheless, the personal factor in preventing infection control remains predominant, and the need continues for a proper understanding of the facts by all members of the hospital staff. Although the subject is complex and involves many disciplines, the basic ideas are simple, and many of the details of asepsis can be made easier by forms of standardization based on evidence of effectiveness and practicality. The infection control team and, in particular, the infection control nurse have a major responsibility for staff education.

REFERENCES

Coello, R., Glenister, H., Fereres, J. *et al.* (1993) The cost of infection in surgical patients: a case-controlled study. *Journal of Hospital Infection* 25, 239.

Combined working party of the British Society for Antimicrobial Chemotherapy, Hospital Infection Society and Infection Control Nurses Association (1998) Revised guidelines for the control of epidemic methicillin-resistant

Staphylococcus aureus infection in hospitals. *Journal of Hospital Infection*. 39, 253.

Daschner, F. (1989) Cost-effectiveness in hospital infection control – lessons for the 1990s. *Journal of Hospital Infection* 13, 325.

Department of Health (1995) *Hospital infection control: guidance on the control of infection in hospitals.* Paper prepared by the DHSS/PHLS Hospital Infection Working Group. London: HMSO.

Department of Health and Social Security (1986a) *The Report of the Committee of Inquiry into an Outbreak of Food-Poisoning at Stanley Royd Hospital.* London: HMSO.

Department of Health and Social Security (1986b) *Public Inquiry into the Cause of the Outbreak of Legionnaire's Disease in Staffordshire.* London: HMSO.

Emmerson, A.M. and Ayliffe, G.A.J. (eds) (1996) Surveillance of nosocomial infections. In *Baillière's clinical infectious diseases.* Vol. 3. London: Baillière Tindall.

Emmerson, A.M., Enstone, J.E., Griffin, M. *et al.* (1996) The Second National Prevalence Survey of Infection in Hospitals – overview of the results. *Journal of Hospital Infection* 32, 175.

Garner, J. (1996) Guidelines for isolation precautions in hospitals. *Infection Control and Hospital Epidemiology.* 17, 53.

Haley, R., Culver, D.H., White, J.W. *et al.* (1985) The efficacy of infection surveillance and control programmes in preventing nosocomial infection in US hospitals. *American Journal of Epidemiology*, 121, 182.

Mayon-White, R.J., Ducel, G.I., Kereselidze, T. and Tikhomirov, E. (1988) An international survey of the prevalence of hospital-acquired infection. *Journal of Hospital Infection* 11 **(Supplement A)**, 43.

Medical Research Council (1968) Aseptic methods in the operating suite. *Lancet* 1, 705, 763, 831.

Meers, P.D., Ayliffe, G.A.J., Emmerson, A.M. *et al.* (1981) Report on the national survey of infection in hospitals 1980. *Journal of Hospital Infection* 2 **(Supplement)** 1.

chapter 2

ADMINISTRATION AND RESPONSIBILITY

The administrative arrangements for infection control will vary in different countries, but most will include an Infection Control Doctor or Officer (ICD or ICO), an Infection Control Nurse or Practitioner (ICN or ICP) and a committee (ICC) (Department of Health, 1995). The UK has undergone significant changes in the structure of health-care provision, and this affects the administration and responsibility for management of infection control services, and further changes continue to occur with changes in government and new Department of Health guidelines.

England and Wales are currently divided into Health Authorities (HA) covering the health needs of populations of varying sizes (see Chapter 18). The Health Authorities (purchasers) are responsible for determining the requirements of both structure and content of the health care required and will stipulate what monies are available and how these monies will be allocated to hospital or community Trusts (providers) together with General Practitioners via contracts, service agreements and other financial links.

Each Health Authority has a Department of Public Health with a Director responsible to the Chief Executive of the Health Authority, together with one or more Consultants in Communicable Disease Control (CCDCs) with responsibility for co-ordination of infection-control activities, including outbreaks involving hospital Trusts, the community at large, and adjacent Trusts and Health Authorities.

Trusts will usually cover acute hospital services, or the community and long-term services, or mental health services, although some may incorporate both hospital and community services. Private hospitals are also expected to follow national guidelines.

The ICD retains responsibility for hospital infection control, and is directly accountable to the Chief Executive and Board of the Trust, and will collaborate with the CCDC. In the event of a major outbreak involving both hospital Trusts and the community, overall responsibility for the co-ordination of the outbreak rests with the CCDC (see p. 22 and Chapter 18).

Hospital Trusts are now accountable for the provision and range of infection control services which they provide, although purchasers can enforce reasonable infection control standards through explicit clauses in contracts. Within this structure, the Infection Control Team (ICT) will normally be within the provider arm of the organization, with the costs of the service recouped by the provider from the prices it charges to the purchasers. The cost of providing an infection control service must be considered an essential part of a Trust. In addition to the annual budget for the ICD and ICN for routine control purposes, costs of an outbreak should be borne by a contingency fund. In major outbreaks, additional funding may be provided by the purchaser.

There are also ICNs working within the Health Authorities, advising them of the measures required for effective infection control within the Trusts and stipulating ways of monitoring the effectiveness via audit of infection control standards.

It is the responsibility of the Chief Executive of the Trust and the Board to ensure that adequate arrangements are made to control hospital infection (Department of Health, 1995). These arrangements should include the setting up of an Infection Control Committee, and the appointment of an ICD and adequate ICN cover in every Trust.

The Trust Board should be responsible for the implementation of the recommendations of the ICDs and ICC. Within each Trust, a Directorate structure exists for different services (e.g. surgical or medical services), usually with a Clinical Director, Business Manager and Senior Nurse Manager. Each Directorate has budgetary control and has to work within an agreed business plan of services and care to be provided.

The ICD and committee should have access to these Directorates via the Chief Executive to ensure that infection control recommendations are communicated to them and implementation is then supported through the planning process. It is the responsibility of all members of staff within the Trust to inform the ICD or ICN of potential hazards of infection. Without this co-operation, the Infection Control Team cannot be fully effective. In addition to the official responsibilities of the Chief Executive and Infection Control Team, the individual clinician in charge of each patient's care and the senior nurse in a unit have a personal responsibility for preventing infection.

INFECTION CONTROL TEAM (ICT)

The team consists of members of staff with a specialist knowledge and interest in infection control in hospitals. The head of the team will usually be a physician (ICD). The Infection Control Team will include the microbiologist (who will usually be the ICD), ICNs and (where available) members of the scientific or technical staff with responsibilities in infection control. The ICD and ICN should meet frequently, preferably daily.

More than one ICD and ICN may be appointed in a large Trust, depending on the size and also the type of patient. The Trust Operations or Hospital Manager or a representative may be a member of the team, attending meetings when a major problem arises. If they are not a member of the team, they (or a representative) should always be available to the ICD for discussion of problems.

The role of the ICT is to implement the annual programme and policies and to be responsible for providing advice to the Trust or hospital staff on a 24-hour basis.

The team is responsible for the following:
- surveillance of infections and monitoring methods of control;

- rapid identification and investigation of outbreaks or potentially hazardous procedures;
- providing advice on isolation of infected patients and on hazardous or ineffective procedures;
- giving advice, making day-to-day decisions and liaising with staff in all areas where potential risks of infection exist, especially laboratories, occupational health departments and clinical directorates;
- providing, monitoring and evaluating policies for the prevention of infection and its spread;
- audit of infection control procedures as appropriate;
- a staff education programme in collaboration with the occupational health department, including communication and provision of readily available information to staff on measures of infection control;
- preparing the annual infection control programme and reporting to the ICC.

The particular duties of the ICD and ICN are described below, but there is a considerable overlap in duties and responsibilities between the various members of the team.

INFECTION CONTROL DOCTOR (ICD)

The individual holding this appointment should be a senior member of the medical staff with ready access to the Trust Board and Management Committees, and should have sufficient authority to command respect from all categories of staff. They should have a special interest and training in hospital infection, and should be aware of recent developments in the subject. They may be expected to complete the course for the Diploma in Hospital Infection Control in the UK or an equivalent qualification in the future, and they should be appointed by the Trust Board. The medical microbiologist is the logical choice, being suitably qualified and in an ideal position to keep the surveillance and record systems under constant scrutiny and review. The functions of the ICD in conjunction with other members of the team are to assess risks of infection, to advise on preventative measures and to check their efficacy in all parts of the hospital, including the laundry, sterile services department (SSD), domestic, pharmaceutical and engineering departments, as well as clinical and other areas.

Inspection of kitchens and other catering establishments should be regularly carried out (at least every 12 months) by the ICD or their representative, in collaboration with the CCDC and the Local Authority Environmental Health Officer.

Information and advice may be given by the ICD informally or at meetings of the Trust Board, Medical Staff Committee, ICC or Directorate Manager. However, if any immediate action is required, the ICD or Chairman of the ICC (see below) should be empowered to take whatever steps may be necessary without prior reference to the ICC. He or she should have ready access to the Chief Executive, Director of Operations, Directors of clinical services and laboratory facilities, and work closely with the ICN and also the CCDC, especially on notifiable infectious diseases. Some of the duties of the ICD may be delegated to other staff (e.g. the microbiology registrar, ICN (or ICP) or medical laboratory scientific officer, as appropriate).

INFECTION CONTROL NURSE (ICN)

The Infection Control Nurse should be a registered nurse (first level in the UK) with a broad range of clinical nursing experience. They should be experienced in communicating with all grades and disciplines, and able to balance conflicting issues whilst maintaining the individual patient's care needs.

The Infection Control Nurse is the only member of the ICT with a full-time responsibility for infection control, enabling him or her to maintain a clinical input within wards and departments and always to be accessible for advice and support. The nurse responsible for infection control within a Trust should be graded as a Clinical Nurse Specialist or Senior Nurse Manager and have access and links across all clinical directorates. Grading should depend on areas of responsibility and should be reviewed within the Trust's corporate plan. It is recommended that, for the induction of newly appointed ICNs, attendance for a short period at a centre in which there are experienced ICNs working within an established ICT should be included. The principles of hospital microbiology and laboratory procedures, such as specimen collection, should be taught in the new ICN's own hospital to enable development of essential links with laboratory personnel. It is expected that all nurses will complete one of the specialist training courses for ICNs (e.g. English National Board (ENB) 329 in the UK or the equivalent at diploma or university degree level). Many Trusts within the UK normally stipulate that all Clinical Nurse Specialists should be able to function at degree level. The structure of these courses ensures that the ICN will remain within his or her Trust, and that he or she will be able to reflect on the knowledge gained and on practice within the clinical areas.

The attendance of ICNs at the annual conference of the Infection Control Nurses Association (ICNA) and other related specialist conferences (e.g. those of the Hospital Infection Society) should be considered as part of their training, and as mandatory updating required by the United Kingdom Central Council for Nursing, Midwifery and Health Visiting (UKCC 1995). Failure to provide a career structure for ICNs leads to difficulties in recruitment and retention of trained and experienced nurses within the health service.

The ICN is managerially accountable to the ICD and professionally accountable to the Director of Nursing Practice, who should be responsible for advising on attendance by the ICN at conferences, courses and other relevant meetings. If a person other than a nurse is appointed to take on some of these duties, he or she should be on the laboratory staff and may be described, for example, as an 'Infection Control Microbiologist', 'Infection Control Scientific Officer' or 'Infection Control Practitioner'. The appointment is usually in addition to that of a nurse, although in the USA, the Infection Control Practitioner (Professional) is usually a nurse equivalent to an ICN in the UK.

The functions of the ICN are described below. These cover the whole field of infection control and involve co-operation with all of the departments mentioned in the section on the ICC, and particularly with the occupational health department. The ICN is a member of, and shares responsibility with, the Infection Control Team. The nurse should visit all wards regularly and discuss any problems with the staff. The laboratory should be visited every morning by the ICN.

Instruction of nurses and other grades of staff in the practice of infection control is one of the major responsibilities, and should be treated as a priority.

The day-to-day activities of an infection control nurse include the following:

- identifying as promptly as possible potential infection hazards in patients, staff or equipment;
- compiling records of infected patients from ward notifications, case notes, laboratory reports and information collected during routine visits and discussions;
- arranging prompt isolation of infected patients (in co-operation with the ward manager and consultant who have initial responsibility) in accordance with hospital policy, and ensuring that there are adequate facilities for isolating patients, as well as introducing other measures as necessary to prevent the spread of infection or organisms that are highly resistant to antibiotics;
- regular audits of relevant wards in units to ensure that infection control and aseptic procedures are being carried out in accordance with hospital policy (see p. 36);
- liaison between laboratory and ward staff; informing heads of departments and giving advice on infection control problems;
- collaboration with occupational health staff in maintaining records of infection in medical, nursing, catering, domestic and other grades of staff; ensuring that clearance specimens are received before infected staff return to duty;
- collaborating with and advising community nurses on problems of infection;
- promptly supplying information about notifiable diseases by telephone to the public health medical officer (CCDC);
- informing other hospitals, general practitioners and other health-care providers when infected patients are discharged from hospital or transferred elsewhere, and receiving relevant information from other hospitals or from the community where appropriate;
- participation in teaching and practical demonstrations of techniques for control of infection to medical, nursing, auxiliary, domestic, catering, and other professions allied to medicine;
- informing the Director of Nursing and/or Directorate Nurse Managers of practical problems and difficulties in carrying out routine procedures related to nursing aspects of infection control;
- attending relevant committees, usually Control of Infection, Nursing Procedures, Clinical Audit, Risk Management, Equipment Purchase Groups, Health and Safety, Re-Use of Single-Use item Committees etc.;
- produce and update infection control policies and guidelines;
- offer advice on purchase and decontamination of equipment and on planning and capital projects;

- conferring with the sterile services manager about the management of equipment used by patients with certain infections in hospital (e.g. hepatitis B virus).

Much of the ICN's time will be spent providing advice to members of staff on infection control problems.

The nurse will collaborate with other members of the team in investigating outbreaks, conducting surveys, visiting kitchen and catering establishments, monitoring special units, collecting microbiological samples, preparing reports for the ICC, clinicians and Trust management, and assisting in research projects.

INFECTION CONTROL LINK (LIAISON) NURSE

The development of an Infection Control Link Nurse within acute hospital, community and mental health Trusts initially caused concern with regard to the role of such a person. Key to any such role is the responsibility of the link or liaison nurse to a qualified ICN. Ongoing support and education of the link nurses is critical to enable them to be effective communicators and 'agents of change' at ward or department level. Further research is required to identify whether the increased education and knowledge of link nurses results in an improvement in practice throughout the clinical area in which they work. This has to be balanced against the time commitment required by the qualified ICN. Possible considerations could include stability of the work-force within a Trust and the number of ICNs. Link nurses may be particularly useful in specialist departments (e.g. intensive-care units and outlying or non-acute hospitals). Although their role is developing, they should report to the ICN early evidence of outbreaks or infection problems, and any changes in practice and in the use of new equipment relevant to infection control. It is recommended that the link nurse's role should be clearly defined in order to meet local needs, and the placing of excessive demands on individuals should be avoided.

In some hospitals or departments, particularly in developing countries, a Link Doctor could also be useful, but this post has not yet been developed in the UK.

CONSULTANT IN COMMUNICABLE DISEASE CONTROL (CCDC)

This is a relatively new post in the UK (Department of Health, 1995) (see Chapter 18). A CCDC is employed in each Health Authority and is responsible for the surveillance, prevention and control of all communicable disease and infection in the health district. He or she is basically qualified in public health and/or medical microbiology and is specifically trained for the post. The duties of the CCDC and ICD in the hospital overlap, and close collaboration between them is essential. The CCDC advises the health authority on contractual requirements for infection control services and monitoring in the Trusts within the district, and liaises with the ICT in the management of outbreaks of infection in hospital and the community, liaises with adjacent health districts and provides epidemiological advice when required. He or she is a member of the ICT and Major Outbreaks Committee, and if the latter involves the community, he or she may be appointed chairman of the committee. As the shift in health-care delivery moves into primary care, some Trusts and Health Authorities now have a combined medical microbiologist (ICD) and CCDC post which bridges the gap between hospital and community care.

INFECTION CONTROL COMMITTEE (ICC)

The committee of a large hospital Trust should have representatives from all of the major departments which are concerned with control of infection, (e.g. medical, nursing, occupational health, engineering, pharmacy, supplies, domestic, SSD, catering, microbiology, administration and community health), as well as from the Infection Control Team. The chairman of the committee may also be an ICD, but could be a clinician with an interest in infection control (e.g. infectious diseases consultant or surgeon, or a senior ICN). Some hospital Trusts may prefer to appoint a small committee consisting of the Infection Control Team, the CCDC, a senior nurse, clinician and senior manager, and to co-opt others as necessary. The main advantages of a large committee are educational and to ensure adequate communication between the different departments. However, major decisions on hospital problems will be made by the ICT and possibly by a small executive committee as described above.

Meetings should be held 1–12 times a year depending on requirements, but three to four meetings should be adequate for most Trusts, and yearly meetings for small hospitals where problems tend to arise sporadically. The committee should:

- discuss any problems brought to them by the ICD, ICN or other members of the committee and provide support for decisions made by the ICT;
- take responsibility for major decisions;
- be given reports on current problems and on the incidence of infection and evaluate other reports involving infection risk (e.g. kitchen inspections);
- arrange interdepartmental co-ordination and education in control of infection (it is therefore advantageous to have representation of members with various interests);
- introduce, maintain and, when necessary, modify policies (e.g. disinfectant, antibiotic, isolation);
- advise on the selection of equipment for the prevention of infection (e.g. sharps disposal boxes, etc.);
- make recommendations to other committees and departments on infection control techniques;
- advise Trusts on all aspects of infection control and make recommendations for use of resources.

IMPLEMENTATION OF COMMITTEE RECOMMENDATIONS

If the committee or team is to be effective, the results of the investigations and records of infection must be sent to the relevant authorities and recommendations rapidly implemented, especially when the safety of patients or staff is involved. Although the ICT has an overall advisory responsibility to the Trust or hospital, other members of the committee should ensure that recommendations within their own areas of responsibility are carried out as considered necessary by the committee. Heads of departments (e.g. catering, laundry), if they are not members of the committee, should be invited to attend committee meetings when problems concerning their own departments are to be discussed. The Infection Control Committee is a subcommittee of the Trust Board or equivalent. The Chairman and the ICD should have direct access to the Chief Executive, who may also be a member of the committee or team. All recommendations, instructions or procedures involving any aspect of infection in the hospital issued by the Directorates, other committees, the Health and Safety Executive (HSE), environmental health officers or CCDC should be referred for approval to the ICC.

OBJECTIVES OF THE INFECTION CONTROL DEPARTMENT AND IMPLEMENTATION OF POLICIES

The main objective of the Infection Control Team is to reduce preventable infection to the lowest possible level at acceptable cost, and Health Authorities increasingly require evidence that infection control techniques are cost-effective. Although costs can be measured, effectiveness is more difficult to assess, as patients vary in age and other characteristics, as well as undergoing different treatments. Hospitals vary in design and availability of facilities. Comparisons between infection rates in different hospitals or during different periods in the same hospital are of doubtful validity, and require a considerable amount of time for the collection of data. Even if the data can be collected, the numbers of infections over a year in a single hospital are not usually sufficient to provide statistical evidence of efficacy of measures (see Chapter 3). In addition, it is not possible to estimate the infections that might have occurred if early preventative measures had not been implemented.

It is therefore difficult to assess the infection control measures in terms of outcome (e.g. reduced infection rates), but it may be possible to infer the outcome from process measurements. The Study of Efficacy of Nosocomial Infection Control (SENIC) project conducted in the USA showed that a 'reduction in infection rates of about one third could be obtained by intensive surveillance and control methods, the appointment of a physician with expertise in infection control and one Infection Control Nurse to 250 beds' (Haley *et al.*, 1985). It is inferred that if the SENIC criteria are met, a reduction in infection rate will be achieved. However, it is unlikely that the appointment of more infection control nurses will be possible in most hospitals around the world in the foreseeable future, and maintaining a comprehensive clinical surveillance system will often not represent optimal use of the nurse's time. However, the infection control staff should be able to demonstrate to the Trust Board that certain objectives have been achieved. Essential surveillance reports could be presented to the ICC, as well as evidence of audits of policies and appropriate infection control techniques which have proven value. Priorities can be defined and unnecessary rituals eliminated (e.g. wearing of caps and overshoes in intensive-care units, and unnecessary washing of operating-theatre walls).

ACTION DURING AN OUTBREAK OF INFECTION

When an outbreak occurs (e.g. due to the sudden appearance of an increasing incidence of one type of infection in a ward), immediate action is needed to prevent further spread to patients and staff. This action will vary according to the nature and severity of the infection, but certain general principles apply. The ICD or ICN must be notified, and they should take immediate steps (e.g. isolation of suspected cases) in consultation with the microbiologist (if not the same person) and the clinicians and nursing manager whose patients are involved. The CCDC responsible for communicable diseases should be informed if the outbreak is of a notifiable disease or involves the community. If a major outbreak occurs, a meeting of the 'emergencies' or 'outbreak' committee should immediately be arranged by the Chairman of the Infection Control Committee or ICD and the Hospital Operations Manager or his or her representative. Other members of this committee include the ICT, the clinician responsible for affected patients, a senior nurse, the occupational health team and the CCDC. The CCDC has legal responsibility for controlling infection, and may prefer to chair the committee him- or herself.

A major outbreak is difficult to define in terms of the numbers of patients and staff involved. Numbers of cases (e.g. '20 salmonella infections') have been suggested, but two cases – or even one – of a hazardous infection (e.g. diphtheria) might be considered to be a major outbreak. The decision should be made by the ICD, based on factors such as the severity and communicability of infections, the necessity of closing the ward, the need to prevent transfer of staff to other wards, to provide additional staff, to provide additional supplies, linen etc. or to open an isolation ward.

The ICD (or chairman of the Infection Committee) will usually be responsible for co-ordinating infection control arrangements in the hospital. The following steps are suggested:

- arrangements should be made for the clinical care of patients;
- adequate channels of communication should be set up and a decision made as to who will be responsible for communication with the media;
- an assessment of the situation should be made – details of the patients with infection should be recorded, including date of admission and first symptoms, and the nature of the disease; bacteriological samples should be examined and when possible, pathogens typed (or kept on suitable medium for typing) in the hospital or the Public Health Laboratory;
- isolation of infected patients (for appropriate methods see Chapter 8);
- introduction of additional techniques for control of infection in affected wards (e.g. alcoholic hand disinfection), closure of one or more wards (this is rarely required, but may be necessary if the outbreak is extensive, and particularly if the infection involves a hazard of severe illness or even death in some patients); the ward should be closed to further admissions, and thoroughly cleaned after discharge of the last patient before reopening; such a procedure may also apply to an operating-theatre or other affected area;

- the allocation of beds (e.g. the entire isolation unit, side wards, or possibly a larger ward) for care and management of infected patients may be required;
- an epidemiological survey should be undertaken where appropriate in order to provide evidence of the time and place where infection was acquired, including enquiry about the possible admission of patients incubating infection;
- surveillance of contacts (who may be incubating the disease) is sometimes necessary, and this includes clinical surveillance and laboratory screening;
- bacteriological search for the source of infection; examination of all staff and patients for carriage to see whether, for example, the same phage type of *Staphylococcus aureus* is isolated from all infections; search for the infecting strain in the inanimate environment (e.g. fluids if the organism is *Pseudomonas aeruginosa* or other Gram-negative bacilli, or food if the illness is gastroenteritis of possible food origin;
- survey of methods, equipment and buildings – such a survey could include dressing technique, theatre discipline, kitchen hygiene – for evidence of lapses and the 'personal factor', and also for effectiveness of sterilizers, ventilation systems, disinfection, and protection against recontamination of sterilized objects and solutions;
- the ICN or Occupational Health Nurse will discuss the situation with heads of departments (e.g. catering, SSD, laundry and domestic departments) to relieve anxieties and identify any necessary procedures;
- the requirement for assistance should be assessed at each meeting and advice sought as necessary (e.g. from a Public Health Laboratory, Division of Hospital Infection, Colindale, or other specialist physicians or units, such as the Infectious Diseases Physician, Hospital Infection Research Laboratory, Birmingham, or the Communicable Disease Surveillance Centre, Colindale).

Check-lists of practices should be prepared for investigation of infection arising in surgical, maternity and general medical wards and in special departments (e.g. operating suites, kitchens, laundries, SSD) (e.g. Williams *et al.*, 1966).

PATIENT VISITORS

Infection may be brought into hospital by visitors, or transferred by them from one patient to another, or acquired by them from infected patients. Although visitors do not appear to play an important role in hospital infection, some precautions are required to meet recognized hazards.

Many volunteer organizations now offer hospital visiting to patients without family and friends to support them during their hospital stay. The volunteer may visit more than one patient and assist in feeding or mobilizing the patients whom they visit. Such volunteers should be co-ordinated via the Trust and the volunteers should receive basic infection control information, (e.g. about immunization, hand-washing and use of plastic aprons, and that they should refrain from visiting if they have a bad cold, a sore throat, diarrhoea or other communicable disease). Such advice should also be given to individual visitors of patients with enhanced susceptibility to infection (e.g. neonates, adult critical-care patients, patients receiving chemotherapy or those who are immunocompromised). Visits by non-immune individuals (especially children and pregnant women) to patients in isolation with highly communicable diseases (e.g. chicken-pox) should be prohibited. Trusts have a responsibility to offer reasonable protection to anyone who visits the premises (see p. 26). Therefore notices (which maintain the patient's right to confidentiality) at the entrance to a ward or isolation cubicle should be used to allow the ward manager to control access to patients in isolation. For example:

> **Please contact
> nurse in charge
> before visiting**

LEGAL ASPECTS OF INFECTION CONTROL

Legal regulations have increased considerably in recent years and have had a major impact on infection control staff. Many of these are the consequence of European Directives and Standards, and particularly apply to medical devices, waste disposal and the health and safety of staff. National guidelines and standards have been produced to improve quality of patient care, and most hospitals have written policies for procedures. Claims for negligence have increased to costs of millions of pounds per year for Health Authorities and NHS Hospital Trusts.

REGULATIONS, GUIDELINES, STANDARDS AND POLICIES

Statutes and statutory regulations (i.e. Acts of Parliament and subsidiary regulations) may be used as a basis for either civil or criminal prosecution. They are usually less detailed than guidelines or standards, which are often used to add specific detail to the regulations. For example, the guidance produced by the Health Services Advisory Committee interprets and expands upon the Controlled Waste Regulations 1992 and the Environmental Protection Act 1990 for disposal of clinical waste. Other important Acts and Regulations are the Health and Safety Act (1974) and the Control of Substances Hazardous to Health Regulations (COSHH) Act of Parliament (1988).

However, medical negligence is often dealt with by common law based on previous court judgements. Medical negligence due to failure in the duty of care owed to patients usually involves a civil action unless the negligence is gross (e.g. if it is responsible for the death of a patient), and might then be associated with a criminal prosecution.

Guidelines and standards produced by national professional organizations, health departments and government agencies are usually advisory and not legally enforceable (Hurwitz, 1995). Nevertheless, they are frequently used as a basis for a civil action in claims of negligence, and when produced by a government agency may be used as a basis for criminal prosecution. Any deviation from national guidelines or standards requires careful consideration, although it must be accepted that a consensus decision reached by a group of experts does not always arrive at the only or necessarily the correct solution (see p. 30). National standards produced by professional organizations or the British Standards Institute tend to be stronger in their requirements than guidelines, but usually allow some local deviations. For instance, the standards on 'Infection Control in Hospitals', prepared by four national organizations, mainly include managerial requirements and state that 'the proposed standards might be used as a point of reference in discussions between the Infection Control Team and managers about the arrangements needed to deliver a high quality infection control service' (Infection Control Working Party, 1993).

Clinical guidelines have been defined as 'systematically developed statements which assist healthcare staff and patients in making decisions about appropriate treatment or courses of action for specific conditions or procedures (modified from *Clinical Guidelines*, NHS Executive 1996). Wherever possible, these (as well as legal requirements, standards and policies) should be evidence based. The NHS Executive describes three categories of evidence:

1 randomized controlled trials;
2 other robust experimental or observational studies;
3 more limited evidence, but the advice relies on expert opinion and is endorsed by respected authorities.

For many years the control of infection has whenever possible been based on scientific evidence (e.g. Medical Research Council, 1968; see Chapter 11). The Centers for Disease Control have produced guidelines, on most infection control procedures, and categorize them as follows (Garner, 1996):

1A strongly recommended for all hospitals, and strongly supported by well-designed experimental or epidemiologic studies;
1B strongly recommended for all hospitals, and reviewed as effective by experts in the field and consensus of the Hospital Infection Control Practices Advisory Committee (HICPAC), based on strong rationale and suggestive evidence, even though definitive scientific studies have not been performed;
2 suggested for implementation in many hospitals; recommendations may be supported by suggestive clinical or epidemiologic studies, a strong theoretical rationale or definitive studies applicable to some, but not all, hospitals;
3 no recommendation – unresolved issue; practices for which insufficient evidence or consensus regarding efficacy exists.

Those responsible for preparing national guidelines should take into account variations in structure, resources, and particular problems of individual hospitals, and should ensure that recommendations are practicable, reasonable and achievable. The guidelines should not inhibit advances made by practitioners who are prepared to take some risks, but deviations should be backed by research if possible. The same requirements apply to local guidelines and policies. Hospital policies should be included in an infection control manual available on all hospital wards and units. Manuals and policies or guidelines have been published and can be used as a guide to reduce the amount of work in an individual hospital (Damani, 1997; Ward *et al.*, 1997). The recommendations in the manual should be implemented, or changed if they are not practicable, and should be subject to occasional audit. If a Health Authority or NHS Trust is sued for negligence, local guidelines and policies will be closely examined even if they are not legally enforceable. However, 'courts are unlikely to adopt standards of care advocated in clinical guidelines as "gold standards" because the mere fact that a guideline exists does not of itself establish that compliance with it is reasonable in the circumstances, or that non-compliance is negligent' (Hurwitz, 1999).

Failure to follow legal regulations, national guidelines or standards may be associated with the following:

- health-care purchasers (i.e. Health Authorities in the UK) obtaining their medical services from another hospital (provider), or refusal by insurance companies to fund treatment in a particular private hospital;
- sanctions against the hospital by the NHS Executive or appropriate government authority;
- civil proceedings against the hospital Trust concerned for medical negligence;
- criminal proceedings against the hospital or health-care worker taken by national or local government agencies because of failure to comply with official regulations, or in the event of possible gross negligence.

LEGAL RESPONSIBILITIES OF HOSPITAL AUTHORITIES, STAFF AND PATIENTS

The legal responsibilities of hospital authorities and staff, visitors and patients depend upon the application of general common law principles and some statute law to the particular circumstances of each case.

Under the Occupiers Liability Act (1957), hospital authorities must provide safe premises, so that if patients are admitted to wards or hospitals where there is a known outbreak of infection, the hospital authorities might be made responsible for the death of a patient or for injury suffered by a patient as a result of such infection. Nursing and medical staff therefore have a duty to report such infection at the earliest possible opportunity when it is discovered, and the Infection Control Doctor or Team must decide immediately what steps should be taken to prevent a spread of the infection. There is a further duty of the hospital authorities to ensure that no staff are employed at the hospital who may transmit serious infection to others. If it becomes known to the hospital authorities that a particular member of staff is a carrier of organisms that may cause a dangerous infectious disease, then the hospital authorities must take steps either to terminate that person's employment (if appropriate) or to deploy him or her where there is minimal risk of infection to other members of staff or to patients. These restrictions must not be applied in the case of less dangerous organisms (e.g. *Staphylococcus aureus*) which are often carried by healthy persons. However, special precautions should be taken when these apparently less dangerous organisms cause an outbreak of clinical infection, but routine screening for symptomless carriers is not usually recommended.

In the case of tuberculosis, tuberculin testing of staff should be carried out routinely and BCG should be given if necessary when there is a possibility of nursing and other staff coming into contact with patients suffering from the disease. If this is not done, the hospital may be sued by a nurse or other member of staff who contracts tuberculosis, on the grounds that the hospital is not providing a safe system of work. Immunization against hepatitis B should similarly be offered to all staff involved with the use of invasive procedures or the handling of materials contaminated with blood or body fluids. Immunization against other diseases which can be prevented in this way should, in some circumstances, be offered.

A patient in a hospital cannot be held liable either for introducing infection or for spreading it in the hospital, but it is clear that the hospital authorities must take care, by all reasonable precautions, including some kind of isolation if necessary, to prevent the spread of infection. Similarly, a claim against the hospital authorities in respect of infection caused by a member of the hospital staff, either to another member of the staff or to a patient or visitor, would only be likely to succeed if the hospital had known (or should have known) about it and had failed to take any appropriate action.

If it is known that a visitor is suffering from an infection which he or she is likely to communicate to hospital staff or patients, there might be a responsibility upon the hospital to stop the visiting, but the hospital authorities cannot really be held responsible for every infection which may be either caused or spread by a visitor. A hospital authority can be, and has been, held legally responsible when a patient was discharged from a hospital suffering from a specific infectious disease which he subsequently communicated to another person. In that case it was held that there was negligence on the part of the hospital authorities in discharging someone into the community who was likely to infect other members of that community. Such a patient should have been kept in hospital and isolated until he was judged to be no longer infectious (see section on balance of risks on p. 30).

When a patient becomes infected through some error in aseptic techniques or hospital hygiene, the hospital authorities may be held responsible. For example, if it could be demonstrated that it was the accepted practice to sterilize certain containers (e.g. of saline solutions) and the hospital fails to sterilize and maintain sterility of the fluid in the bottle before distribution to patients, then the hospital authorities may be held liable if contamination of the fluid has taken place at any time before it is actually used. On the other hand, if a practice is not universally adopted (e.g. provision of 'ultraclean' air systems for total hip replacement operations) and the hip becomes infected, it could be argued that the hospital authorities should not be liable, as their failure to provide such an enclosure (if antibiotic prophylaxis was used) did not constitute a failure to provide a reasonable standard of care in the treatment of the patient in accordance with current practice in this country.

HEALTH AND SAFETY AT WORK ACT (1974)

Under this Act responsibilities are placed upon health authorities to provide and maintain plant and systems of work that are, so far as is reasonably practicable, safe and without risks to the health of employees and to arrange to ensure, as far as is reasonably practicable, safety and absence of risks to health of employees in connection with the use, handling, storage and transport of articles and substances. Safety representatives may be appointed by staff and, if staff require this, hospital authorities must establish safety committees under the Safety Representatives and Safety Committees Regulations (1977). If this has not been done, it should be undertaken immediately as there are additional responsibilities on Health Authorities under the Act towards patients so that they are not exposed to risks to their health and safety. The Department of Health and Social Security Act (1974) circular HC(78)30 states that, in view of the liabilities imposed by the Act on health authorities and their employees, each authority should establish a general structure of responsibility which makes it clear who is responsible for the discharge of particular aspects of the general duties imposed by the Act. It also sets out the responsibilities of management to have advisers and safety officers for specialist departments, safety liaison officers and, where staff require them, safety committees.

CONTROL OF SUBSTANCES HAZARDOUS TO HEALTH (COSHH) REGULATIONS (1988)

These regulations have been in force since October 1989 and introduce a framework for controlling exposure of personnel to hazardous substances arising from work activity (Department of Health, 1989; Harrison, 1991). It includes micro-organisms as well as toxic substances. The employer is responsible for assessing the health risks created by the work, and the substance, and the measures required to protect the health of the workers. These regulations are particularly relevant to infection control staff, and are likely to involve such hazards as glutaraldehyde in endoscopy units, ethylene oxide sterilizers in the SSD, disinfectants and detergents, transport of laboratory specimens, and protection of staff against blood borne infection, tuberculosis and Legionnaire's disease. The regulations will obviously have a major application in hospital laboratories. Most hospitals will already have guidelines for the control of infection which should be adequate for the regulations involving infection in the clinical units, but there is a continual need for risk assessments.

EUROPEAN REGULATIONS AND MEDICAL DEVICES

At present European regulations do not usually directly involve the clinical aspects of control of infection, but they may cover some associated aspects, such as consumer safety, environmental hygiene, medical devices, tests for disinfection and sterilization, pharmaceuticals, use of toxic agents and laboratory diagnostic tests. European regulations are issued in the form of Directives. A European Council Directive must be incorporated into the national legislation of all countries in the European Community within a defined period of time. The Directives provide a framework only and, if met, products can be identified with a CE mark that allows them to be sold throughout the European Community.

The Directives are expanded into standards produced by Comité European Normalisation (CEN). Member countries of CEN are bound to comply with CEN/CENELEC International Regulations which stipulate conditions for giving the standard the status of a national standard. A CEN standard in the UK replaces the national standard (i.e. British Standard). The CEN standard would usually have to be met for a manufacturer to use the CE mark, although a different but equivalent standard could still meet the requirements of the European Directive. The effects of these standard requirements in individual hospitals often remain unclear. Sterile Services Departments are technically manufacturers, but do not usually 'sell' their products to their own hospital, and would not require a CE mark. However, if they 'sell' products to another hospital Trust or General Practitioner, they will have to meet the requirements of the Directive (Medical Devices Directive 93/42/EEC) and obtain a CE mark for these products (Medical Devices Agency 1999, see also SSDs, page 335). The Directive does not apply to other hospitals or health centres in the same Trust, but nevertheless every effort should be made by processing departments to reach the standards of *Good Manufacturing Practice* or its replacement European Guidance documents for all sterile products, although this may not be possible, or even necessary, in small health centres or doctors' surgeries, carrying out their own processing of basic surgical instruments, provided that the procedures are safe. It is important that drafts of European standards are widely distributed for comment, so that problems, which are often peculiar to individual countries, can be detected at an early stage. Whenever possible, recommendations in standards should be based on evidence of effectiveness as discussed for national guidelines.

The European Community Directive on liability for unsafe products resulted in the Consumer Protection Act 1987 in the UK. Under this Act, a supplier of goods, including dressings, drugs, devices or servicing contractor, can be sued for negligence if a patient dies or suffers a personal injury from the item concerned. This applies to a hospital reprocessing a reusable item which is not legally covered by the Medical Devices Directorate, or reprocessing an item labelled 'single-use'. Legal liability is transferred from the manufacturer to the hospital if an item labelled 'single-use' is reprocessed, but the responsibility for safe reprocessing is the same for the hospital as for any reusable item. However, an item marked 'single-use' would require particular care if it was reprocessed, as in some instances there may be a genuine reason for the 'single-use' label. The decision to reprocess single-use items should be taken by a hospital Devices Assessment Group (Central Sterilizing Club, 1999), and the requirements of the Medical Devices Agency (1995) should be followed. The manufacturer of a reusable item is responsible for providing instructions on reprocessing that are effective and which do not affect the performance of the device (Medical Devices Agency, 1999). The legal liability remains complex.

MEDICAL NEGLIGENCE

Patients now have a greater expectation from treatment than previously, and are often unwilling to accept any risk at all from medical procedures or treatment.

Media publicity (e.g. articles on 'superbugs') may influence their actions and therefore increase their willingness to make claims. It is important that patients are informed of risks prior to treatment (e.g. that wound infection rates are normally 5–10%, depending on the operation, and that an operation always carries some risk).

Medical negligence is dealt with in the civil courts, unless the degree of negligence amounts to a criminal offence and the standard of proof depends on the balance of probabilities (i.e. whether it is more likely that there was negligence which caused a particular injury).

To demonstrate negligence, proof of all of the following must be obtained:
- the practitioner (doctor, nurse or other health-care worker) owed the patient a *duty of care*;
- the defendant was negligent by breaching that duty of care and the plaintiff *suffered an injury*;
- the negligence actually *caused* the injury.

The standard of care required is the duty to exercise reasonable skill and care in the treatment of a patient. The standard of reasonable skill would be that of a competent practitioner in that speciality (e.g. an Infection Control Doctor (consultant microbiologist) would be expected to exercise greater skills in the management of an infection control problem than a junior doctor).

Negligence is usually due to the following:
- outdated knowledge and skills.
- not adopting safety measures that are known to be necessary.

It is not always necessary to follow national guidelines (Hurwitz, 1995, 1999; NHS Executive, 1996; British Medical Association, 1997). In the Bolam case, it was stated:

> that a doctor is not guilty of negligence if he has acted in accordance with a practice accepted as proper by a responsible body of opinion of medical men skilled in that particular art; a doctor is not negligent if he is acting in accordance with such a practice merely because there is body of opinion that takes a contrary view.

Recent authority indicates that the opinion held by a responsible body must be a logical one (Bolitho).

Nevertheless, it is advisable to have a hospital manual of policies and to follow these if possible. It is also important to ensure that all relevant comments and recommendations are written in the patients' and ward records (e.g. doses of antibiotics and times of starting and completing courses of treatment, or measures taken in a ward to combat an MRSA outbreak if the patient becomes infected or colonized with MRSA). The procedures introduced for the infected patient (e.g. isolation, nasal or skin treatment) should be written in the patient's records.

RISK ASSESSMENT AND MANAGEMENT

Balance of Risks

Assessment of risk of spread should be based as far as possible on scientific evidence. A source, a route of spread and a portal of entry of sufficient numbers of organisms to a susceptible host are required for an infection to occur. If these conditions are not met, spread is not possible. For example, a surgical dressing from a patient with an HIV infection is not a risk if it is sealed in a plastic bag or handled with gloves. If the HIV seropositive rate in a hospital is low (e.g. 0.1%), the risk of acquiring infection is extremely low. Only 0.4% of personnel who receive a needlestick injury from a known HIV infected person will acquire infection, and even less from exposure of mucous membrane or skin.

Measures to control infection can be expensive and time-wasting for staff and patients, and should not be introduced unless evidence of their potential value is available or there is consensus agreement by experts.

The application of the Health and Safety at Work Act to infection in hospitals may create problems which are not present in factories or in the general community. The interpretation of the Act in terms of infection in patients is sometimes uncertain, as it is not intended to interfere with the clinical responsibility of medical or nursing staff. The interpretation 'as far as is reasonably practicable' is difficult to define. Hospitals are establishments for treating sick people, many of whom are admitted with an existing infection or will acquire an infection during their stay. The diagnosis of an infection may take several days, and non-infective conditions can closely mimic infection. Susceptibility of the patient and techniques of treatment are important factors in the emergence of infection. Most hospital infections are unlikely to be transferred to staff, and the incidence of acquired infection in staff is usually very low (if the common upper respiratory infections are excluded). Although every effort is made to minimize risks, staff should accept that a high standard of personal hygiene is necessary, and they must also acknowledge that there is some risk of acquiring an infection during the course of their normal duties.

It is important that infected patients, irrespective of the infection (e.g. AIDS), receive the best possible treatment and that this is not impaired because of their infection. The spread of infection between patients and staff cannot be eliminated, but it can be reduced by simple methods such as handwashing. Expensive measures which involve uneconomic use of staff and resources may in fact achieve little more than these simple basic measures. All grades of hospital staff are responsible for adopting measures to reduce the likelihood of spread of infection, and this personal responsibility cannot necessarily be passed on to the employing authority. Some departments, (e.g. intensive care or isolation units) may be potentially more hazardous to patients and staff than others due to the types of patient treated and the methods of treatment required. All patients and equipment should be considered to be potentially infective and require a basic standard of care or treatment to prevent transmission of infection.

Special measures may be recommended by infection control staff for known transmissible infections. The increased risks of infection should also be recognized by visitors and, where appropriate, visitors should be made aware of these possible hazards. Decisions on the measures that are required in a particular situation must be made in terms of possible benefit to patients, benefit to the hospital community, and the cost of the measures. Cost benefit is obviously not a term to be used lightly when considering infection in patients or staff, but it is unfortunately a necessity. The occasional failure of soundly based, commonly accepted measures is not necessarily due to negligence. Some infections in hospitals are inevitable irrespective of preventative measures, and there is an irreducible minimum (Ayliffe, 1986). If legal or other authorities criticize staff in the absence of well-founded evidence, infection control staff are likely to adopt a defensive approach which is detrimental both to patient care and to the NHS as a whole. Some examples of difficult decisions for infection control staff are described below.

A common problem is the management of a chronic salmonella carrier – either a member of staff or a patient. Person-to-person spread of salmonella is rare except in infant nurseries. The staff carrier can still, with reasonable safety, return to work after the cessation of symptoms provided that he or she does not handle food or drugs, and is conscientious in matters of personal hygiene (Pether and Scott, 1982). A patient can with reasonable safety be sent home or to a long-term care unit while still excreting salmonella if he or she is otherwise fit to be discharged, and provided that suitable instructions about personal hygiene are given. If spread of infection occurs in either of these situations, the hospital could be held legally responsible, but the risk was assessed as low and any other course of action would have been unrealistic.

Staphylococcus aureus is the commonest cause of infection of clean operation wounds, and it is carried in the noses of 20% of healthy individuals. Most of these strains are sensitive to antibiotics (except usually to penicillin) and rarely cause infection, but strains that cause infections in hospitals are often resistant to several antibiotics, which may include methicillin. Strains of methicillin-resistant *Staphylococcus aureus* (MRSA) have been present in hospitals world-wide for many years, and are not usually more virulent than antibiotic-sensitive strains. They are usually resistant to several antibiotics, including the penicillinase-resistant penicillins and cephalosporins, but most infections are still treatable (see Chapter 9). Some strains tend to spread more easily than most antibiotic-sensitive strains, but they present little risk to the families and friends of infected patients. Patients are exposed to them in most hospitals, and they are not 'superbugs'. MRSA strains are often present in the noses of patients and staff without causing any symptoms, and they should be treated like any other multi-resistant organism. Efforts to eradicate them from hospitals in most countries have been unsuccessful without considerable use of resources. Although every effort should be made to prevent their spread in high-risk wards (e.g. intensive care), established preventative measures are not always successful (Combined Working Party of the British Society for Antimicrobial Chemotherapy, Hospital Infection Society and Infection Control Nurses Association, 1998; see also Chapter 9). However, full preventative measures may not be cost-effective if many wards are affected (i.e. if MRSA strains are endemic in the hospital). Staff should always make every reasonable effort to prevent the spread of MRSA (and other antibiotic-resistant strains) by hand-washing and good hygiene, but the detection and isolation of all symptomless carriers in general hospital wards is rarely cost-effective or realistic, and failure to achieve this does not constitute negligence by the hospital. The acquisition of

MRSA is one of the risks taken by patients in hospital today, and should be explained to all patients on admission. It should also be explained to the relatives of patients infected with MRSA.

Another of the major risk decisions is the deployment of staff carriers of HBV, HCV and HIV (see Chapter 9). The incidence of carriage is generally low and transmission is rare, so routine screening of staff is therefore not indicated. However, carriers of HBeAg have transmitted infection when performing certain invasive procedures, but risks of transfer from an HBsAg carrier are very low, and the carrier who is e-antigen negative should be able to continue with normal work. The direct transmission of HIV infection from an infected health service staff member during a procedure has not been reported in the UK, and infected health staff members should also be able to continue with normal work. These low risks may still be unacceptable to the public, and patients might expect to be informed and to make their own choice. It is therefore important that the staff carrier receives impartial advice on these problems in line with national guidelines (e.g. UK Health Departments, 1998).

Routine screening of staff involves keeping them unnecessarily off duty without evidence that the organisms they are carrying are likely to infect others. A large proportion of the staff will, if screened, be found to carry *Staphylococcus aureus* in their noses, and a much smaller proportion may be found to carry Group A/β-haemolytic streptococci in the throat or salmonella in the faeces. However, most of them are unlikely to cause clinical infection in patients with whom they have contact.

The inanimate environment is not a major factor in the spread of infection, and structural alterations can be costly. Care should be taken not to embark on expensive structural changes on the basis of infection hazard because of an apparent requirement in a guidance document, rather than on the basis of evidence of efficacy in the prevention of infection. A good selective surveillance system is likely to be more cost-effective in the prevention of infection than routine environmental monitoring, or routine screening of the faeces of catering staff or the noses of theatre staff. Routine monitoring of air or surfaces in operating-theatres, pharmacies or SSD clean rooms is an example of a test method which is not related to the risk of infection.

The risks of acquiring an infection caused by a spore-bearing organism from a properly cleaned and disinfected operative endoscope are small, despite the fact that spores are not killed by routine disinfection processes. Disinfection should therefore be considered to be a reasonable process even if a case of tetanus has occurred, as a chemical 'sterilization' process (e.g. exposure to glutaraldehyde for 3–10 hours) is not a practical possibility for routine decontamination, and in itself may pose an unnecessarily high risk to the health-care worker who would be exposed to higher levels of the substance.

Risk management

Risk management is described as a practical approach to prevention of the possibility of incurring risk (incurring misfortune or loss). Within the context of the NHS, this is reflected in the management of potential financial loss, personal injury, loss of life, staff availability, buildings, equipment and reputation.

Risk management requires consideration of the activities of the organization by, for example:
- identifying the risks that exist;
- assessing their potential frequency and severity;
- eliminating risks if possible;
- reducing the risks that cannot be eliminated and putting in place financial mechanisms to absorb the financial consequences of the risks that remain.

The NHS Management Executive (1993) have stated that effective infection control is vital for the successful operation of all health-care premises, and discusses the following four specific sections.
- organization, policies and information;
- training and awareness;
- food;
- separating 'clean' and 'dirty' matter.

It includes the following action points:
- policies and procedures for infection control must be known to all staff;
- staff must be aware of whom they should approach for advice on infection control issues;
- all staff should receive appropriate training on infection control;
- all staff should be made aware of the importance of good hygiene in the handling and storage of food;
- there should be clear guidance to staff on the separation of clean and dirty materials and adequate facilities to put this into practice.

Although the above requirements are important, the main infection risks involve the management of patients, which often requires balancing risks against necessary treatment.

QUALITY, CLINICAL AND INFECTION CONTROL AUDIT

Rebecca Evans

Since the introduction of the NHS, the need to provide a high-quality, cost-effective service has been evident. Measurements of quality in health-care provision are still evolving. Today, in pursuit of quality, health-care organizations are actively encouraged to monitor and critically evaluate the practices and resources used, through audit and resource management (Baggot, 1994). This has resulted in purchasing or commissioning authorities stipulating pre-determined or negotiated standards of service. Providers, as part of the contractual process for patient services, should, in response to internal standard-setting, adhere to agreed quality standards. The adoption and internalization of the audit process should be viewed as essential activities in providing a quality service.

In parallel with industry and business outside the NHS, where attainment of quality measures such as the BS5750, (now also implemented within the NHS) is seen by producers and customers alike as a marker of quality. Within health care, independent audit bodies such as the National Audit Office (1986), the British Standard Institute and the King's Fund Centre all have national reputations. British Standards are used throughout the UK as markers of quality, and many of them are being replaced by European Standards. Within health-care organizations, particularly infection control, the British Standard Institute is recognized in several areas, including the disposal of sharps and medical electrical equipment and sterilizers. The standards on infection control in hospitals that have been produced for national organizations have been discussed above (see p. 29).

The King's Fund Organization Audit (KFOA) aims to stimulate good practice and innovations in health-care management through service and organizational development, education, policy analysis and organizational audit (King's Fund Centre, 1988). The Organizational Audit project was launched in 1989, one week prior to the Government's White Paper entitled *Working for Patients* (Department of Health, 1989b), to determine whether a national approach to standard-setting in health care was appropriate. Although we have seen a change of government and the introduction of a new White Paper, *The New NHS: Modern, Dependable* (Department of Health, 1997), the focus is still on quality, with government directives aimed at providing a high-quality service for patients. The setting of 'National Standards of Excellence' and the introduction of 'Clinical Governance' is aimed at providing new incentives and imposing new sanctions on health-care organizations to improve quality and efficiency whilst also defining clear boundaries of responsibility.

'Clinical Governance' is a term which encompasses many of the fundamental elements used to improve quality (Department of Health, 1999). The principles behind 'Clinical Governance' can be seen as a tool by which infection control teams provide a quality-led service to the patient, since many of the principles of 'Clinical Governance', such as 'evidence-based practice', audit and risk assessment, are essentially those already underpinning the role of Infection Control Teams.

For decades the aim of Infection Control Teams has been to provide a service which is based on good-quality practices and employs credible surveillance systems. Audit tools have been devised and used in various guises both to identify problem areas and to provide evidence for improvement of practice (Millward *et al.*, 1993; Ward, 1995). The audit tool described by Millward and colleagues assesses compliance with infection control practice against specified standards which embody the basic principles of infection control. This tool has been used widely and effectively as a benchmark for good practice, enabling infection control teams to identify and focus on problem areas. However, although audit tools are a valuable means of monitoring quality, Mehtar (1995) suggests that for surveillance to be effective it needs to be relevant, with findings relayed back to all personnel. Both Millward *et al.* (1993) and Ward (1995) reinforce this view, stating that audit tools should have a strong educational element.

In an attempt to improve quality and provide an efficient, cost-effective service, Infection Control Teams involved in clinical audit should be concerned with the processes which are likely to influence the acquisition of infection. The use and monitoring of infection control practices is an obvious requirement for the prevention and control of infection. However, although monitoring infection rates throughout the hospital is regarded by many as a means of audit, it is not generally perceived as practicable or necessarily cost-effective, as many variables exist (e.g. length of stay, type of operation and associated risk factors) which have the potential to introduce bias and impair the accuracy of data (see Chapter 3).

With the increasing demand for infection control teams to produce data, especially infection rates, there should be clear predefined aims and objectives with regard to the value and use of the audit data. To ensure accurate collection and analysis of data, the approach needs to be logical and consistent to enable standardization of results. Equally, when formalizing information it is essential that all of the relevant data collated includes any complications within clinical audit. However, because of the potential inconsistencies it would be more appropriate if the data presented by infection control teams focused on specific elements such as infections in high-risk or other targeted areas, isolation of alert organisms and efficiency measures taken to control infections (see p. 42). Equally, for infection control teams to disseminate the knowledge gained, they should participate in internal audit sessions to gain an insight into other practices being undertaken across health-care organizations which have infection control implications.

When assessing the need for audit, it is important to take other influences into consideration. A recent report from the House of Lords focuses awareness on the emergence of multi-resistant organisms, highlighting the need for Infection Control Teams (ICTs) to audit antibiotic usage within Trusts, with a view to controlling the dispensing of inappropriate antibiotics (Select Committee on Science and Technology Report, House of Lords, 1998).

Information technology should be used as a tool to implement audit. The new Government White Paper entitled *Information for Health* (Department of Health, 1998) aims to improve communication between hospitals and the community by forming strong computer links. If ICTs are engaging in audit, the links between hospitals and the community should be fully utilized in order to enable more accurate collection of data (e.g. the computerization of patient records and results and post-discharge complications such as wound infections). However, it is essential that prior to the input of data there are clearly defined criteria in place to allow standardization of results (see Chapter 3).

The following audit procedures should therefore be considered by the ICT:
- surveillance of infections (see Chapter 3);
- measurement of compliance with infection control policies and practices (e.g. handwashing, clinical practices, the environment, sharps safety and clinical waste). These assessments should both allow identification of areas with good practice and target areas for improvement, enabling the ICNs to focus on problem areas. The infection control team's involvement in the audit of policies and practice should be structured and concerned with processes which are likely to influence the acquisition of infection and not irrelevant testing, such as routine air sampling of operating-theatres and SSD clean rooms;

- taking part in audits of departments with an infection component e.g. laundries, SSDs and catering establishments;
- attendance at clinical audit sessions on a regular basis to discuss infections with clinicians;
- audit of the ICT's own techniques (e.g. speed of response and efficacy of control of an outbreak).

NOTIFICATION OF INFECTIOUS DISEASES

Some diseases are notifiable by law to the CCDC. The doctor who diagnoses the infection is responsible for the notification (see Chapter 18).

Although there is no statutory obligation to notify the detection of symptom-free carriers of bacteria that cause notifiable disease, it is recommended that persistent carriers of typhoid bacilli and other salmonellae should be reported to the CCDC.

REFERENCES

Act of Parliament (1988) *Control of Substances Hazardous to Health Regulations.* London: HMSO.

Ayliffe, G.A.J. (1986) Nosocomial infection and the irreducible minimum. *Infection Control* 7 (Supplement) 92.

Baggot, R. (1994) *Health and healthcare in Britain.* London: St Martin's Press.

British Medical Association (1997) Medical decisions must be logically defensible. *British Medical Journal* 315, 1327.

Central Sterilizing Club (1999) Reprocessing of single-use medical devices in hospitals. *Zentral Sterilization* 7, 37.

Combined Working Party of the British Society for Antimicrobial Chemotherapy, Hospital Infection Society and Infection Control Nurses Association (1998) Revised guidelines for the control of epidemic methicillin-resistant *Staphylococcus aureus* infection in hospitals. *Journal of Hospital Infection* 39, 253.

Damani, N.M. (1997) *Hospital infection control.* London: Greenwich Medical Media Ltd.

Department of Health (1989a) *The Control of Substances Hazardous to Health: guidance for the initial assessment in hospitals.* London: HMSO.

Department of Health (1989b) *Working for patients. Medical audit.* Working Paper No. 6. London: HMSO.

Department of Health (1993) *Risk management in the NHS.* London: Health Publications Unit.

Department of Health (1995) *Hospital infection control. Guidance on the control of infection in hospitals.* Paper prepared by the Hospital Infection Working Group of the Department of Health Public Health Laboratory Service. London: Department of Health and HMSO.

Department of Health (1997) *The new NHS: modern, dependable.* London: HMSO.

Department of Health (1998) *Information for Health*. London: HMSO.

Department of Health (1999) *Clinical governance: quality in the new NHS*. London: Department of Health.

Garner, J.S. (1996) Guidelines for isolation precautions in hospitals. *Infection Control and Hospital Epidemiology* **17**, 53.

Haley, R.W., Culver, D.H., White, J.W. *et al.* (1985) The efficacy of infection surveillance and control programs in preventing nosocomial infection in US hospitals. *American Journal of Epidemiology* **121**, 182.

Harrison, D.I. (1991) Control of Substances Hazardous to Health (COSHH). Regulations and hospital infection. *Journal of Hospital Infection* **17** (**Supplement A**), 530.

Hurwitz, B. (1995) Clinical guidelines and the law. What is the status of guidelines? *British Medical Journal* **311**, 1517.

Hurwitz, B. (1999) Legal and practical considerations of clinical practice guidelines. *British Medical Journal* **318**, 661.

Infection Control Working Party (1993) *Standards in infection control in hospitals*, London: HMSO.

King's Fund Centre (1988) Health services accreditation. London: Kings Fund.

Medical Devices Agency (1995) *The re-use of medical devices supplied for single use only*. London: Department of Health.

Medical Devices Agency (1999) *Guidance on decontamination from the Microbiological Advisory Committee. Part 3. Procedures. Section 1*. London: Department of Health.

Medical Research Council (1968) Aseptic methods in the operating suite. *Lancet* **i**, 705, 763, 831.

Mehtar, S. (1995) Infection control programmes – are they cost-effective? *Journal of Hospital Infection* **30** (**Supplement**), 26.

Millward, S., Barnett, J. and Thomlinson, D. (1993) A clinical infection control audit programme: evaluation of an audit tool used by infection control nurses to monitor standards and assess effective staff training. *Journal of Hospital Infection* **24**, 219.

National Audit Office (1986) *Value for money: developments in the NHS*. London: HMSO.

NHS Executive (1996) *Clinical guidelines*. London: Department of Health.

Pether, J.V.S. and Scott, R.J.D. (1982) Salmonella carriers. Are they dangerous? Study to identify finger contamination with salmonella by convalescent carriers. *Journal of Infection* **5**, 81.

Select Committee on Science and Technology Report, House of Lords (1998) *Resistance to antibiotics and other antimicrobial agents*. London: HMSO.

United Kingdom Central Council for Nursing, Midwifery and Health Visiting (UKCC) (1995) Post-registration education and practice (PREP). London: UKCC.

UK Health Departments (1998) Guidance for Clinical Health Care Workers: protection against infection with blood-borne viruses. London: Department of Health.

Ward, K.A. (1995) Education and infection control audit. *Journal of Hospital Infection*. **30** (**Supplement**), 248.

Ward, V., Wilson, J., Taylor, L. *et al.* (1997) *Preventing hospital-acquired infection. Clinical guidelines.* London: Public Health Laboratory Service.

Williams, R.E.O., Blowers, R., Garrod, L.P. and Shooter, R.A. (1966) *Hospital infection: causes and prevention*, 2nd edn. London: Lloyd Luke.

chapter 3

SURVEILLANCE, RECORDS AND REPORTS

In most hospitals the overall incidence of infection is unknown and the methods of surveillance (i.e. discovery and recording of infection) are variable. Surveillance has been defined as 'the continuing scrutiny of all aspects of occurrence and spread of a disease that are pertinent to effective control' (Benenson, 1990). Surveillance of infection in hospital is necessary for the following reasons:

- to detect changes in the pattern of disease and measurement of outcome;
- to recognize, by any unusual level or change in level of incidence, the existence or impending spread of an outbreak, and to identify the appearance of any particularly dangerous organism;
- to judge the desirability of introducing special measures to control an outbreak, or threatened outbreak, and to assess the efficacy of such measures;
- to assess the efficacy of the regular preventative measures in use in the hospital and provide information for planning and services and use of resources;
- to reduce the level of avoidable infection and to identify high-risk patients so that selective measures can be introduced, and to ensure that control efforts have their maximum and most cost-effective outcome.

Surveillance consists of the following:

- data collection;
- analysis of the data;
- feedback of the results to medical and nursing staff and others involved in decision-making.

Surveillance and record-keeping must not be regarded as an end in themselves, but as an instrument for measuring the effectiveness of an infection control programme and for giving an early indication of outbreaks or problem areas. The main purpose of recording infections is to provide information to enable action to be taken. Administrative managers should not expect infection rates to be recorded for the whole hospital, as this is not a cost-effective procedure and it does not necessarily improve quality control. Keeping records is time-consuming and should be kept to the essential minimum unless more detailed records are required for a particular purpose (e.g. investigation of an outbreak). However, the Study on the Efficacy of Nosocomial Infection Control (SENIC) conducted in the USA indicated that a highly efficient surveillance and infection control system could reduce the infection rates by one-third. Feedback to clinicians was considered to be of particular importance in reducing wound infection (Haley *et al.* 1985a). This reduction in response to feedback has been reported by other authors, but there have been exceptions (Wilson *et al.*, 1998).

Some surveillance is therefore necessary in every hospital (Department of Health, 1995), but the short hospital stays of many patients mean that surveillance must be extended to the community if accurate data is to be obtained. Several methods of surveillance of infections in patients will be described (Glenister *et al.*, 1993; Emmerson and Ayliffe, 1996; Glynn *et al.*, 1997; for further information see Haley *et al.*, 1992).

In addition to patients, surveillance of staff, the environment and certain equipment will be discussed, but routine screening of staff or routine sampling of the environment is not generally recommended.

METHODS OF SURVEILLANCE OF INFECTION IN PATIENTS

DAILY SCRUTINY OF LABORATORY REPORTS

This is a minimal requirement in all hospitals. It is simple and does not consume much additional staff time. It is aided by computerized laboratory records that allow specified organisms to be 'flagged' up every day.

Examination of the laboratory reports should enable the presence of 'Alert' organisms to be detected (Department of Health, 1995), i.e. those organisms which are likely to spread and cause outbreaks (see Table 3.1). This method can also be usefully supplemented by including all organisms from special units (e.g. intensive care units) or from infections that are particularly severe or difficult to treat (e.g. bacteraemia or meningitis). Evidence of several related wound or urinary tract infections in one ward might also be identified from laboratory reports.

The incidence of infection cannot be calculated from laboratory reports alone, as not all infections will be sampled bacteriologically. Nevertheless, useful tabulations of antibiotic-resistant and other organisms (with unit of origin) can be produced. The laboratory method should be supported by ward staff reporting potential outbreaks (e.g. several cases of diarrhoea) by telephone to the laboratory or ICN before laboratory reports on the patient samples are available. Link nurses can be useful in implementing this procedure.

Similarly, managers of relevant departments (e.g. SSD, catering, or occupational health) should contact the ICN if a member of staff develops an infection which might spread in the hospital.

LABORATORY RECORDS AND ROUTINE VISITS TO THE WARD

The ICN examines the laboratory records every morning (as described above) and discusses the results with the biomedical scientists and ICD. The nurse completes the necessary information on relevant infected patients by visiting the ward, and determines whether they are true clinical infections and whether they are hospital acquired.

Table 3.1 Examples of infections routinely recorded

'Alert' organisms

1   *Streptococcus pyogenes, Salmonella* and *Shigella* species, enteropathogenic or toxigenic strains
    of *E. coli* (e.g. 0157), *Mycobacterium tuberculosis,* rotavirus, RSV, *Pseudomonas aeruginosa,*
    Neisseria meningitidis, Legionella species
2   Highly resistant strains of *Staphylococcus aureus* (e.g. resistant to methicillin, gentamicin, fusidic
    acid, mupirocin)
    Highly resistant strains of Gram-negative bacilli (e.g. resistant to gentamicin, third-generation
    cephalosporins, quinolones)
    Highly resistant enterococci (e.g. resistant to vancomycin, β-lactamase-producing strains)
3   Strains showing unusual resistance (e.g. penicillin-resistant *Streptococcus pneumoniae*)
4   Blood-culture isolates, CSF isolates

Clinical infections

1   All infections from the special-care baby unit, intensive-care unit, paediatric wards and other
    high-risk areas.
2   Communicable diseases ('Alert' conditions) (e.g. food poisoning, diarrhoea and vomiting, enteric
    fever, tuberculosis, childhood infectious diseases, diphtheria, legionellosis, meningitis)
3   Wound or other selected infections (e.g. urinary tract infection)

If the ward staff do not send samples to the laboratory, this method may be no more effective than laboratory surveillance alone, but if frequent visits are made to the ward, the nurse can encourage ward staff to send samples from all patients with suspected infections, and he or she can also obtain information on possible infections which cannot be sampled (e.g. deep infections). In addition, the ward sister or link nurse could be encouraged to keep a daily record of any infection-related problems. This can be examined by the ICN if the sister is busy at the time of the visit. Special-risk units (e.g. intensive-care units) should be visited regularly, even if none of the patients are known to be infected.

LABORATORY-BASED WARD LIAISON

This is an extension of the above method that enables infection rates to be recorded. It is one of the most sensitive methods, detecting 76% of infections when compared to the continuous surveillance method which provides information on all infections (Glenister *et al.,* 1993), but it is still time-consuming, requiring 45 hours per week for 500 beds. The ICN follows up patients as described above, and he or she also visits all wards at least twice weekly to review the notes of all patients considered by the ward staff to be infected. However, it is not a cost-effective method in some wards, particularly if patients are discharged from hospital rapidly, or in wards with few cross-infection problems. It is preferable to use a selective method (e.g. by surveillance of certain wards only). The surveyed wards can be rotated at regular intervals or monitored closely if there is a particular problem, but high-risk wards (e.g. ICUs, transplant units and special-care baby units) should always be routinely surveyed. Other targeted approaches could include surveillance of surgical wounds, bacteraemias, pneumonias, invasive procedures (e.g. urinary tract catheterized patients) and patients receiving antibiotics. However, some of these involve considerable effort (e.g. peripheral IV sites are often poorly recorded and have low infection rates) for limited benefit.

PREVALENCE SURVEYS

The prevalence of infection refers to the number of cases of infection present in a ward or hospital over a defined period of time (e.g. 1 week) (*period prevalence*), or a specified point in time (e.g. 1 day) (*point prevalence*). Prevalence differs from incidence, which refers to the number of new cases of infection in a defined population over a defined period of time, usually at least several months. In a prevalence survey, all patients (or a defined subsample) in a hospital are visited on one occasion only and the presence of infection is recorded. Other information (e.g. antibiotic therapy, possible risk factors and microbiology results) is collected at the same time.

The prevalence rate is usually higher (e.g. 10%) than the incidence rate (e.g. 5%) because it takes into account the length of stay, and infected patients tend to stay in hospital longer than non-infected patients.

A prevalence survey is useful for assessing the rate of infection nationally (Meers *et al.*, 1981; Emmerson *et al.*, 1996). It is also useful in that it enables a recently appointed ICN to acquire knowledge of the hospital and its problems (Jepson, 1996). Some hospitals conduct an annual survey to supplement other surveillance techniques. Such a survey provides an infection rate, but the numbers of infections are usually too small for a statistical comparison between surveys, and it is not adequate for routine day-to-day control of infection. However, repeated surveys may be a convenient method for assessing changes in infection throughout the hospital over several years (Ayliffe, 1986; French *et al.*, 1989; Vaqué *et al.*, 1990). A prevalence survey in a ward or hospital (e.g. taking nasal and lesion swabs from all patients and possibly staff, as well as information on infections) may also be useful for determining the extent and spread of antibiotic-resistant organisms, or to ensure that these have been eliminated.

RECORDS OF INFECTION

Card index systems (e.g. Kardex) have been widely used. If a separate page is used for patients in each ward or unit, this enables problems in a particular area to be detected over a period of time (see Table 3.2). A board showing all of the wards in a hospital can be kept in the ICN's office. Coloured flags can be used to indicate the location of infections, the different shapes and colours of the flags denoting the different organisms. This approach is particularly useful during an outbreak. However, these methods are now being replaced by computerized records with a daily printout (Kelsey, 1996), and infection control computer packages are available (e.g. WHO-CARE). This system has been used to compare infection rates in Belgium and The Netherlands, with some success (Mertens, 1996).

Although computer printouts are usually available for laboratory reports, and in many hospitals patient data are computerized, the merging of data is more

Table 3.2 Example of a card index record

Ward	Date and specimen	Patient's name	Date of birth	Date of admission	Consultant	Operation/diagnosis	Date of operation	Type	Organism	Antibiotic resistance	Comments
A	1/1 W/S	John Smith	1/1/01	1/1	RS	Varicose ulcers	–	–	*Streptococcus group A*	Sens	Present on admission
A	10/1 W/S	John Jones	10/10/10	1/1	RS	Appendectomy	6/1	C/C	*Bacteroides*	Sens	
A	25/1 W/S	John Doe	2/2/22	20/1	RS	Lumbar sympathectomy	23/1	Clean	*Staphylococcus aureus*	PT	Phage type 80/81 drained

W/S,   wound swab;
Sens,   sensitive to all antibiotics tested;
C/C,   clean/contaminated;
P   penicillin-resistant;
T   tetracycline-resistant.

difficult. Hospital infection information often has to be added separately, and this can be time-consuming, added to the fact that the required data may not be available in the patient's records. Patients' notes are frequently incomplete, but the requirements for clinical audit should improve their accuracy. In many instances, clinicians will be responsible for records of infection as part of the audit system, but the infection control team should also be involved in the collection and analysis of data. Computerized data will not necessarily produce accurate infection rates unless possible risk factors can be incorporated and post-discharge infections are included (McGowan, 1996). Variations in interpretations of definitions of infection are also responsible for differences in reported rates between hospitals, and scoring systems are sometimes used to improve the accuracy of definitions (Wilson et al., 1990, 1998). A computerized program, in addition to detecting 'Alert' organisms and other special pathogens, can also be used to detect changes in infection rates over long periods which might otherwise go unrecognized, but there are problems in adjusting the sensitivity of the method if only small numbers of infection are recorded each week.

SURGICAL WOUND INFECTION

A wound is a break in an epithelial surface which may be surgical or accidental. A wound infection should have either a purulent discharge in or exuding from the wound, or a painful spreading erythema indicative of cellulitis (Spencer, 1993). Records of wound infections are commonly kept and are particularly useful for audit purposes.

The wound infection rate must be defined if comparisons are to be made either within a hospital or between hospitals. A list of all operations performed may be obtained from the operating-theatre or from computerized patient records, and should at least be classified into clean, clean–contaminated or contaminated (see below), but even in these categories there can be wide variation in infection rates for different types of operations. A meaningful single overall infection rate for all types of wound is not possible, as the likelihood of infection differs in each of these categories and the numbers involved may be too small for comparison. It is also useful to record the severity of infection for each type of wound, and whether the wound was drained or not. Accuracy may be further improved by comparing individual types of operation (e.g. hernia), and introducing 'risk' factors into the calculation (Cruse and Foord, 1973). Using a computer model, the incidence or prevalence rate can be corrected for 'risk' factors such as age, sex, type of operation (clean, clean–contaminated or contaminated), pre-operative stay, wound drainage and special factors such as diabetes (Bibby et al., 1986, Garibaldi et al., 1991). However, other models are available and differ in some respects (see, for example, Simchen et al., 1984, 1988). Haley et al., (1985b) have suggested the following four factors:
- operation on abdomen;
- length of operation over 2 hours;
- contaminated or dirty wound;
- three or more underlying diagnoses.

These have been further modified (Culver *et al.*, 1991; Wong, 1996) as follows:
- an American Society of Anaesthesiologists pre-operative assessment of 3, 4 or 5;
- an operation classified as contaminated or dirty/infected;
- an operation having a duration of >75th percentile of operation durations noted nationally for the specific procedure.

Infections that occur after discharge from hospital must also be included if accurate rates are to be obtained. The infection rate should be based on clinical and not bacteriological findings. Only operations in which there has been a breach in the skin should be included in the assessment. Non-operative endoscopies, manipulations and examinations under anaesthesia, vaginal operations and also incisions of abscesses, should not be included in the total operations at risk for acquired infection. Ulcerations and pressure sores should also be excluded, but should be recorded separately. When recording the incidence or prevalence of wound infection, the following descriptions, definitions and information are useful.

1 The type of operation, and whether the wound is drained or not.
   Operations are further classified as:
   - clean (e.g. a hernia repair) – an operation not transecting gastrointestinal, genito-urinary or tracheobronchial systems, and not performed in the vicinity of any apparent inflammatory reaction;
   - clean–contaminated (e.g. operations on the stomach or gall-bladder) – an operation transecting one of the above systems where bacterial contamination could occur but is usually not abundant, and where evidence of definite contamination is not available;
   - contaminated (e.g. operations on the colon, mouth or perforated appendix) – an operation transecting systems where bacteria are known to be present (and are usually abundant), or in the vicinity of apparent inflammatory reactions.

   Note In some classifications a dirty/infected category is included where an incision is made through an infected area (e.g. abscess) or where there is gross contamination (e.g. perforated viscus).

2 The presence or absence of pus or cellulitis.
3 Sepsis and degree of severity:
   - mild sepsis – small or superficial area of inflammation with minimal discharge;
   - moderate sepsis – superficial inflammation of the whole wound (or over one-third of it) with a serous or small amount of purulent discharge, or a deeper infection involving a small area (one-third or less) usually with a purulent discharge;
   - severe sepsis – a deep purulent infection, with or without sinuses or fistulae, or widespread cellulitis, or wound breakdown with an obvious inflammatory reaction and pus.

Alternatively, the severity may be classified as major or minor (Spencer, 1993). A major infection is present when the purulent discharge is accompanied by partial or complete dehiscence of the fascial layers of the wound, deep tissue destruction, or spreading cellulitis and lymphangitis that requires antibiotic therapy.

A minor infection is present when there is a discharge of pus without lymphangitis or deep tissue destruction.

The infections can also be classified as primary or secondary. Infections are primary if there are no predisposing conditions. Secondary infections may follow a complication which results in the discharge of bile, serum, gastric or intestinal contents, urine, cerebrospinal fluid (CSF) or a haematoma.

4 Organisms and antibiotic sensitivity.
5 Other information – which can be collected as required by the individual hospital (e.g. operating-theatre, surgeon, length of operations, number of primary diagnoses, use of operative endoscope, antibiotic treatment, probable origin of infection, time of dressing of wound, etc.)

PROBABLE LOCATION OF WOUND INFECTION

It is advantageous to know where the infection was acquired, and the following points may be helpful in determining this.

INFECTION ACQUIRED IN OPERATING-THEATRE

This may be indicated by the following:
1 deep infection in a clean, undrained wound at any time;
2 infection occurring within 3 days of the operation, or prior to first dressing in a clean wound;
3 supporting evidence includes the following:
   ● pyrexia;
   ● staphylococcus of the same type not isolated from any patient in the ward;
   ● staphylococcus of the same type isolated from a member of the operating staff and not present in the ward;
   ● staphylococcus of the same type in different wards from patients operated on in the same operating-theatre.

INFECTION ACQUIRED IN THE WARD

This is indicated by superficial infection in a wound (usually drained), occurring after first dressing. Culture of discharge may initially be negative, and deep infection may develop later in a drained wound. Supporting evidence is staphylococcus of the same type isolated from other patients or members of the staff in the ward.

PLACE OF ACQUISITION OF INFECTION NOT KNOWN

This applies when there is superficial infection in any wound after first dressing and no available evidence from bacteriology in support of theatre or ward infection.

INFECTION ACQUIRED FROM PATIENT'S OWN BACTERIAL FLORA

These include infections due to *Staphylococcus epidermidis* or *Staphylococcus aureus* that was present in the patient's nose or on their skin prior to or at the time of surgery. However, resistant strains may have been acquired by the patient in the ward before the operation.

Infections that are due to antibiotic-sensitive Gram-negative bacilli usually involve *E. coli* or *Bacteroides* species.

POST-DISCHARGE INFECTIONS

Now that many patients are being discharged rapidly from hospital, acquired infections commonly manifest themselves in the community (Department of Health, 1995; Mertens, 1996). This is particularly the case with day surgery. The estimates available suggest that 21–70% of surgical wound infections become apparent after leaving hospital. The accurate detection of these can be difficult and time-consuming. Although infection rates will be of little value without this information, the cost-effectiveness of collecting the data requires consideration. As severe infections will be readmitted to hospital, is it really necessary to know the number of minor infections?

Methods of collection of data on post-discharge infections include the following:

1 A form may be completed by community health-care workers. Community nurses may be prepared to do this, but it is an additional task in an already busy daily schedule. However, it is probably the most appropriate method.
2 The patient may report to their general practitioner, but may only do this if the infection is severe.
3 The patient may complete a form and return it to the hospital in a stamped addressed envelope. Some patients will not bother to do this and will use the stamp for other purposes!
4 The patient may return to the hospital out-patient clinic after a fixed period (e.g. 6 weeks). This post-operative review is now often the responsibility of the general practitioner. This is often the most effective method.
5 Telephone surveys. However, many patients (particularly in inner cities) do not have telephones.

A combination of methods is likely to yield the most reliable results, particularly if data on wound infection alone are collected.

OTHER INFECTIONS

Some of these are defined in Appendix 3.1. It is important to take 'risk' factors into consideration when comparing the incidence rates of infections other than wounds. Indwelling catheterization, duration of catheterization and antibiotic therapy should all be recorded when investigating urinary tract infection. Patient factors (e.g. chronic bronchitis, smoking and mechanical ventilation) will influence hospital-acquired respiratory infection (Haley, 1995; McGowan, 1996).

PRESENTATION OF REPORTS

Information on infections (e.g. wound and neonatal infections) is presented to the infection control committee at monthly or 3-monthly intervals. Although the incidence rate is usually based on infections per 100 patients discharged over 1 month or some other defined interval, a more realistic result can be obtained by using patient-days. The latter may be calculated by dividing the number of infections by the number of days spent by patients in hospital to obtain for example, the rate per 100 patient-days. Data on infections should be presented to clinical directorates for audit purposes, and the infection control team should be involved.

Individual results may be presented to surgeons on their own operations. The infection rate in clean undrained wounds is useful as a measure of acquired infection in the operating-theatre, and the total operations in each category (i.e. clean, clean-contaminated and contaminated) can usually be obtained from operating-theatre records. However, these are not always accurate, and must sometimes be supplemented from the patients' notes. This can be time-consuming, and if computerized data are not available, it may be sufficient to report the total number of infections in each category, provided that the number of operations remains reasonably constant.

Reports should be simple and the data preferably presented graphically, so that the current situation in wards or theatres can be immediately assessed and outbreaks can be monitored (see Figure 3.1). This is more readily achieved if the data is computerized. Commercially produced software packages are now available, but comparisons between surgeons or hospitals can be invalid unless risk factors are taken into consideration. Many hospitals will prefer to develop their own systems.

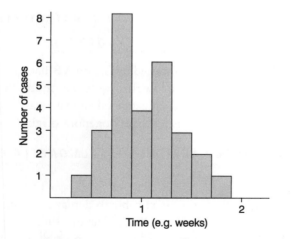

Figure 3.1 Example of an outbreak: number of infections occurring over a 2-week period.

Ward staff are always interested to know the results of studies made on their wards, and particularly the results of their own nasal or other swabs. Reports should always be sent to the ward concerned, following a bacteriological survey. As antibiotic therapy for individual patients is often required before the results of sensitivity tests are available, the medical staff should be provided with information on prevalent pathogens and their sensitivity patterns in the hospital (see Chapter 13).

SURVEILLANCE OF INFECTION IN STAFF

Surveillance of infection among members of staff – in close co-operation with the occupational health department – is also important. This includes enteric and other community-acquired infections, septic lesions and hospital-acquired infections (see Chapter 14).

Treatment and management of these infections can usually be decided by discussion between the ICD and the occupational health (or staff) medical officer and general practitioner.

DETECTION OF STAPHYLOCOCCAL CARRIERS

As approximately 20–30% of healthy staff are nasal carriers of *Staphylococcus aureus,* and as there is no accepted laboratory test for the virulence of this organism, routine nasal swabbing of staff in wards and operating-theatres is rarely indicated. Routine nasal swabs may be required from staff during outbreaks of infection and as a follow-up after treatment of a carrier on the staff. If an identifiable strain of known virulence or a strain with unusual resistance to antibiotics is responsible for an outbreak of infection, routine nasal swabbing may be required for a limited time as part of a programme to eradicate the organisms from the unit (see section on MRSA on p. 186). It is of greater importance to exclude staff with skin lesions or sepsis from wards or theatres than to spend time unnecessarily on the routine examination of nose swabs or swabs from other carriage sites.

DETECTION OF CARRIERS OF GROUP A β-HAEMOLYTIC STREPTOCOCCI (*STREPTOCOCCUS PYOGENES*)

The incidence of puerperal infection caused by Group A β-haemolytic streptococci (formerly the major hazard) is now so low that routine nose and throat swabbing is not required in maternity units. Swabs must be taken from staff and patients when an infection occurs in the unit that is not of endogenous origin (see Chapter 9).

DETECTION OF FAECAL CARRIERS OF *SALMONELLA* OR *SHIGELLA* SPECIES

Experience has shown that it is not practicable to demand routine bacteriological examination of faeces of food-handling staff. This measure is not recommended unless it is specifically indicated by past history or possibly recent visits to areas where enteric infections are endemic (see Chapters 9 and 12).

DETECTION OF HBV AND HCV CARRIERS AND PATIENTS WITH HIV ANTIBODIES

As carriers may not necessarily be excluded from working, routine screening is inadvisable. However, there can be problems with staff involved in invasive procedures (see Chapter 10). If tests for HIV are required, permission should be obtained from the staff concerned. Arrangements should be made for counselling before tests are carried out, and again afterwards if the results are positive.

ROUTINE MONITORING OF ENVIRONMENT AND EQUIPMENT

ENVIRONMENT

Unless there is an outbreak of infection, routine bacteriological sampling of floors, walls, surfaces and air is rarely indicated. If sampling is done, quantitative or semi-quantitative techniques should be used. The results should be reported as numbers of organisms per unit area or volume. Random swabbing of areas of unspecified size will yield results which are not comparable either with each other or with previous results and that are difficult to interpret. The non-quantitative isolation of even known pathogens may also be misleading. Selective and/or indicator media should be used to count pathogens such as *Staphylococcus aureus* or *Clostridium perfringens*. Standards for counts on surfaces are rarely valid; the numbers of organisms on a surface vary according to the amount of recontamination from the air, and on floors also from recontamination from shoes and trolleys. In addition, total bacterial counts in conventional operating-theatres and clean rooms in sterile services departments and pharmacies are of little or no value in assessing infection risks. However, counting of organisms on a surface may be useful for teaching and research purposes. The number of organisms in the air of wards or theatres depends mainly on the number of people in the room and their activity, and also on the airflow (air changes per hour), which is rarely standardized except in operating-theatres. Males often disperse more skin organisms than females.

Routine checking of airflow in a ventilated area is a more reliable guide to the efficiency of a ventilation system than bacteriological tests. However, if air to the theatre is recirculated, as in laminar-flow systems, filters must be checked regularly and occasionally bacteriological tests may be required. A total count of not more than 35 colony-forming units (cfu)/m^3 in the supply air of an empty operating-theatre is suggested as acceptable (Arrowsmith, 1985). Inspection of ducts, and testing of air flows and patency of filters are more accurate criteria (Holton and Ridgway, 1993). Airflows within the operating-room should also be checked using smoke tubes. Slit-samplers or other samplers should be operated by remote control to avoid sampling of organisms dispersed by the sampler operator. In an ultra-clean air theatre with walls, the airflow at 2 m above floor level should not be less than 0.3 m/s, and not less than 0.2 m/s in a unit without full walls. It is often recommended that routine micro-biological tests should be carried out on commissioning, after changing filters, after maintenance and annually (or possibly every 3 months) (Department of Health, 1994; Gosden *et al.*, 1998). However, ensuring that the filters continue to function correctly and the airflow is correct is of greater importance. It could be argued that microbiological sampling is too infrequent (even every 3 months) to be of practical value, but it might provide evidence in cases of wound infection associated with a possible claim for negligence. It is recommended that air sampled at 300 mm from the operation site in the ultraclean unit should contain less than 10 cfu/m³ and less than 1 cfu/m³ if occlusive clothing or a body exhaust suit is used (Department of Health, 1994). This may be difficult to test, and counts at the periphery of the walled enclosure should not exceed 20 cfu/m³, or should be less than 10 cfu/cm³ when using occlusive clothing or body exhaust systems. Air sampling (settle plates, or more quantitative methods, such as slit-sampling) may be useful for detecting the presence of staphylococcal dispersers in a ward or theatre and for testing individuals who are suspected of being dispersers. Contact plates from floors, other surfaces or bedding, may similarly be used to detect dispersers. Contact plates from floors are also useful for determining whether a ward is free of staphylococcal dispersers at the end of an outbreak, but will not necessarily exclude the presence of carriers.

EQUIPMENT

Routine monitoring of sterilization and some disinfection processes is necessary (see Chapter 4). Physical or chemical measurement of the efficiency of the process is generally preferable to bacteriological assessment. The results of bacteriological tests are only available after 1–5 days, depending on the organisms and the method of treatment. Sampling of treated equipment or fluids is of less value than process control, as initial contamination may be low and a large proportion of samples may be sterile. If sampling of the treated product is required, tests should be made by laboratories skilled in this type of work and statistically valid data produced.

Sterilization or disinfection by heat is preferable to chemical methods and, whenever possible, monitoring should be carried out with correctly placed thermometers or thermocouples. Records of temperature and time should be obtained for every cycle. Thorough and regular maintenance of equipment is as important as routine tests for efficiency.

Monitoring of sterilization processes is described in Chapter 4. Disinfection processes are often less well controlled. Heat disinfection of infant feeds, crockery, cutlery, laundry and bedpans, as well as pasteurization processes, should if possible be controlled by regular temperature-time measurements (see Chapter 6).

Disinfection by chemical methods also requires regular process-monitoring. Chemical tests of the process may sometimes be made (e.g. to assess the presence and amount of hydrogen peroxide, formaldehyde and ethylene oxide). Occasional bacteriological in-use testing may be necessary, as disinfectants vary in stability and may be inactivated to a varying extent by materials; dilutions and time of application are less readily controlled than are heating methods. After chemical disinfection of certain specialized equipment (e.g. respiratory ventilators) it may be advisable to confirm by bacteriological sampling that no pathogens can be detected, but this is not necessary if the process is well controlled. Prevention of contamination of equipment by the use of filters or heat decontamination is preferable, and is usually possible.

APPENDIX 3.1 DEFINITION OF HOSPITAL-ACQUIRED INFECTION

Hospital-acquired infection is an infection found to be active or under active treatment at the time of the survey, which was neither present nor incubating on admission to hospital. (In the case of recently admitted patients it is necessary to assess whether any infection was being incubated on admission, and to mark any such infection as not hospital acquired, (i.e. as 'community-acquired'.) Similarly, a patient who is readmitted with established infection which has resulted from an earlier admission is recorded as suffering from hospital-acquired – not community-acquired – infection.

Definitions

Although definitions are required for accurate surveillance, an agreed set is not available. Infections have been defined by many organizations (e.g. Garner et al., 1988; Glynn et al., 1997; Spencer, 1993). Nationally (or preferably internationally) agreed definitions are necessary. The problems of international comparisons have been described by Mertens (1996).

The commonest infections are those of the urinary tract, the respiratory tract and surgical wounds (Emmerson et al., 1996). The definitions, some of which are included below, are those used in the National Prevalence Survey of 1995 (Spencer, 1993).

Urinary tract infection. A patient being treated for a bacteriologically or clinically diagnosed infection, or in whom a bacteriological diagnosis has been made without treatment being given.

Notes.
1 A urinary tract infection should be diagnosed by the presence of micro-organisms in the urine accompanied by one or more of the following: dysuria, loin pain, suprapubic tenderness, pyrexia ($> 38°C$) or pyuria.
2 A bacterial count of $\geqslant 10^5$ organisms/mL is generally considered to be significant in a midstream specimen of urine.
3 If the specimen is obtained from a suprapubic puncture/catheter or there is a pure growth of the common pathogens, a bacterial count of $> 10^3$ organisms/mL can be considered significant.

Lower respiratory tract infection. New or increased production of purulent sputum and/or fever of $> 38°C$ with appropriate chest signs and/or new or progressive X-ray evidence of chest infiltrates not attributed to embolus or heart failure.

Notes.
1 For pneumonia, X-ray changes indicate definite infection; clinical diagnosis without supporting X-ray findings indicates probable or other lower respiratory tract infection.

2 Other lower respiratory tract infections include empyema, lung abscess, tracheitis, bronchitis and mediastinitis. Lung abscess and empyema are defined as the collection of pus within the lung or pleural cavity, respectively, supported by positive bacterial cultures.

Surgical wound infections. (see p. 45).

REFERENCES

Arrowsmith, L.W.M. (1985) Air sampling in operating theatres. *Journal of Hospital Infection* 6, 352.

Ayliffe, G.A.J. (1986) The irreducible minimum. *Infection Control* 7 (**Supplement**), 92.

Benenson, A.S. (1995) *Control of communicable diseases in man,* 16th edn. Washington, DC: American Public Health Association.

Bibby, B.A., Collins, B.J. and Ayliffe, G.A.J. (1986) A mathematical model for assessing postoperative wound infection. *Journal of Hospital Infection* 8, 31.

Cruse, P.J.E. and Foord, R. (1973) A five-year prospective study of 23 649 surgical wounds. *Archives of Surgery* 107, 206.

Culver, D.H., Horan, T.C., Gaynes, R.P. *et al.* (1991) Surgical wound infection rates by wound class, operative procedure and patient risk index. *American Journal of Medicine* 91 (**Supplement 3B**), 152S.

Department of Health (1994) *Health Technical Memorandum 2025* (1994) Ventilation in healthcare premises. London: HMSO.

Department of Health (1995) *Hospital infection control. Guidance on the control of infection in hospitals.* Paper prepared by the Hospital Infection Working Group of the Department of Health and the Public Health Laboratory Service. London: Department of Health.

Emmerson, A.M., Enstone, J.E. and Griffin, M. (1996) The Second National Prevalence Survey of infection in hospitals. Overview of results. *Journal of Hospital Infection* 32, 175.

Emmerson, A. M. and Ayliffe, G.A.J. (eds) (1996) *Surveillance of nosocomial infections.* Baillière's *Clinical infectious diseases.* Vol. 3. No. 2. London. Baillière Tindall.

French, G.L., Wong, S.L., Cheng, A.F.B. and Donnan, S. (1989) Repeated prevalence surveys for monitoring effectiveness of hospital infection control. *Lancet* 2, 1021.

Garibaldi, R.A., Cushing, D. and Lerer, T. (1991) Predictors of intraoperative acquired surgical wound infections. *Journal of Hospital Infection* 18 (**Supplement A**), 289.

Garner, J. S., Jarvis, W.R., Emori, T.G. *et al.* (1988) CDC definitions for nosocomial infections, 1988. *American Journal of Infection Control* 16, 128.

Glenister, H.M., Taylor, L.J., Bartlett, C.R. *et al.* (1993) An evaluation of surveillance methods for detecting infections in hospital inpatients. *Journal of Hospital Infection* 23, 229.

Glynn, A., Ward V., Wilson, J. *et al.* (1997) *Hospital-acquired infection. Surveillance policies and practice,* London: Public Health Laboratory Service.

Gosden, P.E., MacGowan, A.P. and Bannister, G.C., (1998) Importance of air quality and related factors in the prevention of infection in orthopaedic implant surgery. *Journal of Hospital Infection* 39, 173.

Haley, R.W. (1995) The scientific basis for using surveillance and risk factor data to reduce nosocomial infection rates. *Journal of Hospital Infection* 30 (Supplement), 3.

Haley, R.W., Culver, D.H., White, J.W., *et al.* (1985a) The efficacy of infection surveillance and control programs in preventing nosocomial infections in US hospitals. *American Journal of Epidemiology* 121, 182.

Haley, R.W., Culver, D.H., Morgan, W.M. *et al.* (1985b) Identifying patients at high risk of surgical wound infection: a simple multivariate index of patient susceptibility and wound contamination. *American Journal of Epidemiology* 121, 206.

Haley, R.W., Gaynes, R.P., Aber, R.C. and Bennett, J.V. (1992) The surveillance of nosocomial infections. In Bennet, J.V. and Brachman, P.S. (eds), *Hospital infections,* 3rd edn, Boston, MA: Little Brown and Co.

Holton, J. and Ridgway, G.L. (1993) Commissioning operating theatres. *Journal of Hospital Infection* 23, 153.

Jepson, O.B. (1996) Surveillance of hospital infection with limited resources. In Emmerson, A.M. and Ayliffe, G.A.J. (eds) *Surveillance of nosocomial infections.* Baillière's *Clinical infectious diseases. Vol. 3.* No. 2. London: Baillière Tindall, 211.

Kelsey, M.C., (1996) The use of computers in routine surveillance of hospital-acquired infections. In Emmerson, A.M. and Ayliffe, G.A.J. (eds) *Surveillance of nosocomial infections.* Baillière's *Clinical infectious diseases. Vol. 3.* No. 2. London: Baillière Tindall, 253.

McGowan, J.E. (1996) Risk factors and nosocomial infection control. In Emmerson, A.M. and Ayliffe, G.A.J. (eds) *Surveillance of nosocomial infections.* Baillière's *Clinical infectious diseases. Vol. 3.* No. 2. London: Baillière Tindall, 225.

Meers, P.D., Ayliffe, G.A.J., Emmerson, A.M. *et al.* (1981) Report on the National Survey of Infection in Hospitals, 1980. *Journal of Hospital Infection,* 2 (Supplement) 1.

Mertens, R. (1996) Methodologies and results of national surveillance. In Emmerson, A.M. and Ayliffe, G.A.J. (eds) *Surveillance of nosocomial infections.* Baillière's *Clinical infectious diseases. Vol. 3.* No. 2. London: Baillière Tindall, 159.

Simchen, E., Stein, H., Sacks, T.G. *et al.* (1984) Multivariate analysis of determinants of postoperative wound infection in orthopaedic patients. *Journal of Hospital Infection* 5, 137.

Simchen, E., Wax, Y. and Pevsner, B. (1988) The Israeli Study of Surgical Infections (ISSI). II. Initial comparisons among hospitals with special focus on hernia operations. *Infection Control and Hospital Epidemiology* 9, 241.

Spencer, R.C. (1993) National prevalence survey of hospital-acquired infections: definitions. A preliminary report from the steering group. *Journal of Hospital Infection* **24**, 69.

Vaqué, J., Rosselló, J., Arribas, J.L. and EPINE Working Group (1999) Prevalence of nosocomial infections in Spain. EPINE study 1990–1997. *Journal of Hospital Infection* **43**, 5105.

Wilson, A.P.R., Weavill, C., Burridge, J. and Kelsey, M.C. (1990) The use of the wound scoring method 'ASEPSIS' in postoperative wound infection surveillance. *Journal of Hospital Infection* **16**, 297.

Wilson, A.P.R., Helder, N., Theminimulle, S.K. and Scott, G. M. (1998) Comparison of wound scoring methods for use in audit. *Journal of Hospital Infection* **39**, 119.

Wong, E.S. (1996) Surgical site infections. In Mayhall, C.G. (ed.), *Hospital epidemiology and infection control*, Baltimore, MD: Williams & Wilkins, 154.

chapter 4

STERILIZATION

Nigel Cripps

Microbial contaminants can be removed with a detergent and water, or destroyed by sterilization or disinfection (Gardner and Peel, 1998). Cleaning followed by drying of surfaces other than those of the body can be almost as effective as the use of a disinfectant.

Sterilization refers to a validated process used to render a product free from viable micro-organisms. It achieves the complete killing or removal of all types of micro-organisms, including the spores of tetanus and gas-gangrene bacilli which are resistant to most disinfectants and more resistant to heat than non-sporing micro-organisms (British Standards Institute (European Standard), 1994c).

Disinfection is a process used to reduce the number of viable micro-organisms on a surface or in a load, but which may not necessarily inactivate some microbial agents (e.g. spores and prions). It may not achieve the same reduction in microbial contamination as sterilization (modified from Medical Devices Agency, 1993/1999). High-level disinfection is a term used to include mycobacteria and enteroviruses, but not necessarily spores. A *disinfectant* is a chemical or physical agent which can destroy vegetative micro-organisms and viruses. The word *antiseptic* is often used to refer to disinfectants which are applied to the skin or to living tissues, but as the purpose of antiseptics is to disinfect (one speaks of 'skin disinfection'), the word antiseptic is less frequently used. However, it is useful as an indication that the compound can be safely applied to tissues (Russell *et al.*, 1999). The word *sterilant* has sometimes been used to refer to the small range of chemical compounds (ethylene oxide, gas plasma, formaldehyde and glutaraldehyde) which, under controlled conditions, can kill sporing bacteria. All products to be sterilized should be physically cleaned before they are subjected to a standard sterilization process (Department of Health, 1999). Methods of sterilization are summarized in Appendix 4.1. (see also Appendix 6.2 in Chapter 6).

All surgical instruments, dressings and other objects or solutions which are introduced into traumatic or operation wounds or by injection must be provided sterile (i.e. have completed a sterilization process and be adequately protected against subsequent contamination). The same applies, in general, to materials introduced into other areas that are normally sterile, although disinfection by pasteurization or boiling, which destroys vegetative bacteria and most viruses, is accepted as adequate for cystoscopes and some other endoscopes that cannot tolerate heat sterilization. However, there is a slight possibility of clostridial infection arising after operations on the genito-urinary tract, and manufacturers should be encouraged to develop equipment that is able to withstand autoclaving.

Laboratory discard materials should be transported in robust containers without spillage and stored in a safe manner while awaiting sterilization. The Advisory Committee on Dangerous Pathogens (1990) recommends four levels of containment for discard material, the method of disinfection and sterilization being dependent on the level of microbiological risk associated with the discarded materials. An autoclave with an effective containment system for high-risk items has been described (Oates *et al.*, 1983; see also British Standards Institute, 1988).

METHODS OF STERILIZATION (see also Appendix 4.2 and Medical Devices Agency 1993/1999)

Sterilization can be achieved by moist heat at raised atmospheric pressure, by dry heat at normal pressure, by ionizing radiation (gamma radiation or electron beams), by 'sterilants' (e.g. ethylene oxide, gas plasma, glutaraldehyde) or by filtration. It can also be obtained by steam and formaldehyde at sub-atmospheric pressure. If the article to be sterilized is not damaged by heat, heat-sterilizing methods should always be used in preference to other methods because they are more reliable and can be more effectively monitored.

HEAT STERILIZATION

Heat sterilization depends on the temperature to which articles are exposed and on the time of exposure, such that the higher the temperature, the shorter the time period required for sterilization. Two factors must be taken into account when deciding the time of exposure:

1 the equilibration time, i.e. the time which elapses between the chamber and the least accessible part of the load reaching the selected sterilization ('holding') temperature;
2 the holding time, i.e. the time period for which the temperature in all parts of the load is exposed within the selected sterilization temperature band. These times will vary with different sterilization temperatures.

Dry heat is less effective than moist heat, and therefore requires a higher temperature and longer time at that temperature.

Dry heat

Red heat from a Bunsen burner is of value in the laboratory, but is not suitable for sterilizing surgical instruments – the 'flaming' of a scalpel dipped in spirit is not satisfactory. Dry heat was extensively used for sterilization of hospital supplies, but its use is declining except for some medicinal products. Few products can only be sterilized by this process. There are two main types of dry heat sterilizers, namely the fan oven and the conveyor fan.

Fan oven. Heat is produced by electric elements in the walls of the oven and a fan circulates the hot air evenly. The oven works at 160 – 180°C with a holding time of 30 – 120 min, and with a total cycle of 2.5 – 5 hours depending upon the degree of cooling. It can be used for mixed loads of glass and metal instruments and also for some sharp instruments used in ophthalmic surgery. Medicinal products (e.g. fats, oils and powders) which are impervious to steam are also sterilized by this method. The main disadvantage is the long cycle time. All dry-heat sterilizer ovens should be fitted with a door lock and a temperature chart recorder, which are mandatory requirements in the UK (British Standards Institute, 1966; Department of Health, 1994). A bacteria-retentive filter may be needed on the air inlet for sterilizers with a cooling stage. Ovens without a fan are unsatisfactory.

Conveyor fan. This was formerly popular for sterile syringe services but, since the general introduction of disposable syringes, this method has been little used. The articles to be sterilized pass slowly along a conveyor system under an infra-red heat source.

Moist heat

To ensure the destruction of bacterial spores by moist heat, a temperature above 100°C is required. In the pressure steam sterilizer or autoclave, the boiling point of water and the temperature of the steam produced are raised in proportion to the increase in pressure (British Standards Institute, 1990; British Standards Institute, (European Standard), 1994b, 1996). At a pressure of 1.03 bar above atmospheric pressure the boiling point of water is 121°C, and at a pressure of 2.2 bar the boiling point is 134°C. Steam of appropriate quality (Department of Health, 1997) at these temperatures will sterilize objects in 15 min and 3 min, respectively.

In order to sterilize effectively, steam must come into direct contact with the surfaces to be sterilized. The latent heat which is given out when steam condenses to water increases the sterilizing efficiency of steam, but this effect only occurs if the steam is not superheated, i.e raised to a temperature higher than that at which water boils under the pressure present in the autoclave. It is essential to remove all air from the sterilizer chamber. This can be done by admitting steam into the upper part of the chamber, from which it will descend, pushing the air through an outlet in the floor of the chamber. Admitting or generating steam in the base of the chamber and displacing air upwards is also satisfactory. This 'downward displacement' method is suitable for simple unwrapped instruments, bowls and with suitable door interlocks, and bottled fluids. Air can be removed effectively from a sealed chamber and the load by creating a vacuum before the admission of steam. The high-vacuum autoclave was commonly used for sterilization of porous loads (packs) (British Standards Institute, (European Standard), 1997c), but has now been largely superseded by porous load processes. These utilize an improved air removal process which uses pulsed steam (i.e. alternating vacuum with steam injection for 5 – 8 pulses). This method is especially useful when a small load is being sterilized in a large chamber or unwrapped items with long small-bore lumens. Removal of steam and drying of the load in a sterilizer with a vacuum pump is achieved by drawing a vacuum after the sterilization stage. This utilizes the residual heat in the load to 'boil off' any remaining condensation. The complete cycle for a porous load sterilizer is approximately 30 min.

Small bench-top downward-displacement or porous-load sterilizers are available for clinics and doctors' and dentists' surgeries (see Chapter 18).

IONIZING RADIATION

These methods are not suitable for use in hospitals, but are commonly used commercially. The process may damage some plastic materials, and advice should always be sought before reprocessing any item. Equipment made of or containing metal, polythene, paper, wool, cotton, polyvinyl chloride, nylon, terylene or poly-styrene is usually unaffected. Rubber varies in its response, but butyl and chlori-nated rubber are not suitable for sterilization by these methods. Electron beams (β-particles from a linear accelerator) or gamma radiation (from cobalt-60, at a dosage of 2.5 Mrad (25 000 Gy) is used. This dosage gives good penetration and leaves no residual radioactivity. Units used for radiotherapy in hospital are not suitable for sterilization purposes.

CHEMICAL METHODS

Ethylene oxide

Heat-sensitive articles may be sterilized by ethylene oxide gas. Ethylene oxide (EO) is extremely penetrative, non-corrosive and an effective sterilizing agent (Medical Devices Agency, 1993/1999). Unfortunately, it is toxic, irritant and explosive when mixed with air at concentrations higher than 3%. It is also odourless, and leaks may therefore go unnoticed. Despite these disadvantages, EO is widely used commercially for sterilizing heat-sensitive items. It is also used in some hospitals, especially by those offering a specialist or regional facility for processing heat-sensitive items. During a typical cycle, air is removed from the load by creating a vacuum, and the chamber and its contents are heated to the desired temperature (37°C or 55°C). As air removal reduces the humidity, which is an essential prereq-uisite for sterilization, sub-atmospheric steam is introduced to rehumidify the load. Gas is then introduced from a cylinder or single-use canister, and the temperature and pressure or vacuum are maintained for the sterilization period. Finally, gas is removed and the chamber and its contents are flushed with filtered air. The holding time is dependent on the temperature, pressure, humidity and gas concen-tration. The design of sterilizers is therefore related to these parameters and the requirements of the user (i.e. temperature/pressure tolerance of the items processed, size of load, time available for processing, etc.).

The most commonly used hospital EO sterilizers in hospitals in the UK are those of the sub-atmospheric type. High-pressure types, which are commonly used in industrial processes, are also available. By adopting a higher pressure (5.5 bar), it is possible to maintain lethal concentrations of EO using mixtures of EO and inert substances (e.g. carbon dioxide). This reduces the risk of flammability or explosion, but the high pressure increases the risk of leaks. Sub-atmospheric steril-izers utilize pure EO, but the risk of leaks is minimized as the entire cycle is below atmospheric pressure (Babb *et al.*, 1982). Sub-atmospheric EO sterilizers are usually much smaller than high-pressure models, but they may be used to sterilize items which are sensitive to high pressures (e.g. flexible fibre-optic endoscopes).

The effectiveness of EO as a sterilizing agent may be influenced by other factors (e.g. the presence of salt crystals and packaging). All items must therefore be scrupulously clean. For packaging, paper, polypropylene or polyethylene bags are suitable, but nylon must not be used. Packages should be heat-sealed or sealed with tape. Indicator tape or packaging should be used to indicate those items which have been processed. The sterilizing process must be controlled by spore tests supplemented by indicator tests (British Standards Institute, (European Standard), 1994a).

Ethylene oxide and its residues are toxic and irritant, and materials exposed to it should be thoroughly aerated before use. Aeration time is dependent on the absorbency of the items processed, the temperature, and the air-exchange rates in the storage facility. Those with high-capacity sterilizers or a larger throughput should use a separate aeration room with exhaust ventilation and open shelving to allow good air circulation. Very absorbent items, or those required soon after sterilization, may be aerated in a heated, exhaust-ventilated cabinet. Aeration at 55°C greatly enhances the elution of EO, and consequently much shorter aeration periods may be used. Where practicable, aeration is carried out in the chamber itself in order to protect staff from exposure during removal of the load. For aeration outside the chamber, a temperature of 55°C for 24 hours, or 3 – 7 days at room temperature, is normally considered to be adequate.

As much concern has recently been expressed about the toxicity of EO, the Health and Safety Executive (1999) has adopted a control limit of exposure of individuals at work to 5 ppm EO over an 8-hour time-weighted averaged period, but further reductions in acceptable levels are possible in the future. The short-term (15-min) limit is 15 ppm.

Exposure can be minimized by installing the sterilizer in a separate exhaust-ventilated suite of rooms, by carrying out aeration in the chamber, and by installing an exhaust hood above the sterilizer door. It is recommended that access to the sterilizer, plant room and aeration facility be restricted to trained personnel who are fully conversant with the hazards associated with the process and emergency procedures. Notices on emergency procedures should be clearly displayed in the work area.

Irradiated articles should not be subsequently treated with ethylene oxide unless they are known to be safe after such treatment.

Chemical sporicidal fluids

Glutaraldehyde. Immersion of equipment in a fluid is generally a less reliable method of sterilization (or disinfection) than exposure to heat or EO, and it has the disadvantage that thorough rinsing is necessary after processing. All materials must be clean, and only surfaces wetted by glutaraldehyde will be satisfactorily treated.

Alkaline glutaraldehyde, when used in a 2% solution, can be relied upon to sterilize in 10 hours, but for all practical purposes 3 hours should provide an adequate sporicidal effect (Babb *et al.*, 1980). Treatment for shorter periods (e.g. 20 min) only disinfects, but some spores (e.g. those of *Clostridium difficile*) are rapidly killed (Dyas and Das, 1985). The rinse used to remove residual chemicals needs careful control to avoid recontamination or depositing of particulate on the load. Atmospheric pollution due to glutaraldehyde is subject to strict regulatory control, it is potentially toxic, and appropriate precautions are required when it is used (Campbell and Cripps, 1991). Other sterilants include peracetic acid, chlorine dioxide and 'Sterilox' (see Appendix 4.2 and Chapter 5).

Low-temperature steam and formaldehyde (LTSF). This method is an alternative to EO and may be preferable, as it is a much safer process and prolonged aeration is not required. Formaldehyde alone is unacceptable for sterilizing heat-labile items because of its poor penetration and its slow sporicidal activity. However, if it is used in conjunction with sub-atmospheric steam (Hurrell, 1980; Alder, 1987) it becomes a far more reliable process, and sterilization is more rapidly achieved. Most LTSF sterilizers operate at a temperature of 73°C, and a period of 3 – 5 hours is required for the sterilizing process. A vacuum of 40 mbar is generally required during the air removal and pulsing stages to ensure adequate penetration, removal of formaldehyde, and a dry load. Steam is usually pulsed, but the best conditions for admitting formaldehyde at its optimal concentration have not been clearly established. Commissioning and routine testing methods are not available (British Standards Institute, 1990; Department of Health, 1994) which, if satisfactory, ensure a high probability of sterilization. Many machines need careful monitoring and maintenance to reach the required standard, and require considerable attention from skilled engineers and microbiologists. Problems include excessive condensation, poor temperature control, variable formaldehyde concentrations in the chambers, and inadequate removal of residual formaldehyde at the end of the cycle. Temperature variability tends to be less in smaller machines, and the inclusion of a complete heated jacket may be necessary. As some of the equipment processed is expensive and heat-sensitive, it is particularly important that a high temperature cut-out mechanism is fitted. This is usually set at a maximum value of 80°C.

Formaldehyde is an irritant substance, and care should be taken to avoid undue exposure, especially during filling of the reservoir, on removing the load and during maintenance, particularly if an operating-cycle failure occurs. Gloves should be worn to protect against skin contact and, as the eyes are particularly vulnerable, protection is advised when filling reservoirs from stock solutions. Fortunately, formaldehyde is detected by smell at relatively low concentrations, and well below the 2 ppm maximum exposure limit recommended by the Health and Safety Executive (1999). Formaldehyde is rarely absorbed into processed items, provided that they are suitably packed (foam and textiles are not to be used) and condensate is not allowed to accumulate. This can be achieved by placing packages vertically and processing tubing in an arc with the open ends pointing downwards. Processing should be carried out by trained personnel who are fully conversant with the risks and emergency procedures.

Most of the difficulties with LTSF sterilizers are associated with the use of formaldehyde. However, LTS without formaldehyde is a very reliable disinfection process, and treatment for 10 min at 71 – 75°C will meet most requirements in the hospital service (British Standards Institute, 1990). An advantage over the use of disinfectants is that equipment is dry at the end of processing and may be wrapped. There is also no problem with residual disinfectant. Routine microbiological tests are required for the use of LTSF, but not for LTS alone. A daily chamber leak test is required for both processes.

Low-temperature steam, with or without formaldehyde, is a suitable process for heat-sensitive items which will tolerate moisture, a vacuum of at least 40 mbar, and temperatures of 80°C.

Note. Washer disinfectors complying with BS2745 of the British Standards Institute (1993) may be more cost-effective than LTS as a means of disinfection if wrapping is not required (see Chapter 5).

Gas plasma sterilization

Gas plasma has been introduced as a possible alternative to ethylene oxide or low-temperature steam/formaldehyde. The process is relatively short (e.g. 45–80 min) and the end-products are non-toxic. Gaseous hydrogen peroxide is commonly used (e.g. 'Sterrad' machines). Gas plasma consists of a gas excited by radiofrequency or microwave energy under a vacuum at low temperature (below 55°C). Its antimicrobial activity is due to the production of free radicals, electrons, ions and excited radicals.

The 'Sterrad' process is actively sporicidal (Kyri *et al.*, 1995; Rutala *et al.*, 1999) and is as effective as EO. The items to be processed must be clean and dry, and packaging must be compatible with the process. There is some uncertainty about the ability of the process to penetrate narrow-lumen tubing, particularly if it is closed at one end, and a special adaptor may be required.

Bacterial spores (e.g. *Bacillus subtilis* or *Bacillus stearothermophilus*) are dried on carriers for microbiological testing. These are placed in the chamber or in test pieces as for EO. However, the Line–Pickerill test piece is unsuitable for the present 'Sterrad' machine.

Some machines are in use in the UK, but no official commissioning and testing programme has yet been published by the Department of Health.

VALIDATION TESTS FOR STERILIZATION

Validation tests are undertaken to demonstrate the effectiveness of sterilization, and to show that machinery operates in accordance with the manufacturer's specifications (British Standards Institute (European Standard), 1994c). The complete validation process includes commissioning and performance qualification. Performance qualification is required when the production load presents a greater challenge to the process than the challenge of the standard test loads. For example, a surgical instrument box may present a greater challenge than a Bowie-Dick pack (standard test pack) used in the validation of porous-load sterilizers.

STERILIZERS – STEAM AT HIGH TEMPERATURE (POROUS LOADS)

On commissioning a new sterilizer and at regular 3-monthly intervals the chamber temperature and steam penetration should be checked with standard temperature sensors (thermocouples) (Department of Health, 1994). A load dryness test should be performed when new sterilizers are commissioned (British Standards Institute, 1990; British Standards Institute (European Standard), 1994b; see also Appendix 4.1). The temperature and pressure records for each cycle should be examined, and a Bowie-Dick test and a vacuum leak test should be performed daily on all porous-load autoclaves (see also Appendix 4.1). Although a weekly vacuum leak test is sometimes suggested, a daily test is preferable. The satisfactory functioning of the automatic device for detecting the presence of air or gas should be checked weekly and its performance verified annually (see Appendix 4.1). These tests may be supplemented with chemical indicator systems (e.g. Browne's tubes and indicator tape, which should be stored under the manufacturer's recommended conditions and not used if out of date). It must be recognized that these chemical indicator tests provide evidence of physical conditions required for sterilization, not of sterilization. However, they are useful process indicators (British Standards Institute (European Standard), 1997b) enabling the user to undertake a visual inspection to identify that the pack has been processed before it is used. Spore tests (British Standards Institute (European Standard), 1997a) are not recommended for routine use in the UK, but are routinely used (e.g. weekly) in the USA and some European countries. However, tests with biological indicators may be of use in checking packages where penetration may be in doubt, and if there is any suspicion of infection occurring due to the failure of an autoclave. Spore strips used for high-temperature steam sterilizers should comply with BS EN 866 Part 3 (British Standards Institute (European Standard), 1997a). They contain approximately 10^6 *Bacillus stearothermophilus* spores produced by a recognized method, and if well controlled they should be reasonably reliable.

BOTTLED FLUID STERILIZERS

Packages (British Standards Institute (European Standard), 1997c) need to be carefully inspected to ensure that they are intact and the sterility is not compromised. Detailed commissioning and regular testing of loads with multiple temperature sensors (thermocouples) are required. Charts or hard-copy printouts for each cycle should record temperature from a thermocouple in the load, as well as from the active chamber drain and/or chamber space. These records must be compared with master charts of that particular load made during commissioning (Department of Health, 1994).

Modern bottle fluid sterilizers often utilize an air-stream mixture which is intended to over-pressurize the chamber, preventing damage to plastic containers which are weakened by sterilizing temperatures. The manufacturer will advise on how to monitor the performance of these machines, but at the very minimum heat exchangers should be checked to ensure that there is no transfer of mains water into the chamber where it may come into contact with the load. If cooling water is retained between cycles, it should be stored at 80°C and sterilized before use.

There are special requirements for interlocking the doors with a temperature sensor to prevent the door from opening if the load is too hot, namely 80°C for glass containers and 90°C for plastic containers. The performance of the interlocking is monitored quarterly as part of the regular testing procedure (Department of Health, 1994).

DRY HEAT STERILIZERS

These are tested by temperature sensors, and Browne's tubes or other chemical indicators may also be used. A chart recorder or printer is required. Biological indicator tests are not recommended for routine use in the UK, but if used should be *Bacillus subtilis* as specified in BS EN866 Part 6 (British Standards Institute (European Standard), 1997a).

GAS STERILIZERS

The physical and chemical parameters of gas sterilization are difficult to control, and they vary with the type of sterilizer and the nature of the load. Until such time as these can be fully established, biological validation is necessary using bacterial spores as biological indicators.

ETHYLENE OXIDE

Bacillius subtilis var *niger* biological indicators are specified in BS EN866 Part 2 (BS EN550) (British Standards Institute (European Standard), 1994a, 1997a) and should be used to validate EO sterilizers. For commissioning, inoculated carriers are placed in four test helices (Line and Pickerill, 1973) which are double-wrapped and positioned with two each at the front and rear of the chamber. A series of tests is performed, each time increasing the gas exposure stage until all of the biological indicators are inactivated. The gas exposure stage for routine production should be at least double that at which all of the biological indicators are inactivated. It is helpful to include a chemical indicator alongside the biological indicator in each helix. This should give a firm indication of the presence of EO, but does not indicate that sterilization has occurred. In addition to biological indicator tests, the relative humidity must be in the range 40 – 85% at the end of the conditioning stage. Each production load requires a biological indicator test. Chemical indicators may be used to give an early indication of gas penetration. A total of 10 biological indicators are used, evenly distributed throughout the load. A constant technique is needed for preparation of the recovery medium and the procedure for microbiological testing. The procedures described in Health Technical Memorandum 2010 (Department of Health, 1994) are satisfactory.

LOW-TEMPERATURE STEAM AND FORMALDEHYDE

On commissioning, tests should be made for steam penetration and air leakage into the chamber when subjected to a vacuum (British Standards Institute, 1990; Department of Health, 1994). If formaldehyde is used, tests should be made with *Bacillus stearothermophilus* spore biological indicators and produced to BS EN866 Part 1 (British Standards Institute (European Standard), 1997a). For routine testing, biological indicators and chemical formaldehyde indicators are inserted in the capsule of a test helix (Line and Pickerill, 1973) which is placed in the top of the load and centre of the chamber. Following sterilization, this is removed for culture, the temperature recorded compared to the master temperature record, and the paper examined for formaldehyde penetration. Provided that these tests are satisfactory, the cycle is accepted as one of sterilization. Biological indicators should be incubated as described in Health Technical Memorandum 2010 Part 3 (Department of Health, 1994) for at least 7 days for production cycles, but for commissioning and other validation tests incubation for 14 days is recommended.

As with other sterilizers, commissioning and maintenance tests should include electrical and other checks, (e.g. high-temperature cut-out).

Additional tests are necessary both periodically and on commissioning. These include tests of distribution and penetration, hospital load, and environmental and residual formaldehyde vapour tests (Department of Health, 1994).

Distribution and penetration tests

Biological indicators (BI) are removed from their envelopes, mounted on cotton threads and placed at 27 locations within the chambers, at the top, centre, bottom, front, middle and back. Also included are four helices, each containing an inoculated carrier. Two helices are double-wrapped and located with one in the front half and the other in the rear half of the usable chamber space. Formaldehyde-sensitive chemical indicator papers may be included at the site, and may help to identify the reason for BI failures. The test is considered to be satisfactory if no growth is observed from the BIs after 14 days of incubation. Positive and negative controls should be included with each batch. Following sterilization, the biological and chemical indicators are recovered and examined as described previously.

Environmental and residual formaldehyde vapour tests

For this test, two modular cardboard instrument trays (600 mm × 300 mm × 50 mm) are used with a 12mm thickness of high-density open-cell polyurethane foam. Two stainless steel rods are placed inside each tray, the lid is fitted and the trays are placed side by side in the chamber. At the end of the cycle, the door should be opened to a gap of 25 mm and a gas sample taken 100 mm in front of the gap at the operator's breathing zone. This test should be performed without the exhaust-ventilation hood operating. Hospital load test packs should be removed from the sterilizer and left unopened for 10 min. Packs are then opened and left for a further 5 min before measuring the gas concentrations. The load with the highest potential for retaining gas is checked for residual formaldehyde.

The levels of gas measured in the above tests should not exceed those limits laid down by the Health and Safety Executive (1999) in guidance note EH40, namely 2 ppm.

Advice should be sought from sterilizer engineers and microbiologists when contemplating the purchase of new equipment to ensure that it will do the job required and that it is known to operate competently elsewhere.

NOVEL PROCESSES AND LOADS

The validation of a novel sterilization process (e.g. ozone, hydrogen peroxide gas, gas plasma) should confirm that the automatic control system indicated a fault if a condition occurs that may jeopardize the sterilization of the product or the safety of the operator. The satisfactory operation of the sterilizer and its monitoring system can usually be checked by using biological indicators and temperature sensors (thermocouples). Care should be exercised when developing a test protocol. The supplier should advise on the validation procedure undertaken by the manufacturer, and it should be clearly understood how fault conditions are simulated, enabling the monitoring systems to be checked for their correct operation.

EUROPEAN UNION DIRECTIVES

Sterilization and disinfection are now falling within an increasingly strict regulatory requirement. The aim of the regulations is to ensure a constant approach to quality control. The principal regulations are as follows:

1 65/65/EEC – Council Directive of 26 January 1965 on the approximation of provisions laid down by law, regulation or administrative action relating to proprietary medicinal products. *Official Journal of the European Community* No. 22, p. 3769 (9 February, 1965) (European Union, 1965).

2 90/385/EEC – Council Directive of 20 June 1990 on the approximation of the laws of the Member States relating to active implantable medical devices. *Official Journal of the European Community* No. L189, p. 17 (20 July, 1993) (European Union, 1990). The Directive covers all powered implants; heart pacemakers are the most common example.

3 93/42/EEC – Council Directive of 14 June 1993 concerning medical devices. *Official Journal of the European Community* No. L169, p. 1 (12 July, 1993) (European Union, 1993). The Directive covers most other medical devices, ranging from first aid bandages and tongue depressors to hip protheses, and it has a wide impact on sterilization.

APPENDIX 4.1 AUTOCLAVE TESTS

BOWIE-DICK AUTOCLAVE TAPE TEST FOR POROUS-LOAD AUTOCLAVES (Bowie *et al.*, 1963; British Standards Institute, 1990; Department of Health, 1994)

The principle is very simple. A standard test pack is made up from plain cotton sheets. In the centre is placed a piece of paper on which is impregnated a chemical indicator which has been stored according to the manufacturer's recommendations. This chemical shows a colour change when it is exposed to steam. The test pack is now autoclaved in the usual way. *If all of the air has been removed*, the steam will penetrate rapidly and completely and the chemical will show a uniform colour change. *If all of the air has not been removed,* when steam is admitted for the sterilizing stage the air will be forced into the centre of the pack, where it will collect as a 'bubble'. The chemical indicator will not change colour in the region of the bubble because it has not been exposed to steam, and this will show up when the paper with the indicator is removed at the end of the run. If the test is to be a reliable guide to the safe working of the sterilizer, it must be performed exactly as described.

Performance of the test

Plain cotton sheets (90 cm × 120 cm) complying with BS 5815 Part 1 (British Standards Institute, 1989) are required. The sheets should be washed before being used for the first time, and also whenever they are soiled or discoloured. Conditioning agents should not be used.

Between tests they should be unfolded and hung out to air for at least 1 hour. Each towel should be folded to approximately 20 cm × 30 cm and placed one above the other to form a stack approximately 25 cm high. After being compressed by hand, the towels should be wrapped in similar fabric and secured with tape up to 25 mm wide. The exact number of towels needed will depend on how often they have been used, but the recommended weight of the pack is 7.7 kg. If the weight of a 25-cm-high pack exceeds 7.7 kg, the towels should be discarded. A chemical indicator sheet is placed in the centre of the pack. The original test involved a St Andrew's Cross of appropriate tape on an A4 sheet of paper. This does not have sufficient area of chemical indicator to meet the requirement of BS EN 867, Part 3 (British Standards Institute, 1997b), and special chemical indicator A4-sized papers are available. The test pack must be placed in the sterilizer by itself with appropriate chamber furniture to support it above the base, and subjected to a standard sterilizing cycle. The 'holding' or 'sterilizing' time in the centre of the test pack must be 3.3 – 3.5 min at 134°C. If the automatic cycle is set for a longer holding time, this must be cut short. Some machines have a special Bowie–Dick test cycle for the daily test. Should there be any doubt about how to do this, the engineer should be asked for advice. When the cycle is finished, the pack should be taken out and the chemical indicator should be examined.

After a satisfactory run the indicator will show a colour change which is the same at the centre as at the edges. If the colour at the centre is paler than it is at the edges, this means that there was a bubble of air present and that the sterilizer was not working properly. If this happens, the matter should be reported at once.

The chemical indicator from each test can be marked with the date and other details and kept for reference.

The towels should be aired and folded ready for the next test.

Comments. Unless the test is performed exactly as described above it may not be truly reliable. In particular, the following points should be noted.

1 The more air there is to remove, the more exacting will be the test. That is why the test pack is used by itself in an otherwise empty chamber.
2 The exact colour change shown by the processed indicator may depend on the storage conditions. The requirement is to determine whether the colour change occurs at the centre and differs from the edges.

3 The contrast in colour change from centre to edge will be reduced to an unreadable level if long 'holding' periods are used. That is why the holding period must not be less than 3.3 min and must not exceed 3.5 min, and the temperature must be 134°C. Even an extra 1 or 2 minutes may seriously affect a comparison of results.

4 Because of this, it is important to realize that if a sterilizer fails to pass the Bowie–Dick test as described above, it cannot be made safe merely by increasing the holding time until a uniform colour change is produced. Such a sterilizer is in urgent need of skilled attention.

5 The test should be viewed in parallel with the results of the chamber leak rate test (daily).

Alternative test packs

Alternatives to the Bowie–Dick test packs are available, such as the Lantor cube (Deverill *et al.*, 1987). Only test packs that comply with BS7720 (British Standards Institute, 1995) should be used.

Chamber leak rate test

This test is only applicable to autoclaves, which are capable of creating a vacuum, and it should be performed daily. There are two reasons why air leaking into the autoclave is unacceptable. First, the presence of air prevents penetration of the load by steam, and secondly, the air will not have passed through the bacteria-retentive filter, and therefore there is a potential risk of recontaminating the load.

The test involves the drawing of a vacuum in the chamber, followed by the closure of all valves leading to the chamber, stopping the vacuum-drawing system and observation of the chamber pressure for a timed period. The manufacturer's instructions should be followed and, in case of doubt, the advice of the sterilizer engineer should be sought.

At the start of the leak test the chamber pressure (P1) should be less than 40 mbar. Five minutes after the start of the test, the chamber pressure (P2) should be noted, and the chamber pressure (P3) should be noted again after a further 10-min period. During this 10-min period the chamber pressure (P3 – P2) should not be greater than 13 mbar for porous-load sterilizers or 5 mbar for low-temperature steam disinfectors, low-temperature steam and formaldehyde and 10 mbar for ethylene-oxide sterilizers.

Considerable care and knowledge must be applied in the interpretation of the results (British Standards Institute, 1990). Both the maximum leak rate and the maximum vacuum level (which gives an indication of the performance capability of the air-removal system) should be recorded in the sterilizer log-book.

The leak rate test and the Bowie–Dick tape test for porous-load sterilizers are complementary tests. A sterilizer which fails to meet the requirements of either of these tests must not be used until any faults have been rectified and the sterilizer satisfies both of these tests.

Air-detector test for porous-load sterilizer

The air detector is tested after the satisfactory completion of the leak rate test. For this series of tests a variable air-flow device should be connected to a valved port in a position where the induced air passes through the chamber before reaching the air detector. A suitable position is usually at a high level adjacent to the chamber door.

When the sterilizer is commissioned, and annually thereafter, an air detector performance test should be undertaken with a small and full load with temperature sensors located at:

1 the geometric centre of the pack;
2 the active chamber discharge;
3 the chamber free space.

During an operating cycle the air detector should indicate a fault first if the chamber pressure rise exceeds 10 mbar/min and second at the commencement of the sterilization hold period if the temperature at the geometric centre of the Bowie–Dick pack is more than 2°C below the temperature of the active chamber discharge.

Following the small load test, in addition to the Bowie–Dick pack the chamber is fully loaded with additional fabric sheets containing at least 50% cotton fibre with a surface density of approximately 200g/m^2. The fabric should be freshly laundered without the addition of starch or fabric conditioner as a Bowie–Dick pack.

During an operating cycle the sensitivity of the air detector is demonstrated to be similar to that found during the small load test. The leak must not exceed 10 mbar/min, but some pre-BS3970 (British Standards Institute, 1990) machines will need an increase in the chamber pressure rise to a value greater than 100 mbar in 10 min.

At weekly intervals the operation of the air detector should be checked by undertaking a *function test*. For this test a Bowie–Dick pack is introduced into the chamber and the same air flow leaked into the chamber as was used during the small load function test described above. The result is satisfactory if during an operating cycle the sterilizer indicates a fault. If a fault is not indicated, the sterilizer should be withdrawn from service and the air-detector performance test should be undertaken.

Load-dryness test

The load-dryness test is performed using a Bowie–Dick test pack without test papers or temperature sensors. The test pack should be aired for at least 1 hour as described above. Three towels are selected and marked, and each is placed in a polythene bag constructed in sheets of thickness not less than 250 μm. The minimum bag size should be 350 × 250 mm. Each bag/towel assembled is weighed on scales with an accuracy of ±0.1 g or better and the mass recorded. The towels are removed from the bags and replaced in the Bowie–Dick test pack, one in the centre, and the others as the second towel from either end of the test pack. With the test pack inserted into the chamber, an operating cycle is initiated within 60 s. The operating cycle should not include extended drying.

Within 60 s after the completion of the operating cycle, the test pack is removed from the chamber. The three marked towels are removed and immediately placed in the three corresponding marked bags. Each bag is sealed by turning its open end over several times. The total time from the completion of the operating cycle to sealing the bags should not exceed 3 min.

The towels in the polythene bags are allowed to cool and weighed. The means of the mass gain should not be greater than 1% (m/m).

APPENDIX 4.2 METHODS OF STERILIZATION

Category	Operating conditions (temperature and/or time for sterilizing)	Approximate process time	Application
Steam – DD			
Instrument sterilizer	126°C/10 min 134°C/3 min	20–60 min 5–15 min	Unwrapped instruments and bowls
Bottle sterilizer	121°C/15 min 115°C/30 min	2–12 hours	Bottled fluids
Steam – HVHT			
Porous loads	134°C/3 min	20–25 min	Dressings, wrapped instruments, lumened devices
Steam – HVLT			
Without formalin[a]	73–80°C/10 min	15–30 min	Heat-sensitive equipment
With formalin	73–80°C /1–3 hours	1–3 hours	Heat-sensitive equipment
Hot air			
Fan oven	160°C/120 min 180°C/30 min	2–4 hours	Glass, metal instruments
Ethylene oxide			
Subatmospheric	37–55°C 100% EO	3–5.5 hours	Heat-sensitive equipment
2% Glutaraldehyde	3 hours		Heat-sensitive equipment
Peracetic acid (0.2–0.35%)	10 min		Heat-sensitive equipment
Chlorine dioxide (1000 ppm available chlorine dioxide)	10 min		Heat-sensitive equipment
Gas plasma	45°C	40–80 min	Heat-sensitive equipment

HVHT, high vacuum, high temperature;
HVLT, high vacuum, low temperature;
DD, downward displacement.
[a]Disinfects only.

REFERENCES AND FURTHER READING

Advisory Committee on Dangerous Pathogens (1990) *Categorisation of pathogens according to hazard and categories of containment*, 2nd edn. London: HMSO.

Alder, V.G. (1987) The formaldehyde/low-temperature steam sterilizing procedure. *Journal of Hospital Infection* 9, 194.

Babb, J.R., Bradley, C.R. and Ayliffe, G.A.J. (1980) Sporadical activity of glutaraldehydes and hypochlorites and other factors influencing their selection for the treatment of medical equipment. *Journal of Hospital Infection* 1, 63.

Babb, J.R., Phelps, M., Downes, J. *et al.* (1982) Evaluation of an ethylene oxide sterilizer. *Journal of Hospital Infection* 2, 385.

Bowie, J.H., Kelsey, J.C. and Thompson, D. R. (1963) Bowie and Dick tape test. *Lancet* 1, 586.

British Standards Institute. (1966) *BS 3421. Performance of electrically heated sterilizing ovens.* London: British Standards Institute.

British Standards Institute (1988) *BS 2646. Autoclaves for sterilization in Laboratories.* London: British Standards Institute.

British Standards Institute (1989) *BS 5815, Part 1. Specification for sheeting, sheets and pillowslips.* London: British Standards Institute.

British Standards Institute (1990) *BS 3970. Sterilizing and disinfecting equipment for medical products.*

British Standards Institute (1993). *BS 2745. Washer disinfectors for medical purposes.* London: British Standards Institute.

British Standards Institute (1995) *BS 7720. Non-biological sterilization indicators equivalent to the Bowie and Dick test.* London: British Standards Institute.

British Standards Institute (1997) *BS 7893. Pressure-sensitive adhesive, closing and sealing tapes for use with sterilization packing materials.* London: British Standards Institute.

British Standards Institute (European Standard) (1994a) *BS EN 550. Sterilization of Medical Devices – validation and routine control of ethylene oxide sterilization.* London: British Standards Institute.

British Standards Institute (European Standard) (1994b) *BS EN 554. Sterilization of medical devices – validation and routine control of sterilization by moist heat.* London: British Standards Institute.

British Standards Institute (European Standard) (1994c) *BS EN 556. Sterilization of medical devices – requirements for terminally sterilized medical devices to be labelled 'STERILE'.* London: British Standards Institute.

British Standards Institute (European Standard) (1996) *BS EN 285. Steam sterilizers – large sterilizers.* London: British Standards Institute.

British Standards Institute (European Standard) (1997a). *BS EN 866. Biological systems for testing sterilizers.* London: British Standards Institute.

British Standards Institute (European Standard) (1997b). *BS EN 867. Non-biological systems for use in sterilizers.* London: British Standards Institute.

British Standards Institute (European Standard) (1997c). *BS EN 868. Packaging materials for sterilization of wrapped goods.* London: British Standards

Institute. Part 1. Specification for general requirements. Part 2. Specification for steam sterilizers for aqueous fluids in sealed rigid containers. Part 3. Specification for steam sterilizers for wrapped goods and porous loads. Part 4. Specification for transportable steam sterilizers for unwrapped instruments and utensils. Part 5. Specification for low-temperature steam disinfectors. Part 6. Specification for sterilizers using low temperature steam with formaldehyde. London: British Standards Institute.

Campbell, M. and Cripps, N.F. (1991) Environmental control of glutaraldehyde. *Hospital Estates Journal* 45, 2.

Department of Health (1994) *Health Technical Memorandum No. 2010. Steam sterilizers.* London: HMSO.

Department of Health (1997) *Health Technical Memorandum No. 2031. Clean steam for sterilization* London: HMSO.

Department of Health (1999) LI SC 1999/179. *Controls assurance in infection control: decontaminated medical devices.* London: Department of Health.

Deverill, C.E.A., Cripps, N.F., Roberts, M. *et al.* (1987) The Bowie–Dick test: an alternative way. *Journal of Sterile Services Management* 5, 21.

Dyas, A. and Das, B.C. (1985) The activity of glutaraldehyde against *Clostridium difficile. Journal of Hospital Infection* 6, 41.

European Union (1965) *Official Journal of the European Community* No. 22, p. 369 (9 February 1965). *65/65/EEC – Council Directive of 26 January 1965 on the approximation of provisions laid down by law, regulation or administrative action relating to proprietary medicinal products.* London: HMSO.

European Union (1990) *Official Journal of the European Community* No. L189, p. 17 (20 July 1990). *90/385/EEC – Council Directive of 20 June 1990 on the approximation of the laws of the Member States relating to active implantable medical devices.* London: HMSO.

European Union (1993) *Official Journal of the European Community* No. L169, p. 1 (12 July 1993). *93/42/EEC – Council Directive of 14 June 1993 concerning medical devices. Health and Safety Executive Guidance Note (1999) EH 40/99 Occupational Limits.* London: HMSO.

Gardner, J.F. and Peel, M.M. (1998) *Sterilization, disinfection and infection control,* 2nd edn. Edinburgh: Churchill Livingstone.

Health and Safety Executive (1999) *Occupational exposure limits. EH40/99.* Norwich: HMSO.

Hurrell, D.J. (1980) Low-temperature steam disinfection and low-temperature steam/formaldehyde sterilization. *Sterile World* 2, 13.

Kyri, M.S., Holton, J. and Ridgway, G.L. (1995) Assessment of a low-temperature hydrogen peroxide gas plasma sterilization system. *Journal of Hospital Infection* 31, 275.

Line, S.J. and Pickerill, J.K. (1973) Testing a steam-formaldehyde sterilizer for gas penetration efficiency. *Journal of Clinical Pathology* 26, 716.

Medical Devices Agency (1993/1999) Guidance on decontamination. Parts 1, 2 and 3. London: Department of Health.

Oates, K., Deverill, C.E.A., Phelps, M. and Collins, B.J. (1983) Development of a laboratory autoclave system. *Journal of Hospital Infection* 4, 181.

Russell, A.D., Ayliffe, G.A.J. and Hugo, W.B. (eds) (1999) *Principles and practice of disinfection, preservation and sterilization.* 3rd edn. Oxford: Blackwell Scientific Publications.

Rutala, W.A., Gergen, M.F. and Weber, D.J. (1999) Sporicidal activity of a new low-temperature sterilization technology. The Sterrad 50 sterilizer. *Infection Control and Hospital Epidemiology* **20**, 514.

chapter 5

PHYSICAL AND CHEMICAL DISINFECTION

Christina Bradley

Disinfection can be achieved using moist heat or chemicals. The applications for each method are described in Chapter 6. Wherever possible heat should be used for the decontamination of instruments and equipment. However, if this is not possible due to the thermal tolerance of the item, the time available or the accessibility/availability of processing equipment, chemical disinfectants may be used.

PHYSICAL DISINFECTION

Exposure to moist heat is probably the most effective and controllable method for the disinfection of heat-tolerant items. This method is widely used for respiratory/anaesthetic equipment, surgical instruments and trays, bedpans, urine bottles, linen, crockery and cutlery.

PROCESS TIMES AND TEMPERATURES

These vary between 65°C and 100°C, but generally the higher the processing temperature the shorter the processing time. The recommended times and temperatures in the UK (MDA, 1996) are shown in Table 5.1.

BOILERS

The use of boilers has largely been discouraged due to the lack of controls and the

Table 5.1 Recommended process times and temperatures in the UK (Medical Devices Agency, 1996)

	Temperature °C	Time
Instrument boiler	100	10 min
Automated washer disinfectors[a] for	71	3 min
medical equipment, including bedpans	80	1 min
and urine bottles	90	1 s[b]
Linen	65	10 min
	71	3 min

[a] Lower temperatures are used in washer disinfectors as cleansing accompanies the decontamination process.

[b] 1 s is difficult to measure, so 12 s are recommended.

risk of scalding. However, they are still used in the community and small clinics for instruments such as proctoscopes, vaginal speculae and other non-invasive medical equipment. Very few boilers have thermal interlocks, so it is possible to remove items before they have been effectively disinfected. If they are used correctly and items are added to boiling water and maintained for at least 10 min, therefore achieving 5 min at 100°C, boilers can disinfect reliably. Small bench-top sterilizers that are relatively inexpensive are now widely available and provide a far more reliable decontamination process.

THERMAL WASHER DISINFECTORS

These are used for automatic cleaning and thermal disinfection of surgical instruments and trays, holloware, respiratory/anaesthetic equipment and receptacles for human waste. They have the advantage of cleaning items, in addition to thermally disinfecting them, thereby reducing staff handling of contaminated instruments and equipment.

Washer disinfectors are widely used in hospital sterilization and disinfection units for the decontamination of used instruments and equipment from operating-theatres and other departments. Their use at the recommended temperatures for thermal disinfection has not been adopted for flexible endoscopes due to the damage sustained by these instruments. However, they are suitable for non-invasive heat tolerant rigid endoscopes if sterilization by autoclaving is not possible and disinfection is acceptable. Washer disinfectors vary in design from large tunnel/conveyor machines, which have a rapid throughput and are widely used in SDUs, to smaller cabinet machines that are used in small departments and clinics. They may be a suitable alternative to chemical disinfectants, (e.g. clear soluble phenolics) for instruments used in post-mortem rooms.

Users/purchasers should ensure that the equipment complies with national guidelines/recommendations. In the UK this would be BS 2745 (British Standards Institute, 1993), and HTM 2030 (NHS Estates, 1997). These documents describe design considerations and test methods for the assessment of cycle parameters such as cleansing efficacy, temperature compliance and drying. Other European and international standards are currently under discussion. It is recommended that machines are tested on commissioning, after changing the programme or detergent, on the advice of the infection control team/committee and/or 3-monthly, or if a problem associated with the washer disinfector is highlighted. If the washer disinfector is functioning correctly, it should render processed items free from infection risk and safe for patient reuse. If organic material is not removed from surfaces, it may become baked or fixed on to them during subsequent heat or chemical sterilization, it may cause friction in moving parts (causing accelerated wear) and it may lead to blockages in lumens.

A typical cycle consists of a low-temperature flush/rinse at a temperature which will not fix or bake organic material (usually < 45°C), and a main wash at > 55°C followed by a disinfection rinse at the appropriate temperature as stated in Table 5.1. Optional stages include a final rinse and a drying stage.

CHEMICAL DISINFECTION – TYPES OF CHEMICAL DISINFECTANTS (see Russell *et al.*, 1999)

Most hospitals have produced their own policy for the use of disinfectants, but it is still possible to find inappropriate disinfectants being used at inadequate or inappropriate concentrations. Expensive and ineffective disinfectants are still in use when cheaper or more effective agents are available, or when a disinfectant is not required at all. There remains a need for some degree of regional (if not national) standardization. A sound disinfectant policy should considerably increase the cost-effectiveness of disinfection in hospitals.

PHENOLICS (see Table 5.2)

Phenols and cresols are usually derived from the distillation of coal tar, but mixtures of synthetic phenols may be used. Chlorinated fractions and petroleum residues may also be added.

Black and white fluids

These are crude coal tar derivatives. Black fluids (e.g. 'Jeyes fluid') are solubilized in soap and are toxic and irritant to the skin. White fluids (e.g. 'Izal') are emulsified suspensions and tend to precipitate on surfaces, making subsequent cleaning more difficult. These disinfectants, especially white fluids, are sometimes used for environmental disinfection in hospitals, but have been largely replaced by clear soluble phenolics.

Clear soluble phenolics (e.g. Stericol, Hycolin, Clearsol)

Like other phenolics, these compounds are active against a wide range of bacteria, including *Pseudomonas aeruginosa* and *Mycobacterium tuberculosis*. They are fungicidal, but have limited virucidal activity and poor activity against bacterial spores. They are relatively cheap, stable, and are not readily inactivated by organic matter. However, they often contain a compatible detergent, so pre-cleaning of the surface is not necessary.

Uses are mainly confined to environmental disinfection, particularly in the presence of faeces or sputum, as they are too corrosive for many instruments and

Table 5.2 Phenolic disinfectants for environmental use

Disinfectant	Type	Routine use dilution (%)	Strong concentration (%)	Manufacturer
Stericol	CSPD	1.0	2	Lever Industrial Ltd
Hycolin	CSP	1.0	2	Wm. Pearson Ltd
Clearsol	CSPD	0.625	1	Coventry Chemicals Ltd
Izal	W	1.0	2	Lever Industrial Ltd

CSP, clear soluble phenolic; D, contains added detergent; W, White fluid.

too toxic to be applied to the skin. These and other phenolics should not be used in food preparation areas as they taint food, or on equipment that is likely to be in contact with skin or mucous membranes. Their use has decreased as a result of the growing need for a virucidal disinfectant for bloodborne viruses, and they have been largely replaced by chlorine-releasing agents. However, they are still widely used for instruments in post-mortem rooms when thermal decontamination methods are not available.

CHLOROXYLENOLS (e.g. 'DETTOL', 'IBCOL')

These are non-irritant but are readily inactivated by a wide range of materials, including organic matter and hard water, and high concentrations are required (2.5–5%). Chloroxylenols are effective against Gram-positive bacteria but poorly active against Gram-negative bacteria. The addition of a chelating agent (EDTA) increases the activity of chloroxylenols against Gram-negative bacilli. However, they are non-corrosive and non-irritant. They are not suitable for environmental or instrument use in hospitals.

PINE OIL DISINFECTANTS

These compounds are non-toxic and non-irritant, but are relatively ineffective against many organisms, especially *Pseudomonas aeruginosa*. They should not be used in hospitals.

HALOGENS (COMPOUNDS OR SOLUTIONS THAT RELEASE CHLORINE OR IODINE)

Chlorine-releasing agents

These are cheap and effective disinfectants which act by releasing of available chlorine. They are rapidly effective against viruses, fungi, bacteria and spores. They are particularly recommended for use where special hazards of viral infection exist (e.g. hepatitis B virus or HIV). Solutions are unstable at concentration use and dilutions should therefore be prepared daily. They are readily inactivated by organic matter (e.g. pus, dirt, blood, etc.) and may damage certain materials (e.g. plastics, rubber, some metals and fabrics). Chlorine-releasing agents are not compatible with some detergents, and should not be mixed with acids, including acidic body fluids such as urine, as the free chlorine produced may be harmful, particularly in a confined space. Solutions may be stabilized with alkali or sodium chloride. Chlorine-releasing agents at low concentrations are non-toxic and are particularly useful for water treatment, babies' feeding bottles and food preparation areas, and may also have other uses in the hospital environment. Their uses and recommended concentrations are shown in Table 5.3.

Preparations of chlorine-releasing agents include the following.

1 Strong alkaline hypochlorite solutions (e.g. 'Chloros', 'Domestos', 'Sterite') containing approximately 10% (100 000) ppm available chlorine (av Cl_2). Similar solutions in the USA are supplied at 5% (50 000 ppm av Cl_2). The

Table 5.3 In-use concentrations of chlorine-releasing agents

Uses	Available chlorine (mg/L) (ppm)[a]
Blood spillage from patient with HIV or HBV infection	10 000
Laboratory discard jars	2 500
General environmental disinfection	1 000
Disinfection of clean instruments	500
Infant feeding bottles and teats Food preparation areas and catering equipment	125
Eradication of *Legionella* from water supply system, depending on exposure time	5–50

Hydrotherapy pools
  Routine
  If contaminated
	
	1.5–3
	6–10

Routine water treatment	0.5–1

[a] Undiluted commercial hypochlorite solution contains approximately 100 000 ppm available chlorine.

concentrated solutions are corrosive and should be handled with care. Dilute solutions may be used with a compatible detergent, but will only reliably disinfect clean surfaces.

2 Hypochlorite solutions containing 1% (10 000 ppm av Cl_2) and stabilized with sodium chloride (e.g. 'Milton' or a preparation with comparable properties). These solutions are usually diluted 1: 80 (125 ppm av Cl_2) for the disinfection of infant feeding bottles and catering equipment and surfaces. The low chlorine content is inactivated by very small amounts of organic matter, and in-use solutions have a much narrower margin of safety.

3 Hypochlorite/hypobromite powders (e.g. 'Septonite', 'Diversol BX'). Solutions of these powders (0.5–1.0%) are used in the same way as other hypochlorite preparations, and are rather less corrosive. The powder may be used for cleaning baths and sinks where an abrasive preparation is undesirable.

4 Abrasive powders containing hypochlorites (e.g. hospital scouring powder, 'Vim', 'Ajax', etc.)

5 Non-abrasive powders (e.g. 'Titan', 'Diversey Detergent Sanitiser') containing hypochlorites are now usually preferred to abrasive powders for cleaning and disinfection of hospital baths and sinks.

6 Other chlorine-releasing compounds include sodium dichloroisocyanurate (NaDCC) (e.g. 'Sanichlor', 'Haztab', 'Presept') tablets, powders or granules. These compounds are growing in popularity as the tablets/powders are stable during storage, and solutions can be prepared more conveniently and accurately. However, the stability of prepared solutions is similar to that of

sodium hypochlorite solutions. They tend to be slightly more effective and less corrosive than hypochlorite solutions, but care is still necessary with metals. The cost of preparing solutions with a low concentration (e.g. 100–200 ppm av Cl_2) is comparable to that of liquid hypochlorite preparations, but the use of tablets for preparing high concentrations (e.g. 10 000 ppm av Cl_2) may be slightly more expensive.

NaDCC powders or granules may be applied directly to spillage of blood or body fluids from patients with suspected HBV or HIV, and are convenient and effective alternatives to solutions (Coates, 1988; Bloomfield and Miller, 1989). However, their use may not be suitable for large spills (> 30 mL), when disposable cloths or a mop and bucket with a solution of disinfectant may be more appropriate.

Chlorine dioxide (Tristel)

This has been used for many years for the treatment of drinking and waste water and for slime control, but more recently products have been introduced for instrument disinfection (Babb and Bradley, 1995). Chlorine dioxide is a highly effective compound which is rapidly bactericidal – including activity against mycobacteria (Griffiths *et al.*, 1999) – virucidal and sporicidal, achieving high-level disinfection within 5 min and sporicidal activity within 10 min. The product is supplied at several concentrations which will affect the stability/use life. This compound may be suitable for the decontamination of heat-labile equipment (e.g. endoscopes) provided that user acceptance and instrument and processor compatibility have been established (see Chapter 6).

Iodine and iodophors

A 1% solution of iodine in 70% alcohol is an effective pre-operative skin antiseptic. Skin reactions may occur in some individuals, and for this reason 0.5% alcoholic chlorhexidine or an alcoholic iodophor solution is usually preferred.

Iodophors are complexes of iodine and 'solubilizers' which possess the same activity as iodine, but are non-irritant and do not stain the skin. Iodophors are mainly used for hand disinfection – for example, povidone-iodine (PVP-I) ('Betadine', 'Disadine', 'Videne') detergent preparations or 'surgical scrubs'. These contain 7.5% PVP-I (equivalent to 0.7% available iodine) and are effective for this purpose. Alcoholic preparations containing 10% PVP-I (1% available iodine) are suitable for pre-operative preparation of the skin at the operation site. Some iodophors may also be used for disinfection of the environment, but they are expensive and cannot be recommended for general disinfection in hospital.

Iodine is the only antiseptic which has been shown to have a useful sporicidal action on the skin. When applied as an iodophor it can be left on the skin long enough to remove a large proportion of *Clostridium perfringens* spores when these are present, but this property is of uncertain clinical value (see Chapter 7).

Electrolysed water (Sterilox)

This is a recent introduction to the market for the decontamination of flexible endoscopes. The solution is produced by electrolysing a salt solution and collecting the solution produced at the anode (anolyte). A generator produces the solution at the point of use and pipes it to existing washer disinfectors (provided that they are compatible). The solution is used once only and then discarded. Freshly generated Sterilox is rapidly sporicidal (Selkon *et al.*, 1999) and mycobactericidal (Selkon *et al.*, 1999; Shetty *et al.*, 1999), provided that generation criteria are fulfilled. These criteria are the redox potential (> 950 mV), pH (5.0 – 6.5) and current (9 A). Sterilox is affected by organic matter, so items need to be scrupulously clean, and it is also very unstable. Only freshly generated solution should be used, and the pipework should be purged to remove 'dead' solution if left for a period of time. At present, little data is available on instrument compatibility and field trials are in progress. If these trials show that it can be economically and reliably generated and it can be established that it does not damage instruments or processing equipment, it could improve the processing of endoscopes. Other electrolysed (acid) water systems with varying pH are under development which may also prove useful for the decontamination of endoscopes.

QUATERNARY AMMONIUM COMPOUNDS SUCH AS BENZALKONIUM CHLORIDE (e.g. 'ROCCAL', 'ZEPHIRAN', 'MARINOL' AND CETRIMIDE ('CETAVLON')

These are relatively non-toxic antibacterial compounds with detergent properties. They are active against Gram-positive organisms but much less active against Gram-negative bacilli, and are readily inactivated by soap, anionic detergents and organic matter. Quaternary ammonium compounds (QACs) at higher dilutions inhibit the growth of organisms (i.e. they are 'bacteriostatic') but do not necessarily kill them (i.e. they do not show a 'bactericidal' effect). For this reason, their effectiveness has often been exaggerated. Their use in hospitals is limited because of their narrow spectrum of activity, but they may be useful for cleansing dirty wounds (e.g. cetrimide). Apart from possible uses in food preparation areas, QACs are not widely used in the UK for environmental disinfection. Contamination of a weak solution of a QAC with Gram-negative bacilli is a possible hazard which can be prevented by avoidance of cork closures or of 'topping-up' stock bottles. Incorporating a chelating agent enhances the activity of QACs against Gram-negative bacilli. However, QACs are ineffective against the hepatitis B virus, tubercle bacilli and spores, and show variable activity against HIV. More recently, some QACs have been introduced which show reasonable activity against *Pseudomonas aeruginosa* and other Gram-negative bacilli although their activity against viruses (particularly enteroviruses) and mycobacteria has yet to be established.

CHLORHEXIDINE ('HIBITANE')

This useful skin antiseptic is highly active against vegetative Gram-positive organisms, but less active against Gram-negative bacilli. It also has good fungicidal activity, but shows little or no activity against tubercle bacilli, enveloped viruses and bacterial spores. It is relatively non-toxic, but is inactivated by soaps. Its use in hospitals should be restricted as much as possible to procedures involving contact with skin or mucous membranes. It is too expensive for environmental use.

Detergent solutions containing 4% chlorhexidine gluconate are available (e.g. 'Hibiscrub', 'Hibiclens'). These have been found to be highly effective for the disinfection of surgeons' hands prior to operating, and they have a good persistent effect due to residuals left on the skin after rinsing and drying. Some alternative preparations show inadequate bactericidal effects and may be irritant to the skin. Trials are necessary before new products are introduced even if they contain similar concentrations of chlorhexidine gluconate. Cosmetic acceptability is an important factor when selecting a disinfectant for the skin, particularly that of the hands.

'Savlon' is a mixture of chlorhexidine and cetrimide. The hospital concentrate contains 15% cetrimide and 1.5% chlorhexidine. It is usually used at a concentration of 1%. At this concentration the antimicrobial activity of the chlorhexidine is poor. However, cetrimide is a good cleansing agent and enhances the activity of chlorhexidine. 'Savlon' is expensive and, if used, should be reserved for clinical procedures, such as cleansing dirty wounds, and not used for instruments or environmental disinfection.

Low concentrations of antiseptics are likely to become contaminated during use. The provision of pre-sterilized single-use sachets ('Hibidil',' 'Savlodil') reduces this risk.

'Hibisol' is a 0.5% solution of chlorhexidine in 70% isopropanol, used for disinfection of clean, intact skin (e.g. that of the hands); 0.5% chlorhexidine gluconate in 70% ethanol (or isopropanol) is used for disinfection of the operation site.

HEXACHLOROPHANE

This compound is highly active against Gram-positive organisms but less active against Gram-negative ones. It is relatively insoluble in water, but can be incorporated in soap or detergent solutions without loss of activity. It has a good residual effect on the skin. These solutions are prone to contamination with Gram-negative bacteria unless a preservative is included in the formulation. Potentially neurotoxic levels may occur in the blood if emulsions or other preparations of hexachlorophane are repeatedly and extensively applied to the body surface of babies. This product, although very effective, is now infrequently used for skin disinfection in hospitals, and can only be obtained for use on medical advice. It may be used for handwashing by staff during staphylococcal outbreaks, or for surgical hand disinfection. Toxic levels are not approached when a hexachlorophane dusting powder (Streak) is used on the umbilical stump of neonates, and this method, which has been found to be highly effective in the control of staphylococcal infection, may still be considered to have a role in hospital practice. It may also be applied to the groin and buttock regions of MRSA carriers.

TRICLOSAN (IRGASAN DP300, e.g. 'STERZAC' BATH CONCENTRATE, 'MANUSEPT', 'PHISOMED', 'ZALCLENSE', 'CIDAL', 'AQUASEPT', 'GAMOPHEN')

Triclosan-containing products have properties and a spectrum of activity similar to those of hexachlorophane, but they show no toxicity to neonates. They are now widely used as an alternative to hexachlorophane in hand rubs, soaps and bath concentrates. In-use concentrations are in the range 0.3–2.0%. Antimicrobial tests and trials for tolerance are required before use of individual products, as these are variable and generally less effective than chlorhexidine preparations. Triclosan-containing products are often used for the treatment of MRSA carriers, as they are better tolerated than some other antiseptic-containing detergents.

ALCOHOLS

Ethyl alcohol 70% (ethanol) and 60% isopropyl alcohol (isopropanol) are effective and rapidly acting disinfectants and antiseptics, with the additional advantage that they evaporate, leaving the treated surfaces dry, but they have poor penetrative powers and should only be used on clean surfaces. They are active against mycobacteria but not against spores. Their activity against viruses is variable, and non-enveloped viruses (e.g. poliovirus) tend to be more resistant, particularly to isopropanol (Tyler *et al.*, 1990). The recommended concentrations of ethanol (70%) and isopropanol (60%) are optimal *in vitro* for killing organisms, and are more effective than absolute alcohol. Alcohol or alcohol-impregnated wipes may be used for the rapid disinfection of smooth clean surfaces (e.g. trolley tops, thermometers, probes and electrical/electronic equipment) which cannot be safely immersed in aqueous disinfectants. They are also useful for irrigating the lumens of bronchoscopes after rinsing if the microbiological quality of the rinse water cannot be guaranteed to eradicate atypical mycobacteria. If the item is contaminated with blood or secretions, prior cleaning is advised.

Alcohol is commonly used for skin disinfection (e.g. without additives for treating skin prior to injection). With the addition of 1% glycerol or other suitable emollients, 60–70% alcohol rubbed on until the skin is dry is an effective agent for the rapid disinfection of physically clean hands, especially if handwashing facilities are unsuitable or not readily available. The addition of other bactericides to alcohol does not appreciably increase its immediate effect as a skin antiseptic, but the repeated use of alcohol solutions may lead to lower equilibrium levels of bacteria on the skin. The addition of non-volatile antiseptics (e.g. chlorhexidine, povidone iodine and triclosan) may provide a residual antiseptic action on the skin.

ALDEHYDES – FORMALDEHYDE, GLUTARALDEHYDE ('CIDEX', 'ASEP', 'TOTACIDE' 28, 'SPORICIDIN') AND SUCCINE DIALDEHYDE ('GIGASEPT')

Although formaldehyde is required in extreme circumstances e.g. for fumigation of rooms following care of a patient with a viral haemorrhagic fever (Advisory Committee on Dangerous Pathogens, 1993) or disinfection of a ventilator not protected by a bacteria-retaining filter and may achieve sterilization if used with sub-atmospheric steam, solutions of formaldehyde are too irritant for use as general disinfectants. However, formaldehyde is still recommended for the fumigation of laboratory safety cabinets (Health and Safety Commission, 1991; Advisory Committee on Dangerous Pathogens, 1995).

Glutaraldehyde is generally used as a 2% activated alkaline solution at room temperature, and is recommended for heat-sensitive items, particularly flexible endoscopes. It is non-damaging to metals, plastics and rubber and is effective against vegetative organisms, viruses (including HBV and HIV) and fungi. Its activity against *Mycobacterium tuberculosis* is relatively slow i.e. 20 min of exposure time may be required (Griffiths *et al.*, 1999), as is its sporicidal activity (> 60 min) (Babb *et al.*, 1980). Glutaraldehyde may be irritant to the eyes, skin and respiratory tract and can cause sensitization, including occupational asthma and contact dermatitis (Cowan *et al.*, 1993). Its use should be restricted to areas where adequate provision has been made for the extraction/total containment of aldehyde vapour and personal protective equipment e.g. gloves, apron, goggles, respiratory masks is available in the event of a spillage. Alkaline solutions require activation, and once activated they remain stable for 2–4 weeks depending on the preparation. However, they may become diluted during use, particularly in auto-mated washers, and may require a more frequent exchange. To ensure sporicidal activity, an exposure period of at least 3 hours is required, although shorter times may be sufficient to kill some pathogenic spores (e.g. *Clostridium difficile* (Dyas and Das, 1985; Rutala *et al.*, 1993). (For further information on contact times for endoscopes, see Chapter 6.)

Acid solutions of glutaraldehyde are more stable and do not require activation, but usually have a slower sporicidal effect. They may be more suitable for the occasional or small user. Their activity is improved by use at a temperature of 50 – 60°C, although this can be associated with an increase in vapour levels and possible damage to instruments. Lower concentrations of aldehydes (0.125 – 2%) have been used at an elevated temperature (45 – 60°C) within an automated endoscope washer disinfector (see Chapter 6). Other aldehydes e.g. succine dialdehyde ('Gigasept') have similar properties to glutaraldehyde. The addition of a phenolic compound to 2% glutaraldehyde ('Sporicidin') improves the sporicidal action, but the advantages are marginal for routine disinfection. Most of the tests have been made on 2% glutaraldehyde solutions, and lower concentrations are less effective over the same time period, although they may offer a longer use life.

HYDROGEN PEROXIDE

Hydrogen peroxide (3% or 6%) is infrequently used as a hospital disinfectant in the UK compared to the USA. It is used for the disinfection of tonometers and soft contact lenses, and also for ventilators not protected by filters. It has also been added to urinary drainage bags. Frequent use has been associated with corrosion of certain metals.

Peroxygen compounds (e.g. Virkon) have variable virucidal activity (Tyler *et al.*, 1990) and little or no activity against mycobacteria (Broadley *et al.*, 1993; Holton *et al.*, 1995; Griffiths *et al.*, 1999). They are less corrosive than hypochlorites, so they may have a role in the disinfection of laboratory equipment and environmental surfaces where the infection risk is low and compatibility with the surface has been established. Virkon powder may be used as a less corrosive alternative for decontamination of spillage (e.g. on carpets).

PERACETIC ACID ('NU-CIDEX', 'STERIS')

Peracetic acid has been used for the disinfection of certain types of equipment e.g. patient isolators and, more recently, for the decontamination of endoscopes. It is rapidly bactericidal, virucidal and mycobactericidal (within 5 min) and sporicidal (within 10 min), and is claimed to be relatively non-toxic and non-corrosive at the concentrations used. It is currently marketed in two forms. 'Nu-Cidex' contains 0.35% peracetic acid which is prepared from a 5% concentrate with minimal user contact during preparation of the dilution, and is used at room temperature. This solution is stable for 24 hours post-preparation and can be used in existing equipment. 'Steris' contains 0.2% peracetic acid solution and has to be used in a dedicated processing machine i.e. a Steris System 1 Endoscope Processor at an elevated temperature of 45°C (Bradley *et al.*, 1995). The disinfectant is supplied as a concentrate which is diluted within the machine and discarded to waste after use (for more information, see Chapter 6). It is important to establish compatibility with instruments and processing equipment before use.

AMPHOLYTIC COMPOUNDS (e.g. 'TEGO')

These compounds combine detergent and antibacterial properties. They are similar to the QACs, and may be of value in the food industry, but they are expensive and there are few indications for their use in hospitals.

OTHER ANTIMICROBIAL COMPOUNDS

Many other antimicrobial compounds have been used. Among these are the acridine and triphenyl methane (crystal violet and brilliant green) dyes, which were once widely used as antiseptics for skin and for wounds. Silver nitrate and other silver compounds (e.g. silver sulphadiazine) have a valuable place as topical antiseptics in prophylaxis against infection of burns. 8-Hydroxyquinoline has been found to be effective as a fungicide. Mercurial compounds have poor bactericidal powers, but they are strongly bacteriostatic. Phenyl mercuric nitrate has been used as an effective preservative for ophthalmic solutions.

Other compounds have been described by Block (1991) and Russell *et al.* (1999).

THE FORMULATION OF A DISINFECTION POLICY

The general principles for formulation of a policy are summarized below (Ayliffe *et al.*, 1993: Coates and Hutchinson, 1994). The hospital infection control committee should prepare the disinfectant policy and decide on the types of disinfectants to be used. This requires consultation between the microbiologist, infection control doctor, infection control nurse, pharmacist, supplies officer and representatives of medical, nursing and domestic staff. Demands for disinfectants come from many departments of the hospital, and there are many sources of supply. All requests for disinfectants should be approved by the hospital pharmacist, who can check whether they are in agreement with the hospital policy.

The selection of a disinfectant depends on many factors, including the following:

1 intended use of the disinfectant – medical equipment, environment, skin and mucous membranes;
2 range of activity;
3 speed of action;
4 inactivation by organic material;
5 compatibility with items processed and processing equipment;
6 user safety;
7 stability;
8 cost.

PRINCIPLES

1 List all of the purposes for which disinfectants are used, then check requisitions and orders to ensure that the list is complete.
2 Eliminate the use of chemical disinfectants when heat can reasonably be used as an alternative, when sterilization is required, when thorough cleaning alone is adequate, or if single-use equipment can be used economically. There should be few remaining uses for chemical disinfectants.
3 Select the smallest practicable number of disinfectants for the remaining uses, i.e. one routine disinfectant for each field of use (the environment, skin and equipment), plus an alternative for use if patients or staff are sensitive to the routine disinfectants, for instruments which may be damaged by the disinfectant, and for use when the routine disinfectant is either unavailable or inappropriate for a particular purpose.
4 Arrange for the distribution of disinfectants chosen at the correct use-dilution, or supply equipment and personal protective equipment for preparing and measuring disinfectants at the site of use.
5 All potential users of disinfectants should receive adequate instruction in their preparation and use. This should include information on the following:
   • the correct disinfectant and concentration to be used for each task;
   • the shelf-life of the disinfectant at the concentration supplied, the type of container to be used, and the frequency with which the solution should be changed;
   • substances or materials which will react with or neutralize the disinfectant;
   • an assessment of toxic or other risks to employees using the disinfectant or detergent is needed, together with the measures required for protection of employees (Control of Substances Hazardous to Health (COSHH)) Regulations 1988). Personal safety measures should be addressed e.g. whether rubber gloves should be worn, how the product can be safely opened and prepared, how the disinfectant should be disposed of, what action is required if the product comes into contact with the skin or eye.

6 The policy should be monitored to ensure that it is effective and continues to be so. Occasional in-use tests and chemical estimations of concentration may be required.

SELECTION OF DISINFECTANTS (see also Rutala, 1990)

Antimicrobial properties

Where this is compatible with other requirements, the disinfectants used should be bactericidal rather than bacteriostatic, active against a wide range of microbes, and not readily inactivated. The manufacturer should supply information on the properties of the disinfectant, but independent antimicrobial tests are also required. The Kelsey Sykes test (Kelsey and Maurer, 1974) was formerly commonly used in the UK, but the EU are now introducing CEN tests to which all disinfectants should be subjected. These will take the form of a standardized suspension test (Council of Europe, 1987), and others which will include surface/carrier tests and more practical 'in-use' tests. The AOAC surface test in the USA has been criticized on account of its lack of reproducibility, and it is hoped that some international standardization of tests will be possible in the future. Manufacturers should also provide Material Safety Data Sheets to enable the user to carry out COSHH assessments, as well as information on material compatibility.

Other properties

The properties of the disinfectants chosen should be considered in terms of acceptability as well as antibacterial activity. Stability, toxicity and corrosiveness should be assessed with the aid of relevant information obtained from the manufacturers. Acceptability and cleaning properties should also be assessed. Cost is clearly important, and a regional contract for one or two generally acceptable disinfectants should considerably reduce costs. A trial period (possibly of 3 months) might be introduced, and an assessment of all relevant factors should be made before the policy is permanently implemented. COSHH assessments should be performed on all chemical disinfectants.

RECOMMENDED DISINFECTANTS AND USE-DILUTIONS

ENVIRONMENT

A chlorine-releasing agent and a phenolic disinfectant should be sufficient for most environmental hospital requirements.

Hypochlorites and other chlorine-releasing agents (see Table 5.3) have the properties already mentioned. They may be incorporated in a powder (abrasive or non-abrasive) for cleaning baths, toilets and washbasins. Solutions (1000 ppm av Cl_2) may be used for disinfecting clean surfaces and, when necessary, for food preparation areas. Chlorine-releasing agents should be used if disinfection of virus-contaminated material is required. However, routine or too frequent use can cause expensive corrosion and damage to equipment and some surfaces, in which case other less corrosive antiviral agents are required. Higher concentrations of chlorine (i.e. 10 000 ppm) are recommended in the presence of organic material e.g. blood/body fluid spillages.

A clear soluble phenolic disinfectant (e.g. 'Stericol', 'Hycolin', 'Clearsol') is often chosen as one of the disinfectants for routine use (see Table 5.2). There is little to choose between these compounds in terms of effectiveness at the recommended use-dilutions. For most purposes the concentration required for light contamination will be adequate (i.e. 'Clearsol' 0.625%, 'Stericol' 1%, 'Hycolin' 1%, 'Izal' 1%). This provides a reasonable margin of safety and should be used unless otherwise indicated. The strong concentrations, (i.e. twofold, should be used for heavily contaminated areas or if contamination with *Mycobacterium tuberculosis* is likely (disinfection by heat or use of single-use items is particularly important for dealing with contamination by *Mycobacterium tuberculosis*). Phenolics are not usually suitable for use against viruses, and the increasing anxiety about HIV is responsible for a reduction in their routine use.

Narrow-spectrum or expensive disinfectants are mainly used for clinical purposes and are not recommended for general environmental use, but may sometimes be required for special equipment. After thorough cleansing with detergent and water items may be immersed in alcohol or cleaned and disinfected using a disposable alcohol-impregnated wipe. This is preferable to the use of glutaraldehyde. NaDCC compounds tend to be less corrosive than hypochlorites.

Instruments

If possible, heat-tolerant instruments should be purchased. However, for heat-labile instruments glutaraldehyde may be used provided that total containment/extraction of vapour is in place. Other alternative agents include peracetic acid and chlorine dioxide, but users are advised to establish instrument and processing equipment compatibility and to ascertain what personal protective equipment is required in relation to COSHH.

Skin

Antiseptics containing chlorhexidine, povidone iodine or triclosan are widely used for the disinfection of the skin i.e. hands and operation site. Alcohol is also widely used for the hands, especially where handwashing facilities are either unavailable or unsuitable. Cosmetic acceptability is an important factor when selecting agents for the skin, particularly the hands. In most instances soap and water are sufficient (see Chapter 6).

DILUTION AND DISTRIBUTION OF DISINFECTANTS

Ineffective cleaning and too low a concentration are the commonest causes of failure of a disinfectant to kill organisms, and survival of contaminants in the disinfectant is unlikely if it is at the recommended use-dilution. It is therefore preferable for the pharmacist to supply departments with containers of disinfectant already prepared at the correct use-dilution, or for departments to prepare their own solutions. Containers should be labelled with the date of issue and the date after which the disinfectant should not be used (e.g. 1 week after issue); they should be clearly labelled with an instruction such as 'do not dilute' or 'use undiluted'. Containers should be thoroughly washed and preferably disinfected by heat before refilling. If heating is not possible, thorough drying after washing should be adequate as this will kill most of the bacteria that are likely to be present. Corks must not be used – containers should have plastic closures which can be easily cleaned.

The main disadvantage of this method of dispensing is the transport of large quantities of fluid (mainly water), particularly if large amounts of disinfectants are used, and as some disinfectants (e.g. chlorine-releasing agents) are unstable when diluted. The alternative method is to supply undiluted disinfectant to the department where dilutions are prepared when required. A suitable and relatively foolproof measuring system is required for both disinfectant and water. A measuring device attached to the container is commonly used, but unless staff are well trained, dilutions will be inaccurate. A measured amount of undiluted disinfectant in a bottle, tablet or sachet is an alternative, but the water must also be measured. The strong disinfectant solution requires careful handling in order to avoid damage to the skin or the eyes of the operator. Gloves and a plastic apron should be worn and eye protection is necessary if splashing is likely.

TRAINING AND STAFF INSTRUCTION

Whichever system of supplying disinfectants is used, all personnel handling or using them must be adequately trained, supervised and regularly updated. Training should include preparation and use of the disinfectant, with particular emphasis placed on safe use and the COSHH regulations.

IN-USE TESTS

As disinfectants are used under a variety of conditions, it is essential to test their effectiveness under the actual conditions of use. Contamination of a disinfectant solution is a particular hazard, and 'in-use' tests (Ayliffe et al., 1993) should be performed when a new disinfectant or different concentration of an existing disinfectant is introduced. Repeat tests should be carried out occasionally to ensure that no changes in the recommended policy have occurred and that resistant bacterial strains are not selected. If the cleanliness of the equipment (e.g. mops and brushes) immersed in the disinfectant is uncertain, the surface of the equipment should also be examined by a microbiological surface-sampling technique (e.g. cotton-wool swabs, contact plates). Routine testing is probably unnecessary if staff are well trained in disinfection procedures.

REVIEW OF POLICY

This should be considered annually. Defects of the current system should be noted and changes introduced where necessary.

REFERENCES

Advisory Committee on Dangerous Pathogens (1993). *Management and control of viral haemorrhagic fevers*. London: HMSO.

Advisory Committee on Dangerous Pathogens (1995) Categorisation of biological agents according to hazard and categories of containment, 4th edn. London: HMSO.

Ayliffe, G.A.J., Coates, D. and Hoffman, P.N. (1993) *Chemical disinfection in hospitals*. 2nd edn. London: Public Health Laboratory Service.

Babb, J.R. and Bradley, C.R. (1995) A review of glutaraldehyde alternatives. *British Journal of Theatre Nursing* 5, 20.

Babb, J.R., Bradley, C.R. and Ayliffe, G.A.J. (1980) Sporicidal activity of glutaraldehyde and hypochlorite and other factors influencing their selection for the treatment of medical equipment. *Journal of Hospital Infection* 1, 63.

Block, S.S. (1991) *Disinfection, sterilization and preservation*. 4th edn. Philadelphia, P.A: Lea & Febiger.

Bloomfield, S.F. and Miller, E.A. (1989) A comparison of hypochlorite and phenolic disinfectants for disinfection of clean and soiled surfaces and blood spillages. *Journal of Hospital Infection* 13, 231.

Bradley, C.R., Babb, J. R. and Ayliffe, G.A.J. (1995) Evaluation of the Steris System 1 peracetic acid endoscope processor. *Journal of Hospital Infection* 29, 143.

British Standards Institute BS 2745 (1993) Washer disinfectors for medical purposes. Part 3. London: British Standards Institute.

Broadley, S.J., Furr, J.R., Jenkins, P.A. and Russell, A.D. (1993) Antimycobacterial activity of 'Virkon'. *Journal of Hospital Infection* 23, 189.

Coates, D. (1988) Comparison of sodium hypochlorite and sodium dichloroisocyanurate disinfectants. Neutralization by serum. *Journal of Hospital Infection* 11, 60.

Coates, D. and Hutchinson, D.N. (1994) Infection control in practice: how to produce a disinfection policy. *Journal of Hospital Infection* 26, 57.

Control of Substances Hazardous to Health Regulations (1988) London: HMSO.

Council of Europe (1987) *Test methods for the antibacterial activity of disinfectants*. Strasbourg: Council of Europe.

Cowan, R.E., Manning, A.P., Ayliffe, G.A.J. *et al.* (1993) Aldehyde disinfectants and health in endoscopy units. *Gut* 34, 1641.

Dyas, A. and Das, B.C. (1985) The activity of glutaraldehyde against *Clostridium difficile*. *Journal of Hospital Infection* 6, 41.

Griffiths, P.A., Babb, J.R. and Fraise, A.P. (1999) Mycobactericidal activity of selected disinfectants using a quantitative suspension test. *Journal of Hospital Infection* 41, 111.

Health and Safety Commission (1991) *Health Services Advisory Committee. Safety in Health Service Laboratories. Safe working and the prevention of infection in clinical laboratories*. London: HMSO.

Holton, J., Nye, P. and McDonald, V. (1995) Efficacy of selected disinfectants against mycobacteria and cryptosporidia. *Journal of Hospital Infection* 31, 235.

Kelsey, J.C. and Maurer, I.M. (1974) An improved Kelsey–Sykes test for disinfectants. *Pharmaceutical Journal* 213, 528.

Medical Devices Agency (1996) Sterilization, disinfection and cleaning of medical equipment: guidance on decontamination from the Microbiology Advisory Committee. Part 1. Principles. London: Department of Health.

NHS Estates (1997) Health Technical Memorandum 2030. Washer disinfectors: design considerations. Leeds: NHS Estates.

Russell, A.D., Hugo, W.B. and Ayliffe, G.A.J. (1999) *Principles and practice of disinfection, preservation and sterilization.* 3rd edn. Oxford: Blackwell Science.

Rutala, W.A. (1990) APIC guidelines for selection and use of disinfectants. *American Journal of Infection Control* 18, 99.

Rutala, W.A., Gergen, M. F. and Weber, D. J. (1993) Inactivation of *Clostridium difficile* spores by disinfectants. *Infection Control and Hospital Epidemiology* 14, 36.

Selkon, J.B., Babb, J.R. and Morris, R. (1999) Evaluation of the antimicrobial activity of a new super-oxidised water, Sterilox®, for the disinfection of endoscopes. *Journal of Hospital Infection* 41, 59.

Shetty, N., Srinivasan, S., Holton, J. and Ridgway, G.L. (1999) Evaluation of microbicidal activity of a new disinfectant: Sterilox® 2500, against *Clostridium difficile* spores, *Helicobacter pylori*, vancomycin-resistant *Enterococcus* species, *Candida albicans* and several *Mycobacterium* species. *Journal of Hospital Infection* 41, 101.

Tyler, R., Ayliffe, G.A.J. and Bradley, C.R. (1990) Virucidal activity of disinfectants: studies with the poliovirus. *Journal of Hospital Infection* 15, 339.

chapter 6

DECONTAMINATION OF THE ENVIRONMENT, EQUIPMENT AND THE SKIN

John Babb

The choice of method of decontamination (i.e. cleaning, disinfection or sterilization) depends on many factors, but the initial choice can be based on infection risks to patients. These can be classified as high, intermediate, low and minimal risks (Ayliffe *et al.*, 1993). However, there is an overlap between these categories, and requirements for decontamination may vary within a category.

INFECTION RISKS TO PATIENTS FROM EQUIPMENT, MATERIALS AND THE ENVIRONMENT

HIGH RISK

For invasive items, those in close contact with a break in the skin or mucous membrane or introduced into a sterile body area (see p. 105) (e.g. surgical instruments, dressings, catheters and prosthetic devices), sterilization is required. If sterilization is not practically achievable, high-level disinfection, although not optimal, may be adequate.

INTERMEDIATE RISK

For items in contact with intact mucous membranes, body fluids or contaminated with particularly virulent or readily transmissible organisms, or items to be used on highly susceptible patients or sites (e.g. gastrointestinal endoscopes, respiratory equipment), disinfection is required.

LOW RISK

For items in contact with normal and intact skin (e.g. washing bowls, toilets and bedding), cleaning and drying is usually adequate. Disinfection is needed if there is a known infection risk (e.g. bath after washing MRSA patient).

MINIMAL RISK

Items not in close contact with the patient or his or her immediate surroundings are in the minimal risk category. For surfaces that are unlikely to be contaminated

with a significant number of pathogens or those transferred t\
(e.g. floors, walls, sinks), cleaning to remove organisms and
adequate.

HOSPITAL ENVIRONMENT

The inanimate environment of the hospital (i.e. usually with minimal risk) is of
little importance in the spread of endemic hospital infection (Ayliffe *et al.*, 1967;
Maki *et al.*, 1982; Collins, 1988), as it is unlikely to make contact with a susceptible site, but it may occasionally have a role in outbreaks. Recommendations for
decontamination are listed in Appendices 6.1 and 6.2.

WARD

A ward surface (floor, furniture, equipment or wall) that is physically clean and dry
is unlikely to represent an appreciable infection risk. A clean environment is
necessary to provide the required background to good standards of hygiene and
asepsis, and to maintain the confidence of patients and the morale of staff (Maurer,
1985). Wet surfaces and equipment are more likely to encourage the growth of
micro-organisms and to spread potential pathogens. Cleaning equipment and used
cleaning solutions may be heavily contaminated with bacteria and should be
removed from patient treatment or food preparation areas as soon as cleaning is
completed. Thorough cleaning will remove micro-organisms and the organic
material on which they thrive. This will render most items relatively free of
infection risk and safe to handle. Disinfectants are not usually required, and should
only be used as part of a properly controlled policy. Disinfectants should be accurately diluted, freshly prepared for each task and disposed of promptly after use.
Antimicrobial agents are sometimes included in cleaning solutions not described as
disinfectants. These may be highly selective and adversely affect the microbial
ecology, and their use should therefore be avoided whenever possible. If cleaning
services are contracted to an industrial organization, the cleaning solutions and
equipment should conform to hospital policy.

DUTIES AND RESPONSIBILITIES OF DOMESTIC SERVICES STAFF

The Domestic Services Manager is usually responsible for hospital domestic staff,
and should ensure that they are properly trained and supervised. Routine cleaning
of the environment, including floors, toilets, baths, wash-basins, beds, locker-tops
and other furniture, should be the responsibility of the domestic service in all
wards and departments. Domestic staff who are specially trained and aware of
possible infection hazards should be available to clean and, if necessary, disinfect
the rooms occupied or vacated by infected patients. The cleaning procedures in use
should be agreed with the infection control staff, and should include a list of the
contents of the room to be cleaned or disinfected, methods for disposal of waste
material, and methods of disinfection of cleaning equipment. Nursing and other
patient care staff should, wherever possible, be relieved of cleaning tasks. Surfaces

...quipment contaminated with potentially infectious material require immediate attention. Nurses should continue to clean and disinfect these items unless specifically trained domestic staff are available. If there is an unusual infection risk associated with the presence of a particular patient (e.g. in cleaning blood spillage from an HBV- or HIV-infected patient, or in a high-risk department), the ward sister should ensure that the domestic staff are aware of that risk. It may be considered that the task could be performed more safely by a trained nurse. Cleaning should be carried out in a carefully planned manner, and cleaning schedules should be drawn up for each area to include all equipment, fixtures and fittings. New items should be added to schedules as they are commissioned. Cleaning schedules should be sufficiently detailed to specify the method, frequency, timing where relevant, equipment to be used, where that equipment is to be stored and how it is to be cleaned and disinfected. The responsibility for each task should be indicated and should include the maintenance of paper-towel cabinets and soap or dispensers, and replacement of cleaning materials and linen. The schedules should be agreed with the individuals in charge of the area to be cleaned and, in high-risk areas, with the infection control staff.

FLOORS

The bacteriological advantages of using a disinfectant rather than a detergent solution, or a wet method rather than a dry one, are marginal in routine hospital cleaning. In a busy ward, recontamination from airborne settlement or transfer from shoes and trolley wheels is rapid. Levels of bacterial contamination on floors may be restored to their original values within 2 hours of cleaning, whether or not disinfectants are used (Ayliffe *et al.*, 1966). Infection rates are not influenced by the use of a disinfectant, and a detergent alone will normally suffice (Danforth *et al.*, 1987). Disinfectants should only be used where there is a known or predictable risk (i.e. removal of potentially infectious spillage such as salmonella, tubercle bacilli, HBV or HIV, or decontamination of cleaning equipment before use elsewhere). Disinfection of floors and other environmental surfaces may also be included in cleaning policies for specific areas (e.g. clean rooms, isolation units, etc.), and where recommended by the microbiologist to deal with a particular risk. However, the risks of acquiring infection from floors and other environmental sites in these areas – including operating-theatres – are low, and cleaning alone is usually adequate.

DRY CLEANING

Brooms re-disperse dust and bacteria into the air and should not be used in patient treatment areas or food preparation and service areas. Suitable methods are a vacuum cleaner or dust-attracting mop. Vacuum cleaners should meet the requirements of BS 5415. The inner paper bag should be checked before use and discarded if it is more than half full. Bags should be exchanged away from patient treatment areas with the minimum dispersal of dust. Filters should be inspected at regular scheduled intervals (e.g. monthly), and must be changed if they are dirty or blocked.

The dust-attracting mop, although less efficient, may be used either as a supplement or as an alternative to a vacuum cleaner. Dust-attracting mops may be either impregnated with or manufactured from a dust-attracting material, and may be disposable or re-processable. If used for an excessive period without replacement, they will fail to retain the dust and may indeed disperse it and adherent bacteria into the air. An acceptable period of use should be decided upon for each area. To avoid dispersal during use, the head should remain in contact with the floor during sweeping and should not be lifted at the end of each stroke. Dry-cleaning removes soil but will not remove stains or scuff marks.

WET CLEANING

Wet cleaning is required at intervals to remove stains and scuff marks. Sluice rooms, toilets and other moist areas require wet cleaning at least once daily. A neutral detergent is usually adequate and should be freshly prepared for each task. Mops and other equipment should be cleaned, drained where appropriate, and stored dry. Buckets should be rinsed and stored inverted to assist drying. Mops are difficult to dry completely and are frequently contaminated with Gram-negative bacilli. Although these may be transferred to the surface during cleaning, they will disappear rapidly as the surface dries. Floors transiently contaminated in this way do not appear to cause infections in general surgical and medical wards. Mops require disinfection after use in the rooms of infected patients, and possibly before use in rooms occupied by immunosuppressed patients. Laundering in a machine with a heat disinfection cycle is the preferred method, but rinsing followed by a soak in 1% bleach or an alternative chlorine-releasing agent (1000 ppm available chlorine) for not more than 30 min, re-rinsing and allowing to dry, is an acceptable alternative. If disinfection is not required, mops should be kept clean, and laundering is the preferred method.

All cleaning equipment should be examined at regular scheduled intervals and cleaned if it is soiled. Worn or damaged equipment should be repaired or replaced. Cleaning solutions should be changed frequently to prevent the accumulation or multiplication of bacteria, and should be discarded or removed from the patient treatment area as soon as cleaning is completed. A two-compartment bucket or a wheeled stand containing two buckets (which allows the used water from the mop to be discarded into a separate bucket or compartment) is an advantage. Surfaces should be left as dry as possible after cleaning. Poorly designed or inadequately maintained mechanical cleaning equipment may increase the bacterial count of the cleaned surface or the surrounding air, and should not be introduced into high-risk areas without consultation with the microbiologist or infection control staff. The cleaning and maintenance of all new equipment should be agreed upon before putting it into use. Protocols should indicate the acceptable area of use for the equipment and any attachments. It may be permissible to use a scrubbing machine in more than one area, but separate pads should be used. It is preferable that scrubbing machines with integral tanks which cannot be totally drained should not be used in patient treatment areas. If a machine has a solution storage tank it should be drained as completely as possible at the end of the day's session and kept dry until it is required.

SPRAY CLEANING

It is important to ensure that solutions sprayed in patient treatment areas are not heavily contaminated with Gram-negative bacilli. Solutions should be freshly prepared and spray bottles that are not in use should be stored clean and dry.

CARPETS (OR OTHER SOFT FLOORING MATERIALS) IN HOSPITAL WARDS

Although bacteria are usually present in large numbers and survive longer on carpets than on hard floors, there is no evidence that carpets are associated with an increased infection risk (Ayliffe et al., 1974). Nevertheless, it is still reasonable to minimize potential infection hazards by selecting carpets with specifically desirable properties. If installed in wards or other clinical areas, the carpets should have a waterproof backing and joints should be sealed. Pile fibres should preferably be water-repellent and non-absorbent. Ease of cleaning and rate of drying are both improved by having a pile of short upright fibres. The carpet should be washable and, if possible, not damaged by the application of commonly used disinfectants. Spillage of blood, particularly from patients at high risk of bloodborne infection, may require disinfection with chlorine-releasing agents which damage most carpets. Alternatives to chlorine-releasing compounds (e.g. peroxygen powders) which are less damaging to carpets are available. However, spillage can usually be safely removed by thorough washing with a detergent solution, provided that gloves are worn by the operator. Before buying a carpet, it is important to ensure that it is resistant to the agents that are likely to be applied in the ward, and that stains can be easily removed. Carpets should be vacuum cleaned daily and periodically wet cleaned with specially designated equipment (e.g. steam cleaners with a vacuum extraction facility).

The decision as to whether or not to fit carpets in clinical areas is a difficult one, and is not entirely based on infection risk, as other factors need to be considered (e.g. appearance, comfort, sound reduction, etc). Carpets in wards with frequent or large-volume spillage (e.g. units for the mentally handicapped) are usually inadequately maintained, and are therefore not recommended in these areas (Collins, 1979). Other clinical areas, such as surgical and obstetric wards, may also frequently be contaminated with blood and other body fluids, and again routine cleaning may be inadequate. Problems of smell and staining have been responsible for the removal of carpets in many clinical areas. In general, it would seem preferable to avoid carpets in these areas as attractive alternative flooring is now available. Washable floors are advisable in isolation wards, as carpets may prolong the survival of certain organisms (e.g. multi-resistant strains of *Staphyloccus aureus* (such as MRSA). If it is still decided to fit carpets in clinical areas, it is of major importance to ensure that, in addition to buying suitable carpets and cleaning equipment, the cleaning schedules are agreed upon before the carpet is bought, and that they are achievable. The cleaning guidelines provided by manufacturers are often impracticable as ward areas need to be evacuated during the procedure. Facilities should also be available for the prompt removal of spillage. Absorbent powders are particularly useful for this purpose, followed by either vacuum cleaning or the spot application of a suitable carpet-compatible detergent. As it is not usually possible to use a disinfectant because of possible damage to the carpet, protective clothing (i.e. gloves and a plastic apron) should be worn when removing spillage.

SPILLAGE

Cleaning with a detergent and water may be adequate for most spillage (e.g. food, urine, etc.). A disinfectant should be used for spillage containing potentially hazardous organisms (Ayliffe *et al.*, 1993; Babb, 1996). Disposable gloves should always be worn when cleaning known contaminated spillage. If there is a risk of contaminating clothing, a disposable plastic apron should also be worn. A sprinkler may be used to cover small amounts of the spillage with sufficient chlorine-releasing granules or powder to absorb any moisture. When the fluid is completely absorbed, a disposable paper wipe should then be immediately used to remove the residue and discarded into a plastic bag. Finally, the surface should be washed using a disposable paper wipe and dried. All waste, wipes, disposable gloves and apron (if worn), should be discarded, sealed and disposed of as clinical waste. Powders or granules should be used on wet spillage only. Liquid disinfectants (e.g. chlorine-releasing agents or clear soluble phenolics) can also be used and may be necessary for larger spillages (> 30 mL). Chlorine-releasing powder, granules or fluids containing 10 000 ppm available chlorine should be used for blood or body fluid spillage that is known or suspected to be contaminated with HIV or HBV. If chlorine-releasing agents are added to hot water, anionic detergents or acidic body fluids (e.g. urine), this may result in a rapid release of toxic levels of chlorine. At these concentrations chlorine-releasing agents are toxic and corrosive and likely to damage or decolorize many surfaces; 1000 ppm can be used for other spillage or precleaned surfaces. Paper towels are useful for absorbing spillage of blood and other body fluids. These should be disposed of as clinical waste and the area wiped or mopped with disinfectant. If the surface is likely to be damaged by chlorine-releasing agents, other agents with antiviral activity (e.g. peroxygen compounds) may be more appropriate. Universal precautions assume that all blood and certain body fluids are potentially infectious, and routine disinfection before cleaning is often recommended. This would seem to be excessive (particularly in hospitals where the infection rate with HBV or HIV is low) and unnecessary, provided that gloves and a plastic apron are worn and hands are washed. Thorough cleaning alone is usually sufficient. Clear soluble phenolics (0.6–2%) are less likely to damage surfaces and are suitable for bacterial contamination (e.g. with enteric organisms or mycobacteria), but they are poor virucidal agents.

Disinfectants should be freshly prepared and accurately diluted for each task. Chlorine-releasing powders, granules and tablets, i.e. sodium dichloroisocyanurate (NaDCC), are stable but solutions are not, and so should be discarded on completion of the task or at the end of the day.

WALLS AND CEILINGS

Only very small numbers of bacteria adhere to clean, smooth, dry, intact walls (Ayliffe *et al.*, 1967). These surfaces are therefore unlikely to be a significant infection hazard. Ceilings have an even smaller number of bacteria. The cleaning of walls and ceilings should be carried out sufficiently often to prevent the accumulation of visible dirt. Intervals between cleaning should not usually exceed 12–24 months in patient treatment areas, or 6 months in operating-theatres.

Disinfection is not required unless known contamination has occurred. Splashes of blood or known contaminated material should be removed promptly. When cleaning walls, the surface should be left as dry as possible. Damaged paintwork exposes plaster which cannot be effectively cleaned or disinfected, and which may become heavily colonized with bacteria if it becomes moist (e.g. through condensation). Damaged wall surfaces should be promptly repaired and redecorated, particularly in operating-theatres. A moist surface may encourage growth of fungi, especially *Aspergillus*.

OTHER SURFACES

Locker-tops should be wiped daily with a freshly prepared detergent solution using disposable wipes. Other furniture should be similarly cleaned as required. Shelves and ledges should be damp-dusted weekly, or more often if dust accumulates. Disinfection is not required unless the surface is contaminated with body fluids and other potentially infectious material.

BATHS, SINKS AND WASH-HANDBASINS

Baths and wash-handbasins should be cleaned at least daily by the domestic staff and, if practicable, patients should be encouraged to clean the bath after each use. Detergent is adequate for routine cleaning. A cream cleaner may occasionally be required to remove scum, but should not be used on fibreglass baths unless its use is approved by the manufacturer. It is necessary to disinfect baths after use by infected patients or those carrying multi-resistant or problematic strains (e.g. MRSA), or before use by patients with open wounds. A non-abrasive chlorine-releasing powder can be used for this purpose. Abrasive powders are effective, but they damage porcelain surfaces and must never be used on fibreglass.

Alternatively, solutions or cream cleaners containing chlorine-releasing agents may be used with a detergent, but only if the detergent is known to be compatible.

Wash-handbasins should be used solely for this purpose. Compliance is more likely if plugs are removed and elbow/wrist-operated mixer taps are installed. Chlorine-releasing agents may also damage the recirculating pumps of some hydrotherapy baths and birthing tubs. Quaternary ammonium compounds are often used but are less effective. Check the suitability of all cleaning agents and disinfectants with the equipment manufacturers before use. No attempt should be made to disinfect sink traps or outlets, as disinfection of these sites is usually ineffective and treatment may disperse potential pathogens.

TOILETS AND DRAINS

Toilet seats and handles should be cleaned at least once daily, and also when they are visibly soiled. A detergent solution should be used for routine cleaning. Disinfection with a chlorine-releasing agent or clear soluble phenolic may be required if the seat is obviously contaminated, or after use by patients with a gastrointestinal infection. If a disinfectant is used, the seat should be rinsed with water and dried before use. Pouring disinfectant into lavatory pans or drains is unlikely to reduce infection risks.

CROCKERY AND CUTLERY

Centralized arrangements for machine washing and drying of all crockery and cutlery are preferable to washing on individual wards (see also Dishwashing in Hospital Wards 2: Domestic Service Management Advice Note 1976). A washing-machine with a final rinse temperature of 80°C for 1 min or other appropriate disinfection time/temperature combination (e.g. 71°C for 3 minutes) is a satis-factory alternative in ward kitchens (see the section on kitchen hygiene in Chapter 12), and is desirable in isolation wards.

CLEANING MATERIALS

Wherever possible, single-use wipes should be used for cleaning surfaces (e.g. baths, sinks, bowls, mattresses, beds, furniture, etc.). They should also be used for mopping up spillages from a known source of infection and for cleaning cubicles occupied by infected patients. If disposables are not available for use in other areas because of cost, the following alternatives can be used.

1 A nylon brush, which can be dried quickly, may be used for cleaning baths. Absorbent cotton mops or bristle brushes become heavily contaminated, are difficult to disinfect and should not be used.

2 If non-disposable cloths are used for cleaning, these should be washed after use, preferably in a washing-machine with a disinfection stage in the cycle, and then dried. Separate cloths should be used in the kitchen, sluice and other ward areas. A colour code may be used to distinguish the different areas of usage.

3 Toilet brushes should be rinsed well in the flushing water of the lavatory pan. After the excess water has been shaken off, they should be stored dry.

Sponges dry slowly, are difficult to disinfect and should not be used.

DISINFECTION OF ROOMS WITH FORMALDEHYDE GAS

Formaldehyde disinfection may be required for rooms that have been occupied by patients with viral haemorrhagic fevers, although the necessity for this is doubtful. Formaldehyde is also used for disinfecting laboratory safety cabinets and for fumigation of Category 3 and 4 handling facilities following spillage. The method is not required or recommended for terminal disinfection of rooms occupied by patients with the common range of infectious diseases or hospital-acquired infections. If required, expert supervision should be available, as formaldehyde is a toxic gas. The windows and other outlets should be sealed and formaldehyde generated from formalin or paraformaldehyde. The amount needed depends on the volume of the room. For formaldehyde fumigation, 100 ml of formalin plus 900 ml of water are required for each 30 m^3 of space. The mixture is boiled away in an electrically heated pan fitted with a timing device. If paraformaldehyde is used, 10.5 g/m^3 is heated in the same way. After starting the generation of formaldehyde vapour, the door should be sealed and the room left unopened for 48 hours. The atmospheric formaldehyde levels should be checked before the room is reoccupied. The maximum exposure limit for formaldehyde is 2 ppm (2.5 mg/m^3) over a 15-min reference period and 8-hour TWA.

DECONTAMINATION OF NON-CLINICAL EQUIPMENT (see also Appendix 6.1)

WASHING AND SHAVING EQUIPMENT

Plastic washing bowls
The bowls should be thoroughly washed with a detergent and hot water after each use and dried. It is important to remove residual fluid remaining in the bowl after cleaning, and if possible the bowls should be stored separately and inverted. Each patient should preferably have their own washing bowl, particularly in intensive-care or other high-risk units. The bowl should be terminally disinfected by heat or with a chlorine-releasing agent or clear soluble phenolic before it is issued to the next patient. Thorough cleaning and drying is probably sufficient in general wards. A hanging basket is convenient for storage of washing bowls under the bed.

Nailbrushes
Nailbrushes frequently become contaminated with Gram-negative bacilli even when they are stored in a disinfectant solution, and their use should be avoided except for special procedures (e.g. first scrub of the day in an operating-theatre). Nylon brushes kept in a dry state are less often contaminated than bristle brushes, but brushes should be avoided if possible. If nailbrushes are required in patient treatment or food production areas, they should preferably be supplied sterilized or heat-disinfected by the SSD.

Soap dishes and dispensers

Soap dishes are rarely necessary, and may encourage bacterial growth. If used, they should be washed and dried daily. The nozzles of liquid soap dispensers should be cleaned daily to remove residues, and the outside should be cleaned and dried. Disposable cartridge-type refills with an integral nozzle are preferred, but they tend to be expensive. If non-disposable reservoirs are used, topping up should be avoided and the inside of containers should be cleaned and dried before refilling. In cartridge-type dispensers the channel and reservoir between the refill and nozzle, if not disposable, require periodic cleaning. Liquid soaps used in hospitals should contain a preservative (e.g. 0.3% chlorocresol), which should prevent bacterial growth during periods of use.

Razors

For pre-operative shaving, a disposable or autoclavable razor is preferred. Communal razors used by the hospital barber should be wiped clean and disinfected after each shave using 70% alcohol. Electric razor-heads should also be immersed in 70% alcohol for 5 min.

BEDS AND BEDDING

Bed frames

Bed frames are rarely an infection risk and, unless visibly soiled, routine cleaning is unnecessary after discharge of a patient. However, bed frames should be included in cleaning schedules and should be wiped with detergent solution and dried. If disinfection is considered necessary, a chlorine-releasing agent (1000ppm available chlorine), or a clear soluble phenolic is usually suitable. Expensive antiseptics should not be used.

Mattresses and pillows

Mattresses and pillows cannot readily be disinfected if they become contaminated. They should be enclosed in a waterproof cover and additional waterproof draw sheets used if contamination with body fluids is likely. Wiping the cover with a detergent solution and thorough drying, usually provides adequate decontamination. Avoid excessive wetting during cleaning. Disinfectants, particularly clear soluble phenolics, can make covers permeable and should be avoided. If disinfection is required, use a chlorine-releasing (1000 ppm available chlorine) solution and then rinse well (Department of Health, 1991).

It may be possible to disinfect some pillows, hoists and patients' supports using hot water laundering at 71°C for 3 min or 65°C for 10 min, or by low-temperature steam (73–80°C). Silver nitrate used for topical treatment of burns will also damage mattress covers. Stained mattress covers are often permeable to fluids and should therefore be changed (Lilly *et al.*, 1982). All mattresses should be routinely inspected for damage.

Duvets

Duvets with a waterproof outer surface and covered with a launderable outer fabric cover are now used in some hospitals, but some patients find them uncomfortable, particularly in hot weather. Provided that the duvet does not become soiled or wet, replacement of the outer fabric cover of the duvet between patients is usually adequate. The plastic surface will need to be cleaned if it becomes soiled or contaminated. Thoroughly wiping the outer surface of the duvet with a detergent solution and allowing it to dry completely will usually be sufficient. If disinfection is required after spillage or use by an infected patient, proceed as described for mattresses and pillows. Launderable duvets without a waterproof outer surface are available, but routine disinfection of the whole duvet in the laundry could be a problem. The possible implications of this should be carefully considered by the infection control team after discussion with the laundry manager before they are introduced (e.g. an outbreak of MRSA may require laundering of all duvets in a ward at the same time). Duvets are not recommended for incontinent patients or if gross contamination with body fluids is likely.

Bedding

Bedding can rapidly become heavily contaminated with colonized skin scales. Frequent changing is therefore of limited value in controlling the spread of infection. Procedures for laundering are described in Chapter 12.

Cotton blankets should be used, and these should be changed on discharge of the patient or if they become soiled or contaminated with potentially infectious spillage.

Sheets should be changed on discharge of the patient and also at least twice weekly and if soiled, wrinkled, stained or contaminated with potentially infectious material.

Curtains

The level of microbial contamination on curtains is related to the level of dispersal by patients in the immediate vicinity and, if changed, will rapidly regain that level. Curtains should therefore be washed when they are obviously soiled or else every 6 months. The curtains in the vicinity of a disperser of an epidemic strain of *Staphylococcus aureus* may remain heavily contaminated for some hours, and should be changed if the area is to be reoccupied by a susceptible patient within 24 hours. The degree of microbial contamination is not usually related to the type of material used or the time since the curtains were last changed.

Bed-cradles

These should be kept clean and maintained in good condition. They only need to be disinfected after use by an infected patient. The cradle may then be wiped with a chlorine-releasing solution or a clear soluble phenolic and rinsed. Bed-cradles should not be stored in patient treatment areas.

TOYS

Disinfection of toys is rarely necessary. Contaminated solid toys may be wiped with a chlorine-releasing agent and rinsed, or else wiped with 70% alcohol. Soft toys may be disinfected using low-temperature steam or hot water. If they are grossly contaminated they should be destroyed.

DRESSING-TROLLEY TOPS

To clean dressing-trolley tops, use a detergent solution and a disposable paper wipe, and then dry them. To disinfect them, wipe with 70% alcohol.

INSTRUMENTS, HOLLOWARE, ETC. FOR CLINICAL PROCEDURES

These should be supplied packed and sterilized by the SSD. Sterilization or disinfection of instruments at ward level should rarely be required. If it is necessary to sterilize instruments at the point of use, a small autoclave should preferably be used. Bench-top autoclaves with vacuum-assisted air removal are now available for packaged, lumened and porous items. Boiling-water baths do not sterilize, but if used correctly are a more reliable method of disinfection than most chemical agents. In an emergency, precleaned instruments can be disinfected, but not sterilized, in boiling water for 5–10 min. Immersion of clean instruments in 70% alcohol, or 2% glutaraldehyde for 10 min will disinfect, but is not as reliably effective as hot water or steam. Instruments immersed in glutaraldehyde should be thoroughly rinsed in water in order to remove irritant residues before use. Sterile water should be used for invasive items. Glutaraldehyde is irritant and sensitizing, and its use in wards or clinics should be avoided if possible unless adequate protection is given to prevent skin, eye and respiratory contact. Wiping with 70% alcohol is a rapid but less certain method of disinfection of instruments such as scissors, and is particularly useful for electrical equipment and other items which cannot be immersed. Cheatle forceps should preferably not be used for aseptic techniques. If there are circumstances requiring their use (e.g. in hospitals without an SSD), the forceps, complete with container, should be cleaned and autoclaved or boiled between uses and stored dry.

Used instruments should be transferred to a paper or plastic bag which is placed in a rigid container and returned without further treatment to the SSD. If a delay is anticipated before processing, gross soiling with blood or other body fluids should be removed under running water, otherwise subsequent removal may prove difficult. Suitable protective clothing (e.g. gloves and apron) should be worn.

THERMOMETERS

Oral thermometers

Oral thermometers should be stored clean and dry, as growth of Gram-negative bacilli is possible if they are kept in a disinfectant. If separate thermometers are used for each patient, they may be disinfected by wiping with an alcohol wipe before returning them to their respective holders. Thermometers should be disinfected by immersion in 70% alcohol or 1–2% clear soluble phenolic solution for 10 min when the patient is discharged. If not kept for individual patients, thermometers may be wiped clean and disinfected with alcohol at the end of the round, and then stored dry.

Rectal thermometers

Disposable sleeves will reduce the risk of contamination and, if used, the sleeve should be removed and the thermometer treated as for oral thermometers. If a sleeve is not used, remove all traces of lubricant by wiping the thermometer clean, and then disinfect as described above.

BEDPANS

To prevent transfer of faecal contamination, the hands should always be washed after handling a used or reusable bedpan, even if it is apparently clean.

Reusable bedpans

Where possible, bedpans should be washed and disinfected in a bedpan-washing machine with a heat-disinfection cycle. Thermal disinfection should ensure that all surfaces reach 90°C or are raised to 80°C and maintained at that temperature for at least 1 min (British Standards Institute, 1993, BS 2745 Part 2). The cycle should be checked regularly to ensure that the required temperature is reached. Washing-machines without a heat-disinfection cycle are acceptable in most situations, but not on urological wards, infectious diseases wards or where enteric infections are likely to occur. In such cases they should be replaced by machines with a heat-disinfection cycle when a new machine is required. If washers are not available, emptying the bedpan into the sluice, washing it and allowing it to dry thoroughly before reuse is also acceptable for noninfected patients.

Alternative methods of disinfection

Bedpans may be placed in boiling water for 5–10 min, but this should rarely be necessary. Chemical disinfection is not usually practicable. Immersion tanks should preferably be avoided, as they may be ineffective if not well maintained, and they can encourage the growth of resistant strains of Gram-negative bacilli. Wiping the entire surface of a cleaned bedpan with a clear soluble phenolic or a chlorine-releasing solution, rinsing it and allowing it to dry is an alternative, but this is not as effective as heat disinfection, and should only be used in an emergency or in countries with limited facilities.

Disposable bedpans

Single-use paper-pulp bedpans that are disposed of in a purpose-built macerator are an alternative to washer disinfectors. To minimize the risk of blockages, the horizontal course of the soil pipe above ground should not be greater than 7 m and should have an overall fall of 1 in 40. Paper-pulp bedpans require a reusable support. These supports become contaminated during use and may require washing after use. If heavily contaminated with faeces, they should be washed and wiped with a chlorine-releasing agent or a clear soluble phenolic. An individual support is recommended for each patient. This may be disinfected if soiled and also on discharge of the patient.

COMMODES

The container used in the commode should be treated as a bedpan. Containers which fit bedpan washers are preferred. If the seat becomes soiled or is used by a patient with an enteric infection, it should be disinfected with a clear soluble phenolic or a chlorine-releasing agent, rinsed and dried before reuse. Disposable wipes should be used for cleaning and disposable gloves and a plastic apron should be worn. Hands must be washed at the end of the task even if gloves are worn.

URINE BOTTLES

Bedpan washers will also accommodate urine bottles, and recommendations are as for bedpans. Washers with a heat-disinfection cycle are strongly recommended for urology and infectious diseases wards. Urine bottles not disinfected by heat should always be regarded as contaminated, and hands should be washed after contact with them. If heat disinfection is not available, a separate labelled urine bottle should be supplied to patients with urinary tract infections. This should be rinsed after each use and disinfected on discharge of the patient as described above for bedpans.

Disposable paper-pulp urine bottles for disposal in bedpan macerators are available, but may not be suitable for urology wards if direct visual examination of the urine is required.

DECONTAMINATION OF MEDICAL EQUIPMENT

See also Appendices 6.1 and 6.2 and Microbiology Advisory Committee to Department of Health Medical Devices Agency, 1996.

HIGH-RISK ITEMS

Most of the items in this category (e.g. surgical instruments, prosthetic devices, dressings, surgical drapes and gowns, parenteral fluids, etc.) can be sterilized by steam at high temperatures. Dry heat can be used to sterilize some delicate sharp instruments used in ophthalmic and dental surgery, glass syringes, oils and powders. Single-use items, (e.g. catheters, plastic syringes, needles, grafts and internal pacemakers) are usually sterilized by the manufacturer using ethylene oxide or irradiation. Inexpensive items, especially those which are heat sensitive and difficult to clean, should not be reused (Central Sterilizing Club, 1999, MDA DB 9501 1995). All reprocessed equipment should be cleaned thoroughly before sterilization prior to reuse. Properly validated, automated washer disinfectors are preferred (British Standards Institute, 1993; NHS Estates, 1997). Under the Medical Devices Directive (1998), manufacturers are required to state which methods of decontamination can be used for any reusable item of equipment. Non-disposable items should preferably be able to withstand autoclaving at 134°C (or at least 80°C). If items are damaged at these temperatures, or if they cannot be cleaned easily, their use should be discouraged. Some expensive items, such as flexible endoscopes, are heat sensitive and must be decontaminated by less effective methods, such as immersion in disinfectants.

Operative endoscopes (e.g. arthroscopes, laparoscopes)

Since an increasing amount of operative surgery will be carried out in the future using an endoscope, autoclavable instruments and accessories are preferred (Ayliffe *et al.*, 1992; Medical Devices Agency, 1996a). However, many of the new instruments are flexible and therefore damaged by heat. They should be cleaned thoroughly and if possible sterilized with ethylene oxide. If this is not available, low-temperature steam and formaldehyde (LTSF) may be used for rigid endo-scopes. As these methods may be unavailable or impracticable, immersion in 2% glutaraldehyde for 3–10 hours is an acceptable alternative, but this method is less reliable due to the possible presence of air bubbles and recontamination on subse-quent rinsing. Shorter immersion times (10–20 min) are usually used because of the limited availability of instruments. There is evidence that these short contact times are effective against some pathogenic spores e.g. *Clostridium difficile* (Dyas and Das, 1985). This process is referred to in the USA as high-level disinfection (it is effective against vegetative bacteria, including *Mycobacterium tuberculosis* viruses and fungi, but not usually all bacterial spores or some atypical mycobac-teria (Rutala, 1990). Provided that the endoscope is well cleaned before disin-fection, the risk of infection is small, although the remote risk of infection due to spore-forming organisms cannot be excluded. All invasive endoscopes immersed in glutaraldehyde should be thoroughly rinsed in sterile or bacteria-free (filtered < 0.45 μ) water to remove toxic residues prior to reuse.

Cystoscopes

Autoclaving is preferred for heat-tolerant rigid cystoscopes, but high-level disin-fection is usually used, i.e. immersion in 2% glutaraldehyde for 10 min (Cooke *et al.*, 1993). The longer exposure time of 20 min is required if an effect against *M. tuberculosis* is required (Best *et al.*, 1990; Griffiths *et al.*, 1999). Solutions should not be used beyond the manufacturer's recommended post–activation use-life (e.g. 14–28 days), or if reuse reduces the concentration to below 1.5%. If sufficient instruments are available, autoclaving or low temperature steam with or without formaldehyde may be used. Pasteurization in a water bath at 70–80°C for 10 min is an alternative to chemical disinfection, but the manufacturer should be consulted on heat tolerance if hot water or steam is used. Thermal disinfection/sterilization is unsuitable for flexible cystoscopes. Another alternative is immersion in 70% ethanol for 5 min, but this may damage the instrument if immersion is prolonged beyond the time limit indicated by the manufacturer.

MISCELLANEOUS HIGH-RISK ITEMS

Catheters

Single use is preferred. Some cardiac catheters are too expensive for single use, and reprocessing may therefore be necessary, although it is not usually recommended by regulating authorities in the wealthier countries (Medical Devices Agency, 1995). They may be resterilized with ethylene oxide provided that the cleaning process is efficient and the structure and function remain unimpaired. Single-use items should only be reused if it is cost-effective and safe to do so. The hospital or

Trust must then take corporate legal responsibility for reprocessing and reuse. Single-use items must not be reused if suitable reusable items are available.

Grafts (heart valves, arterial grafts, joints and other implants)
These should be autoclaved if possible. If they are heat labile, use ethylene oxide. Sterilization of these items in the hospital should not usually be necessary unless the package containing the device has been opened and the device has not been immediately used.

Cryoprobes
These should be autoclaved if possible. If they are heat labile, use LTSF or ethylene oxide. Immersion in 2% glutaraldehyde or 70% alcohol may be necessary if cryoprobes are heat labile and gaseous sterilization facilities are not available.

Transducers and blood-monitoring equipment
These may be a source of infection. Single-use items are preferable, or else ethylene oxide or LTSF should be used. High-level disinfection (e.g. 2% glutaraldehyde or 70% alcohol) may sometimes be necessary.

Haemodialysis equipment
See Chapter 17.

INTERMEDIATE-RISK ITEMS

Non-invasive endoscopes
Pseudomonas aeruginosa and other Gram-negative bacilli, including *Salmonella*, have been transferred from one patient to another on inadequately decontaminated flexible fibre-optic endoscopes (Ayliffe, 1999). Reports on the transfer of mycobacteria and HBV are rare, and there has been no evidence of transfer of HIV. Nevertheless, care is necessary to avoid the possibility of spread of any infection by ineffective decontamination (Spach *et al.*, 1993). Endoscopic retrograde cholangiopancreatography (ERCP) is a particularly vulnerable procedure, and severe Gram-negative infections have been reported. Thorough cleaning and disinfection are important with this procedure. Potential pathogens such as the Gram-negative bacilli can grow overnight in the channels of the endoscope, the water bottle and in processing equipment, and disinfection is required at the beginning of the list as well as after each patient. The time available for processing between patients is often short (20–30 min). However, vegetative bacteria and most viruses are killed or inactivated by 1–2 min of exposure to 2% glutaraldehyde (Hanson *et al.*, 1989, 1990; Sattar *et al.*, 1989; Tyler *et al.*, 1990). Preliminary studies with duck hepatitis B viruses suggest that they are inactivated within 2 min by glutaraldehyde preparations (Murray *et al.*, 1991). A variety of automatic cleaning and disinfection machines are available (Bradley and Babb, 1995). Most of these are effective and protect the user from toxic processing chemicals, but preliminary brushing of the suction/biopsy channel and wiping of the insertion tube are still required. All channels should be cleaned and disinfected. The glutaraldehyde concentration is reduced during repeated use, particularly in automated systems, and the solution

should be changed regularly (e.g. after 20–40 procedures). The rinse water should also be changed regularly, preferably after each instrument, in order to avoid any build-up of glutaraldehyde. Infection has been reported from Gram-negative bacilli growing in the rinse-water tank. This should be routinely disinfected. Bacteria-free filtered (0.2–0.45 μ) or sterile water is recommended for invasive instruments and those used for ERCP and bronchoscopy.

Before changing the method of decontamination, it is advisable to consult the manufacturer and give them details of the method to be used. Many disinfectants are corrosive and may damage the endoscope. It should also be noted that low-temperature steam may reach 80°C and ethylene oxide may reach 55°C with considerable variations in pressure. Furthermore, not all endoscopes and accessories are totally submersible.

Flexible gastrointestinal endoscopes

Alkaline activated glutaraldehyde 2% (e.g. 'Asep', 'Cidex', 'Totacide 28') is the most widely used disinfectant for endoscopes (Babb, 1993). The British Society of Gastroenterology (1998) recommends thorough cleaning of all channels and external surfaces followed by immersion for 10 min in 2% glutaraldehyde at the start of a list and for between-patient decontamination. This will destroy vegetative bacteria and viruses, including HIV and HBV. Endoscopes used on patients who are known to have or suspected of having pulmonary tuberculosis should be immersed for 20 min. Known AIDS patients are managed as immunocompromised patients, and the endoscope should be disinfected for 20 min before and after the procedure. This is to protect patients from opportunistic pathogens, some of which are relatively resistant to glutaraldehyde. Similarly, a 20-min immersion is recommended between cases for ERCP when high-level disinfection is required.

Cryptosporidia are resistant to glutaraldehyde, but thorough cleaning should be adequate. Although glutaraldehyde is recommended, an alternative and less irritant agent may be required. Cleansing with a detergent followed by 70% ethanol is recognized as an alternative, but less effective, between-patient method. Immersion of the endoscope in ethanol for longer than 5 min may damage epoxy lens cements. Other agents are being investigated including peracetic acid, chlorine dioxide and super-oxidized water (Babb and Bradley 1995a and b; Bradley et al., 1995; Medical Devices Agency, 1996a; Selkon et al., 1999).

Many of these agents are more rapidly effective than 2% glutaraldehyde, particularly against mycobacteria (5 min) and spores (10 min). However, they are more damaging to instruments and processing equipment, and their long-term toxicity is not known. Users are strongly advised to inform their infection control team, to seek assurance on compatibility from instrument and processor manufacturers (as use may invalidate guarantees and service-level agreements), to cost the change (bearing in mind the stability of the disinfectant and any personal protective equipment and environmental controls) and to keep those responsible for national guidelines informed of progress whether it is favourable or not (Babb and Bradley, 1995a). In view of the toxic, irritant and sensitizing properties of aldehydes, it is necessary to find an effective, non-damaging and less irritant alternative to glutaraldehyde.

Flexible bronchoscopes

The British Thoracic Society (1989) recommends that bronchoscopes are immersed in 2% glutaraldehyde for 20 min between patients and for 1 hour after a known or suspected case of pulmonary tuberculosis. The risk of recontamination of the instrument with environmental mycobacteria (e.g. *Mycobacterium chelonae*) derived from the rinse water is high in some areas. It is therefore recommended that the instrument is rinsed in sterile water, filtered water (0.2–0.45 μ) or tap water followed by 70% alcohol, particularly before use on an immunocompromised patient.

Endoscope accessories

Many endoscope accessories (e.g. biopsy forceps, brushes, snares, water bottles, etc.) are now autoclavable. These should be dismantled where possible, cleaned thoroughly (preferably using ultrasonics), dried, reassembled and processed, either in the SSD or in a dedicated area of the endoscopy suite. A porous load or vacuum bench-top sterilizer (Medical Devices Agency, 1996b, 1998) should be used for packaged and lumened accessories. Non-autoclavable accessories should be dismantled, cleaned and immersed in 2% glutaraldehyde or a suitable alternative.

Use of 2% glutaraldehyde

Although microbiologically effective, glutaraldehyde is irritant to the skin, eyes and respiratory tract. Impermeable gloves (e.g. nitrile) and aprons should always be worn, as well as eye protection if splashing is likely. Solutions should be stored and used in covered containers, preferably under the influence of extract ventilation. As glutaraldehyde is a respiratory sensitizer, the Health and Safety Executive have imposed a maximum exposure limit (MEL) of 0.05 ppm (0.2 mg/m^3) over a 15-min reference period and 8-hour time-weighted average (TWA) (EH40/99). The use of less concentrated solutions may reduce the irritant effect, but longer immersion times will be required to maintain the antimicrobial effect. Similar irritancy and sensitization problems are also likely with other aldehydes (e.g. succine dialdehyde and formaldehyde). It is important to rinse thoroughly all items immersed in glutaraldehyde. All staff who come into contact with glutaraldehyde should undergo health screening which includes a pre-employment enquiry regarding asthma, skin and mucosal symptoms (e.g. rhinitis and conjunctivitis). Lung function tests by spirometry, an annual completion of a health questionnaire and immediate notification of skin rashes, chest and sinus problems are also recommended (British Society of Gastroenterology, 1998).

Endoscope washer disinfectors

These have become an essential part of endoscopy units, as they increase instrument throughput and reduce staff contact with the disinfectant (Bradley and Babb 1995). The washer disinfectors must be effective, safe, reliable and able to cope with endoscope design and throughput. They do not negate the need for manual cleaning (i.e. insertion tube, suction/biopsy channels, instrument tip, valve recesses). If they are not cleaned and disinfected at least on a sessional basis, they may become a source of recontamination.

RESPIRATORY EQUIPMENT

Ventilators

Many types of ventilator are available, most of which can be adequately protected by filters, thus minimizing the need to decontaminate the ventilator itself (Das and Fraise, 1997). Some ventilators have a removable internal circuit which can be autoclaved or disinfected using low-temperature steam. Chemical disinfection may sometimes be required. Most methods of chemical disinfection are not practicable and will not work efficiently in the presence of organic matter, and none of the methods is entirely reliable. Two methods have been used, namely nebulization with hydrogen peroxide (a modification of the method described by Judd *et al.*, 1968) and the use of formaldehyde vapour. The hydrogen peroxide method is quick, and the peroxide readily breaks down and is not toxic to patients or staff. If the ventilator is visibly contaminated, it must be stripped down and cleaned prior to disinfection. An alternative method of disinfection is by the use of formaldehyde (Benn *et al.*, 1973). This method can only be used on machines with closed circuits, and great care is needed to remove residual formaldehyde and protect SSD staff from exposure to the irritant vapour. Formaldehyde cabinets are also effective provided that the ventilator is kept running during the cycle (Babb *et al.*, 1982). If the patient is known or suspected to be suffering from pulmonary tuber-culosis, and the ventilator is not protected by filters, the use of the formaldehyde method is advisable. Nebulized hydrogen peroxide may be used on machines with single circuits, although these may often be dismantled more easily, washed and disinfected by heat. Small machines, (e.g. infant ventilators) may sometimes be sterilized using ethylene oxide. If gaseous methods are used, care should be taken to ensure that all toxic residues are removed by flushing with air or oxygen before the ventilator is reused.

The preferred method of patient humidification is either with a water bath or a heat-moisture exchanger. Less condensation is produced in the tubing with the latter method, thereby reducing the risk of contamination with Gram-negative bacilli. The ventilator external circuitry and humidifier (if used) can be cleaned and thermally disinfected using a washing-machine or disinfected with low-temperature steam. Some circuits are autoclavable, although this may reduce the life of the equipment. If water humidification is used, it is recommended that the circuits are changed every 48 hours in adult patients (Craven *et al.*, 1982), and between patients or weekly in neonatal units. Although filters are hydrophobic, moisture traps may be incorporated to protect the filter. If heat-moisture exchangers are used, circuits may be changed between patients or weekly (Cadwallader *et al.*, 1990).

Humidifiers

Humidifiers in which water vapour (not an aerosol) is blown towards the patient are not a serious infection hazard. They should be changed, together with the ventilator circuit, every 48 hours. The condensate may contaminate the hands of staff and humidifiers should be cleaned and disinfected, preferably by heat, before refilling with sterile water. Alcohol (70%) may be used to disinfect evaporator-type humidifiers in infant incubators. Antiseptics such as chlorhexidine added to the water are unlikely to be effective, and may select resistant organisms.

Contaminated nebulizers, which produce an aerosol, may be responsible for lung infections caused by Gram-negative bacilli, especially *Pseudomonas aeruginosa*. Their use should be avoided unless they can be disinfected by heat daily. Water should be replaced and not topped up. If the nebulizing part of the machine is liable to damage by heat, it should be flushed through with water and dried. If drying is not possible, it should be rinsed in 70% alcohol and allowed to dry.

Oxygen tents
These should be washed and dried after each patient. Oxygen masks and tubing should be disposable. There is no evidence that piped medical gases become contaminated with bacteria, provided that the lines remain dry.

ANAESTHETIC EQUIPMENT

The anaesthetic machines themselves are unlikely to become significantly contaminated during an operation, and routine decontamination is rarely possible or necessary. However, if filters are not used, decontamination may be required after use on a patient with a known or suspected communicable disease (e.g. pulmonary tuberculosis), when formaldehyde gas may be required. In this case, the equipment should be returned to the SSD. The external surfaces of the machine should be kept clean and dry. Contamination is most likely to occur in the face mask and tubing nearest to the patient. This equipment (i.e. tubing, reservoir, ambu-bags, face masks, endotracheal tubes and airways), if not single-use, should be cleaned and thermally disinfected. The Medical Equipment Cleaning Unit of a SSD is most suitable for this. Items should preferably be disinfected in a washer disinfector (> 80°C) or using low-temperature steam (73°C) as frequent autoclaving at 121°C or 134°C may damage the equipment. It is desirable to provide every patient with a decontaminated set of equipment, but this is not usually possible. Sessional or daily treatment of tubing and the reservoir bag is reasonable unless the patient has a respiratory infection or pulmonary tuberculosis is known or suspected (Deverill and Dutt, 1980). However, all patients should have a decontaminated face mask, airway and endotracheal tube. Disposable face masks, tubing and reservoir bags may be preferred on patients with known or suspected infections such as tuberculosis. If not disposable, all items used on such patients should immediately be autoclaved or disinfected using hot water or sub-atmospheric steam.

Laryngoscope blades
Cleaning and drying may be sufficient. If disinfection is required, immersion in 70% alcohol for 10 min should be effective.

Scavenging equipment
The tubing close to the patient should be autoclaved or, if it is heat labile, disinfected using LTS or a washer/disinfector. It should be changed regularly (e.g. weekly) and after use on an infected patient.

Suction equipment

In the absence of piped suction, a separate machine should be available for each patient requiring suction. After use, the contents should be discarded, the bottle washed and dried and fresh connection tubing attached. Bacterial multiplication may occur in the aspirate if it is allowed to stand for long periods. This can be emptied in the sluice and the bottle washed in detergent solution and dried. Alternatively, a washer disinfector may be used. The bottle should be emptied at least daily irrespective of the amount of fluid aspirated. Non-sterile gloves should be worn and the hands must be washed after handling bottle contents. A fresh catheter should be used each time a patient undergoes suction (e.g. bronchial aspiration). An anti-foaming agent may be used to prevent excessive foaming of the bottle contents (which may wet the filter and enter the pump mechanism). The filter should be changed if it becomes moist or discoloured. The use of a detergent or disinfectant in the bottle may be responsible for excessive foaming. Some disinfectants are ineffective and may be toxic to the patient. Disinfectants are therefore avoided during suction, but if the contents are considered to be hazardous to the staff, or the suction equipment is used to irrigate instruments, sufficient disinfectant (e.g. a chlorine-releasing agent) to give a final concentration suitable for a 'dirty' situation may be drawn through the tubing and added to the bottle and left for at least 10 min. The tubing should then be flushed and the bottle washed and dried before re-use. The machine should periodically be returned to the SSD, where the pump can be checked, the filter changed and the tubing, lid, non-return valve and bottle autoclaved or processed in a washer/disinfector. If a patient requires suction for more than 24 hours, the bottle and tubing should be changed. When the machine is not in use, the bottle should be kept dry and the catheter should not be connected until it is required. Disposable suction bottles are now available, but they are expensive. The container itself is disposable, or a disposable liner is fitted within a container. If these are in use, the waste-disposal policy should take into account the difficulties of transport and incineration (i.e. bursting of the canisters or bags).

Infant incubators

It is preferable for these to be cleaned in the SSD. After discharge of a patient, the inner surface of the incubator should be thoroughly cleaned with a moist paper wipe and detergent and dried. Special attention should be paid to the humidifier, ports and the mattress. As cleaning and drying are usually effective, disinfection is rarely necessary, and it may fail without preliminary cleaning. However, if disinfection is required, the cleaned surface can be wiped with a freshly prepared chlorine-releasing solution (e.g. 125 ppm available chlorine), rinsed and dried. Alternatively, surfaces can be wiped with 70% alcohol. However, care should be taken as alcohol is flammable, and the incubator must be aired thoroughly before reuse.

Formaldehyde cabinets are occasionally used, but these are expensive and involve the use of a hazardous chemical. As prior cleaning of the incubator is still necessary, the routine use of a cabinet is of rather doubtful value (Babb *et al.*, 1982).

Vaginal and other specula and rigid sigmoidoscopes

Single-use instruments may be preferred. If not, the instrument should be thoroughly cleaned and autoclaved. Small bench-top autoclaves are now available and are appropriate for use in clinics (Medical Devices Agency, 1996b, 1998). Boiling water (for 5–10 min) is effective, but care is necessary to ensure that items are thoroughly cleaned and completely immersed, and that the instrument is exposed to boiling water for the required time (i.e. at least 5 min). The boiling-water bath should preferably have a timing mechanism. The use of chemical disinfectants should be avoided if possible, especially for vaginal specula (Royal College of Obstetricians and Gynaecologists, 1997), but immersion in 70% alcohol for 10 min should disinfect adequately. Immersion in 2% glutaraldehyde for 10 min is also effective, including activity against *Clostridium difficile* (Dyas and Das, 1985), but it is irritant and sensitizing, so its use should be avoided in clinics unless suitably contained, exhaust-vented processing equipment is available.

Tonometers

These should initially be rinsed and immersed in a disinfectant solution for at least 5 min. The use of chlorine-releasing agents for 10 min (500 ppm available chlorine) or 3–6% stabilized hydrogen peroxide is recommended by the Centers for Disease Control. Tonometers should be rinsed thoroughly and dried before reuse. Hydrogen peroxide in particular is irritant to the conjunctiva, and thorough rinsing or neutralization is important. Wiping with 70% ethanol is probably effective, although the exposure time is short and alcohol can damage the conjunctiva if it is still present on the instrument when it is used. Immersion in 70% alcohol for 5–10 min should be effective, but care is needed to ensure that this does not damage the instrument, and that the alcohol has completely evaporated before use.

DECONTAMINATION OF EQUIPMENT USED ON PATIENTS WITH CREUTZFELDT–JACOB DISEASE (CJD)

The agent that causes this disease is currently referred to as a prion, and is a self-replicating protein without detectable RNA or DNA. It has not been grown in tissue culture, and is extremely resistant to most sterilization and disinfection procedures. CJD is just one of several rare transmissible degenerative diseases of humans and animals with a long incubation period (10–20 years in humans) and is characterized by progressive dementia. Transmission has occurred from contaminated human pituitary growth hormone, corneal transplants and surgical instruments. It is also likely that transmission of variant CJD (VCJD) to humans has occurred from cows with BSE.

The main risk of spread is from the central nervous system (i.e. brain and spinal cord), although care in handling blood is also advised. The Advisory Committees on Dangerous Pathogens (ACDP) and Spongiform Encephalopathies (SEAC) have jointly prepared guidelines (Advisory Committees on Dangerous Pathogens and Spongiform Encephalopathies, 1998) on safe working practices and the prevention of infection with transmissible spongiform encephalopathy agents (see also NHS Executive, 1999). These unconventional agents are extremely resistant

to physical and chemical agents (Taylor, 1992). They are not significantly susceptible to the disinfectants normally used to disinfect instruments, environmental
surfaces and the skin. They are also resistant to gaseous sterilants (e.g. ethylene
oxide, formaldehyde), ionizing radiation, UV light, microwaves and conventional
steam-sterilization cycles (i.e. 121°C for 15 min and 134°C for 3 min). The advice
given by the Medical Devices Agency (via the Department of Health), ACDP and
SEAC is that instruments used on patients with known or suspected CJD or related
disorders and at-risk patients (i.e. those who are asymptomatic, but have a clinical
or family history which places them in one of the risk groups), and which have
been exposed to brain, spinal cord and eye tissue, must be destroyed by incineration. Instruments used on at-risk patients where there has been no involvement of
brain, spinal cord or eye tissue should be thoroughly cleaned, preferably using a
validated automated system, and sterilized or disinfected using an appropriate
physical or chemical process. The few processes that are currently identified as
suitable are porous-load steam sterilization at 134–137°C for a single cycle of 18
min, immersion in sodium hypochlorite (20 000 ppm available chlorine for 1
hour, immersion in 2 M sodium hydroxide for 1 hour and, for histological specimens, immersion in 96% formic acid for 1 hour. These chemical agents, at the
concentrations and contact times described here, are likely to damage most instruments. Wherever practicable, the use of single-use instruments is advised. If the use
of expensive reusable items is unavoidable, it is essential to confirm the process
compatibility of the device with the manufacturers, and to clean the item
thoroughly first.

CLEANING AND DISINFECTION OF SKIN AND MUCOUS MEMBRANES

PRINCIPLES

There are three principal reasons for removing or reducing the number of micro-
organisms present on the skin or mucous membranes:
1 to reduce the number of micro-organisms present prior to an invasive
   procedure;
2 to remove or destroy potentially pathogenic micro-organisms present on the
   hands of staff;
3 to treat a carrier or disperser of a resistant, virulent or highly communicable
   strain of bacteria.

The bacteria present in healthy skin have been classified for practical purposes as
follows:
1 resident organisms that colonize the skin;
2 transient organisms that are deposited on the skin, but do not usually
   multiply there.

The resident organisms consist mainly of coagulase-negative staphylococci, diphtheroids and occasionally *Staphylococcus aureus*. Gram-negative bacilli (e.g.

Klebsiella) are usually transients, but may be temporary residents for periods ranging from several days to many weeks. *Acinetobacter calcoaceticus* var. *anitratum* has many of the survival properties of staphylococci, and may be considered a true resident.

Most of the transient bacteria can be removed by a wash with soap and water, which may be almost as effective as disinfection. However, the resident bacteria are mostly left on the skin after washing with soap and water, but these can be reduced by disinfection. Some naturally acquired bacteria that do not multiply on the skin (e.g. *Clostridium perfringens* present through faecal contamination) may be difficult to remove by washing with soap and water.

Large numbers of bacteria are found as residents of the mucous membrane in the mouth, nose and vagina, but different organisms predominate in different sites. Antiseptics which are non-irritant or damaging to the tissues have a limited although potentially useful effect in reducing these micro-organisms. The urethra normally has few commensal bacteria, but is liable to become contaminated on passage of catheters or other instruments. Disinfection of the urethra before instrumentation is one of the important features of prophylaxis against infection of the urinary tract (see Chapter 7). The conjunctiva also has few bacteria, but these may include *Staphylococcus aureus*.

CLEANING AND DISINFECTION OF HANDS

Social handwashing is the washing of hands with non-medicated soap or detergent and water. Hygienic hand disinfection entails the killing of transient organisms, and may be associated with removal of organisms if an antiseptic detergent is used. Surgical hand disinfection involves the killing of transient organisms and a substantial number of superficial resident organisms, and may also be associated with removal of organisms if an antiseptic detergent is used (Newsom, 1998).

There is some confusion with regard to these definitions, and many European workers do not accept removal as part of the disinfection process. This means that only alcoholic preparations can be accepted as hand disinfectants (Rotter, 1984, 1996). It would seem reasonable to include the processes of both removal and killing in the definitions, as antiseptic detergents are commonly used for disinfection of the hands in many countries, including the UK and USA.

Washing with soap (or detergent) and water removes dirt and dead skin squames and the bacteria present on them. Non-medicated bar soap is usually adequate, provided that it is not kept in a dish of fluid. Liquid soap or detergent may be preferred, provided that dispensers are regularly cleaned and maintained. Washing without a disinfectant is sufficient for most ward procedures (see Chapter 7). Washing with an antiseptic-detergent preparation is usually more effective in reducing transients than washing with non-medicated soap, but the differences are often marginal. The agents commonly used are 4% chlorhexidine detergent (e.g. 'Hibiscrub', 'Hydrex') or 7.5% povidone-iodine (e.g. 'Betadine', 'Videne'). Triclosan preparations (e.g. 'Aquasept') are also used, and are increasingly popular with staff, but they tend to be less effective.

Repeated applications of these agents, particularly chlorhexidine, show a residual effect against transient organisms, but it remains uncertain whether this effect alone would influence the transmission of infection.

A single application of 60–70% ethanol or isopropanol with an emollient (e.g. 1% glycerol) and with or without an antiseptic (e.g. chlorhexidine, povidone-iodine, triclosan) is significantly more effective against transients than a soap-and-water wash (Ayliffe *et al.*, 1988; Rotter, 1996). A volume of 3 ml is poured on to cupped hands and rubbed to dryness. It is important that the formulation used is popular with staff and that all areas of the hands are covered with the agent, as certain areas (e.g. the tips of the fingers and thumbs) are easily missed (Taylor, 1978).

The following standard procedure is recommended (Ayliffe *et al.*, 1978). The hands are rubbed, with five strokes for each movement, backwards and forwards, palm to palm, right palm over left dorsum, left palm over right dorsum, palm to palm with the fingers interlaced, backs of fingers to opposing palm with the fingers interlaced, rotational rubbing of right thumb clasped in left palm and left thumb in right palm, rotational rubbing with clasped fingers of the right hand in the palm of the left hand, and the left hand in the palm of the right hand, complete hands and wrists (see Figure 6.1).

If the hands are visibly soiled, a preliminary wash with soap or detergent and water is required before application of an alcoholic solution. The same technique may be used for a surgical scrub, but the application should be extended to cover the forearms.

Alcoholic solutions may not be effective against some viruses (e.g. enteroviruses), due to the relatively short exposure time of the agent on the hands, and washing with soap and water prior to the use of alcohol is therefore preferable if contamination with these agents is likely (Davies *et al.*, 1993). However, 70% alcohol is effective against rotaviruses on the hands (Bellamy *et al.*, 1993).

The same antiseptic-detergent or soap preparations (e.g. chlorhexidine and povidone-iodine) are commonly used for surgical hand disinfection as for hygienic hand disinfection (Lowbury and Lilly, 1973; Babb *et al.*, 1991). The main difference in the procedure is the longer application time (2 min instead of 10–30 s for hygienic disinfection). Triclosan or hexachlorophane preparations are less frequently used, but are still useful if hypersensitivity to other agents develops. Repeated applications of all of these agents reduce the superficial residents to low levels.

The antiseptic detergent should be thoroughly applied to the hands and wrists for 2 min and then rinsed off. A brush may be used for the first application of the day, but continual use is inadvisable, as damage to the skin increases the risk of colonization with *Staphylococcus aureus* or with an increase in the number of residents.

An alternative and more effective method is the application of an alcoholic solution with or without an antiseptic (Lowbury *et al.*, 1974).

Two 5 mL amounts are applied, allowing the first to dry before applying the second, to the hands, wrists and forearms using the standardized technique described above and rubbed to dryness. A single application as indicated for hygienic hand disinfection (3 mL applied for 30 s) may be adequate for invasive

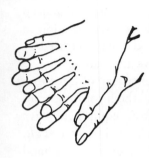

1. Palm to palm

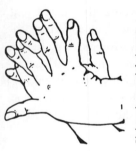

2. Right palm over left dorsum and left palm over right dorsum

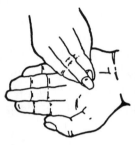

3. Palm to palm fingers interlaced

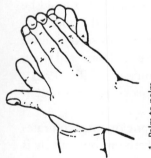

4. Backs of fingers to opposing palms with fingers interlaced

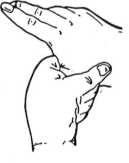

5. Rotational rubbing of right thumb clasped in left palm and vice versa

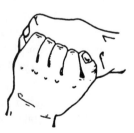

6. Rotational rubbing, backwards and forwards with clasped fingers of right hand in left palm and vice versa. Wrists are similarly rubbed.

Figure 6.1 Handwashing technique (Ayliffe *et al.*, 1978). The hands are moistened and 3–5 mL of soap or detergent are applied to cupped hands. The hands are then rubbed together as shown. This technique, which normally takes 15–30 seconds, is suitable for handwashing and disinfection in all clinical areas and for surgical scrubs, provided that in the latter case the forearms are included. Additional aliquots of soap or detergent may be necessary for the more prolonged surgical scrub (2 min). The wrists are similarly rubbed. The same technique is used for alcohol hand rubs, but no water is used and the hands are rubbed together until dry.

procedures where the resident flora of the hands is a less frequent cause of infection. Alcohol is also useful for the rapid disinfection of clean hands of surgeons following glove puncture during an operation. Alcohol without an added antiseptic surprisingly shows a persistent effect for several hours if gloves are worn. This is probably due to the delayed death of skin bacteria that are damaged but not immediately killed by alcohol (Lilly *et al.*, 1979). Where sensitization to commonly used aqueous formulations is a problem, soap and water followed by the application of an alcohol hand rub is a useful and effective alternative.

The hands are considered to be one of the main routes of spread of infection. Effective handwashing or disinfection is therefore probably the most important infection-control measure. Studies using electronic counting equipment have found handwashing frequency to be much lower than that claimed (Ayliffe *et al.*, 1988). To improve compliance it is essential that the soaps, detergents and hand rubs used in clinical areas are acceptable to staff, or else they will not be used. A thorough wash at the right time with a cosmetically acceptable formulation is more important than the agent used. Dedicated wash-basins and soft paper towels should be readily available. Alcoholic hand rubs are ideal for disinfecting clean hands where wash-basins are unavailable or inconveniently placed (e.g. during ward rounds or in the community). Guidance should be given by the infection control team on when to wash or disinfect the hands (e.g. before aseptic or invasive procedures or preparing food, and after contact with secretions and excretions, going to the lavatory, cleaning duties or bedmaking) (Infection Control Nurses Association, 1988). Gloves should be worn when handling heavily contaminated materials, and the hands should be washed on removal of the gloves.

CLEANING AND DISINFECTION OF OPERATION SITE

A rapid reduction of the skin flora is required in pre-operative preparation of operation sites. For this purpose, a quick-acting antiseptic is desirable. Alcoholic solutions containing chlorhexidine, povidone-iodine or triclosan are preferable to aqueous solutions for intact skin (Davies *et al.*, 1978). The antiseptic should be applied with friction, on a sterile gauze swab, over and well beyond the operation site for 3–4 min. If a gloved hand is used to apply the antiseptic, a second glove should be worn by the surgeon over his or her operating glove, and removed when the preparation of the operation site is complete (Lowbury and Lilly, 1975). Alcoholic solutions must be allowed to dry. This is especially important if diathermy is to be used.

The effect of repeated washing or bathing with an antiseptic on infection rates remains controversial (see Chapter 11). A single antiseptic bath pre-operatively is unlikely to reduce the risk of infection. Repeated washing and bathing with chlorhexidine-detergent does reduce the level of the resident flora on the skin, and could be of value in cardiovascular or prosthetic surgery. However, a single application of alcoholic chlorhexidine rubbed on until the skin is dry, as described above, will reduce the number of resident bacteria to levels approaching the low equilibrium obtained on repeated applications of chlorhexidine detergent.

Before operations on hands with ingrained dirt (e.g. in gardeners) or on the legs of patients with a poor arterial supply (e.g. amputations for diabetic gangrene of the foot), the application of a compress soaked in povidone-iodine solution to the operation site for 30 min will greatly reduce the numbers of spores of gas-gangrene bacilli that present a special hazard in such patients. Ordinary methods of disinfection are ineffective against bacterial spores. However, some spores may remain and antibiotic prophylaxis is still required. Washing with detergents and grease-solvent jellies (e.g. 'Swarfega', 'Dirty Paws') helps to remove ingrained dirt and the dead skin scales on which organisms are carried.

CLEANING AND DISINFECTION OF MUCOUS MEMBRANES

Repeated applications (three or four times a day) of a cream containing 0.5% neomycin and 0.1% chlorhexidine ('Naseptin') to the inside of the nostrils has been shown to remove *Staphylococcus aureus* from a fairly large proportion of nasal carriers. Possible alternatives include neomycin-bacitracin ointment or 1% chlorhexidine cream (Williams *et al.*, 1967). Mupirocin cream ('Bactroban') is more rapidly effective and more likely to eliminate the staphylococci than other preparations, and is particularly useful for treating carriers of methicillin-resistant *Staphylococcus aureus* (MRSA) (see Chapter 9).

Resistance to mupirocin has been described, and its widespread use should be avoided as it is the only useful agent for treating carriers of MRSA. *Streptococcus pyogenes* can usually be cleared from the throat by a course of penicillin (injected or given by mouth, but not by local application). Erythromycin is effective and should be used in patients who are sensitive to penicillin.

Applications of aqueous solutions of chlorhexidine or povidone-iodine are effective for disinfection of oral mucous membranes, but some dental surgeons consider disinfection to be of doubtful value. Treatment of the vaginal mucosa with obstetric creams containing chlorhexidine or chloroxylenol is considered to have little disinfectant action. An application of a povidone-iodine solution reduces the number of organisms, but the effect on clinical infection is uncertain.

APPENDIX 6.1 SUMMARY OF METHODS FOR DECONTAMINATION OF EQUIPMENT OR ENVIRONMENT

Heat	Autoclave if materials are not likely to be damaged by high temperatures, otherwise use washer disinfectors or low-temperature steam
Chemical disinfection	(a) Chlorine-releasing agents
	(b) Clear soluble phenolics at concentrations recommended for light contamination, unless otherwise specified
	(c) 2% glutaraldehyde
	(d) alcohol (use either 60–70% ethyl or isopropyl alcohol)

Equipment or site	Routine or preferred method	Acceptable alternative or additional recommendations
Airways and endotracheal tubes	1 Heat sterilize 2 Heat disinfect	3 Chemical disinfection (a). For patients with tuberculosis use disposables or heat
Ampoules	Wipe neck with (d)	Do not immerse

Baths and hoists	Non-infected patients
	Wipe with detergent solution or cream cleaner and rinse
		Infected patients and patients with open wounds
		Chemical disinfection (a):
		    chlorine-releasing detergent solution
		    non-abrasive chlorine-releasing powder or granules

Bedding	See section on laundering
	Heat disinfection:
	    65°C for 10 min
	    71°C for 3 min
		Heat-sensitive fabrics, low-temperature wash and chemical disinfection (a)

Bed frames	Wash with detergent and dry or (b)	After infected patient/spillage disinfectant (a)
Bedpans	Washer disinfector or use disposables Wash carriers for disposable pans if soiled	Patients with enteric infections: if washer disinfector or disposables are not possible, chemical disinfection (a) or (b) 1–2%. Individual pan for infected patient
Bowls (surgical)	Autoclave	

Bowls (washing)	Wash and dry	For infected patients use individual bowls and disinfect on discharge
		    heat disinfection
		    chemical disinfection (a) or (b)

Carpets	Vacuum daily; clean periodically by hot-water extraction	For known contaminated spillage, cleaning, chemical disinfection with suitable agent if available, then rinse and dry
Crockery and cutlery	1 Machine wash, heat disinfect and dry 2 Hand wash by approved method	For patients with enteric infections or open pulmonary tuberculosis, heat disinfect if possible, or use disposables
Duvets	Heat disinfect or wash with detergent solution and dry	Heat disinfect or disinfect (a) if contaminated, do not soak or disinfect unnecessarily, as this may damage the fabric
Endoscopes	1 Clean and heat disinfect or sterilize 2 If heat sensitive, clean and disinfect with (c)	See p. 108 for alternatives to (c)
Feeds, bottles and teats	1 Pre-sterilized or heat-disinfected feeds	2 Use teats and bottles sterilized and packed by SSD 3 Disinfectant (a) should only be used in small units where other methods are unavailable
Floors (dry cleaning)	1 Vacuum clean 2 Dust-attracting dry mop	Do not use broom in patient areas
Floors (wet cleaning)	Wash with detergent solution Disinfection not usually required	Known contaminated spillage and terminal disinfection, chemical disinfection (a) or (b)
Furniture and fittings	Damp dust with detergent solution	Known contaminated and special areas, disinfectant (a) and (b)
Infant incubators	Wash with detergent and dry with disposable wipe	Infected patients – after cleaning, wipe with (d) or 125 ppm available chlorine (a)
Instruments	1 Heat 2 If heat sensitive, (a), (c), (d)	Contaminated surgical instruments should be cleaned before sterilization, preferably in a washer disinfector
Locker-tops	See furniture and fittings	

continued overleaf

APPENDIX 6.1 (*continued*)

Equipment or site	Routine or preferred method	Acceptable alternative or additional recommendations
Mattresses	Water impermeable cover, wash with detergent solution and dry	Disinfect (a), if contaminated; do not disinfect unnecessarily as this may damage the mattress
Mops (dry – dust-attracting)	Do not use if overloaded or for more than 2 days without reprocessing or washing	Vacuuming after each use may prolong effective life between processing
Mops (wet)	Rinse after each use, wring and store dry; heat disinfect chlorine) for 30 min, rinse and store dry	If chemical disinfection is required, rinse in water, soak in (a) (1000 ppm available
Nailbrushes	Use only if essential	A sterile or heat decontaminated brush should be used for all clinical procedures
Pillows	Treat as mattresses	
Razors (safety and open)	Disposable or autoclaved	Chemical disinfection (d)
Razors (electric)	Chemical disinfection (d) Immerse head only	
Rooms (terminal cleaning or disinfection)	Non-infected patients: wash surfaces in detergent solution and allow to dry	Infected patients: wash with detergent solution and allow to dry Use (a) or (b) if required Fogging not recommended
Shaving brushes	Do not use for clinical shaving	Autoclave. Use brushless cream or shaving foam
Sputum container	Use disposable only	Non-disposable – should be emptied with care and heat-disinfected or sterilized
Suction equipment	1 Clean and dry 2 Heat disinfection or sterilization	If chemical disinfection is required, clean and soak in (a)
Thermometers	1 Individual thermometers: wipe with (d), store dry, terminally disinfect as 2, or use disposable electronic probe	2 Collect after round, wipe clean and disinfect with (d) for 10 min and store dry

Thermometers (electronic clinical)	1 Use disposable sleeve 2 Wipe probe with (d) 3 Disposable	Do not use without sleeve for oral or rectal temperatures
Toilet seats	Wash with detergent and dry	After use by infected patient or if grossly contaminated, chemical disinfection (a) or (b), rinse and dry
Tooth mugs	1 Disposable	2 If non-disposable, heat disinfection

Toys	Clean first but do not soak soft toys. If contaminated disinfect:
	   heat
	   chemical; wipe surface with (d)
	   or (a)
		Expensive or treasured toys may withstand low-temperature steam or ethylene oxide; the latter needs a long aeration period. Heavily contaminated soft toys may have to be destroyed

Trolley-tops	1 Clean with detergent and wipe dry	2 Clean first, then chemical disinfection (d) or (a) and wipe dry

Tubing (anaesthetic or ventilator)	Heat disinfection:
	   washer disinfector or
	   low temperature steam
		Disposable tubing

Urinals	1 Use washer disinfector or use disposables	2 Chemical disinfection (a) or (b)
Ventilator (mechanical)	Heat disinfection or disposable circuit Protect machine with filters	If machine is unprotected by filters, disinfect with hydrogen peroxide or formaldehyde (for tuberculosis)
Wash-basins	Clean with detergent. Use cream cleaner for stains, scum, etc. Disinfection not normally required	Disinfection may be required if contaminated. Use non-abrasive agent (a)
X-ray equipment	Damp dust with detergent solution; switch off, do not over-wet, allow to dry before use	Wipe clean and disinfect with (d)

APPENDIX 6.2 DECONTAMINATION OF EQUIPMENT

HEAT

Method	Temperature (°C)	Holding time (min)	Level of decontamination
Autoclave	134	3	Sterilization
	121	15	Sterilization
Sub-atmospheric steam (LTS)	73–80	10	Disinfection
Boilers and pasteurizers	65–100	5–10	Disinfection
Washing-machines			
Bedpans	80	1	Cleaning/disinfection
Linen	65	10	Cleaning/disinfection
	71	3	
Others	71–100	Variable	Cleaning/disinfection

CHEMICAL

Method and equipment	Holding time at room temperature (min)	Level of decontamination
2% glutaraldehyde[a]		
Gastroscopes	10	Disinfection
Bronchoscopes	20	Disinfection[b]
	60	Disinfection (known or suspected atypical mycobacterial infection, e.g. MAI)
Cystoscopes	10	Disinfection
Arthroscopes	10–20	Disinfection[b]
Laparoscopes	10–20	Disinfection[b]
70% Alcohol		
Instruments (not endoscopes)	10	Disinfection

[a] Alternatives include peracetic acid, chlorine dioxide and superoxidized water.

[b] High level to include *M. tuberculosis* (20 min).

REFERENCES

Advisory Committees on Dangerous Pathogens and Spongiform Encephalopathies (1998) *Transmissible encephalopathy agents: safe working and the prevention of infection*. London: HMSO.

Ayliffe, G.A.J. (1999) Nosocomial infections associated with endoscopy. In Mayhall C.G. *Hospital Epidemiology and Infection Control*, 2nd edn. Baltimore, MD: Williams and Williams.

Ayliffe, G.A.J., Collins, B.J. and Lowbury, E.J.L. (1966) Cleaning and disinfection of hospital floors. *British Medical Journal* ii, 442.

Ayliffe, G.A.J., Collins, B.J. and Lowbury, E.J.L. (1967) Ward floors and other surfaces as reservoirs of hospital infection. *Journal of Hygiene* (London), 2, 181.

Ayliffe, G.A.J., Babb, J.R. and Collins, B.J. (1974) Carpets in hospital wards. *Health and Social Services Journal* 84, 12.

Ayliffe, G.A.J., Babb, J.R. and Quoraishi, A.H. (1978) A test for hygienic hand disinfection. *Journal of Clinical Pathology* 31, 923.

Ayliffe, G.A.J., Babb, J.R., Davies, J.G. and Lilly, H.A. (1988) Hand disinfection: a comparison of various agents in laboratory and ward studies. *Journal of Hospital Infection* 11, 226.

Ayliffe, G.A.J., Babb, J.R. and Bradley, C.R. (1992) Sterilization of arthroscopes and laparoscopes. *Journal of Hospital Infection* 24, 265.

Ayliffe, G.A.J., Coates, D. and Hoffman, P.N. (1993) *Chemical disinfection in hospitals*. 2nd edn. London: Public Health Laboratory Service.

Babb, J.R. (1993) Disinfection and sterilization of endoscopes. *Current Opinion in Infectious Diseases* 6, 532.

Babb, J.R. (1996) Application of disinfectants in hospitals and other health care establishments. *Infection Control Journal of Southern Africa* 1, 4.

Babb, J.R. and Bradley, C.R. (1995a) A review of glutaraldehyde alternatives. *British Journal of Theatre Nursing* 5, 22.

Babb, J.R. and Bradley, C.R. (1995b) Endoscope decontamination: where do we go from here? *Journal of Hospital Infection* 30 (**Supplement**), 543.

Babb, J.R., Bradley, C.R. and Ayliffe, G.A.J. (1982) A formaldehyde disinfection unit. *Journal of Hospital Infection* 3, 193.

Babb, J.R., Davies, J.G. and Ayliffe, G.A.J. (1991) A test procedure for evaluating surgical hand disinfection. *Journal of Hospital Infection* 18 (**Supplement B**), 41.

Bellamy, K., Alcock, R., Babb, J.R., Davies, J.G. and Ayliffe, G.A.J. (1993) A test for the assessment of 'hygienic' hand disinfection using rotavirus. *Journal of Hospital Infection* 24, 201.

Benn, R.A.V., Dutton, A.A.C. and Tully, M. (1973) Disinfection of mechanical ventilators: an investigation using formaldehyde in a Cape ventilator. *Anaesthesiology* 27, 265.

Best, M., Sattar, S.A., Springthorpe, V.S. *et al.*, (1990) Efficacies of selected disinfectants against *Mycobacterium tuberculosis*. *Journal of Clinical Microbiology* 28, 10.

Bradley, C.R. and Babb, J.R. (1995) Endoscope decontamination: automated vs manual. *Journal of Hospital Infection* 30 (Supplement), 537.

Bradley, C.R., Babb, J.R. and Ayliffe, G.A.J. (1995) Evaluation of the Steris System 1 peracetic acid endoscope processor. *Journal of Hospital Infection* 29, 143.

British Society of Gastroenterology (1998) Working Party Report. Cleaning and disinfection of equipment for gastrointestinal endoscopy. *Gut* 42, 585.

British Standards Institute (1993) *British Standard BS2745. Washer-disinfectors for medical purposes. Part 1. Specification for general requirements. Part 2. Specification for human waste container washer-disinfectors. Part 3. Specification for washer-disinfectors except those used for processing human waste containers and laundry.* London: British Standards Institute.

British Thoracic Society (1989) Bronchoscopy and infection control. *Lancet* ii, 270.

Cadwallader, H.L., Bradley, C.R. and Ayliffe, G.A.J. (1990) Bacterial contamination and frequency of changing ventilator circuitry. *Journal of Hospital Infection* 15, 65.

Central Sterilizing Club. (1999) Reprocessing of single-use medical devices in hospitals. *Central Service,* 7, 37.

Collins, B.J. (1979) How to have carpeted luxury. *Health and Social Services Journal* 28 September.

Collins, B.J. (1988) The hospital environment: how clean should a hospital be? *Journal of Hospital Infection* 11 (Supplement A), 53.

Cooke, R.P.D., Feneley, R.C.L., Ayliffe, G.A.J. *et al.* (1993) Decontamination of urological equipment: interim report of a Working Group of the Standing Committee on Urological Instruments of the British Association of Urological Surgeons. *British Journal of Urology* 71, 5.

Craven, D.I., Connolly, M.G., Lichtenberg, D.A. *et al.* (1982) Contamination of mechanical ventilators with tubing change every 24 or 48 hours. *New England Journal of Medicine* 306, 1505.

Danforth, D., Nicolle, L.E., Hume, K. *et al.* (1987) Nosocomial infections on nursing units with floors cleaned with a disinfectant compared with detergent. *Journal of Hospital Infection* 10, 229.

Das, I. and Fraise, A.P. (1997) How useful are microbial filters in respiratory apparatus? *Journal of Hospital Infection* 37, 263.

Davies, J.G., Babb, J.G., Ayliffe, G.A.J. (1978) Disinfection of the skin of the abdomen. *British Journal of Surgery* 65, 855.

Davies, J.G., Babb, J.R., Bradley, C.R. and Ayliffe, G.A.J. (1993) Preliminary study of test methods to assess the virucidal activity of skin disinfectants using poliovirus and bacteriophages. *Journal of Hospital Infection* 25, 125.

Department of Health (1991) Hospital mattress assemblies: care and cleaning. *Safety Action Bulletin* 91, 65.

Deverill, C.E.A. and Dutt, K.K. (1980) Methods of decontamination of anaesthetic equipment: daily sessional exchange of circuits. *Journal of Hospital Infection* 1, 165.

Dyas, A. and Das, B.C. (1985) The activity of glutaraldehyde against *Clostridium difficile. Journal of Hospital Infection* 6, 41.

Griffiths, P.A., Babb, J.R. and Fraise, A.P. (1999) Mycobacterial activity of selected disinfectants using a quantitative suspension test. *Journal of Hospital Infection* 41, 111.

Hanson, P.J.V., Gor, D., Jeffries, D.J. *et al.*, (1989) Chemical inactivation of HIV on surfaces. *British Medical Journal* 298, 862.

Hanson, P.J.V., Gor, D., Jeffries, D.J. and Collins, J.V. (1990) Elimination of high-titre HIV from fibre-optic endoscopes. *Gut* 31, 657.

Infection Control Nurses Association (1998) *Guidelines for hand hygiene.* London: Infection Control Nurses Association.

Judd, P.A., Tomlin, P.J., Whitby, J.L. *et al.* (1968) Disinfection of ventilators by ultrasonic nebulisation. *Lancet* 2, 1019.

Lilly, H.A., Lowbury, E.J.L., Wilkins, M.D. *et al.* (1979) Delayed antimicrobial effects of skin disinfection by alcohol. *Journal of Hygiene* 82, 497.

Lilly, H.A., Kidson, A. and Fujita, K. (1982) Investigation of hospital infection from a damaged mattress. *Burns* 8, 408.

Lowbury, E.J.L. and Lilly, H.A. (1973) Use of 4% chlorhexidine detergent solution (Hibiscrub) and other methods of skin disinfection. *British Medical Journal* 1, 510.

Lowbury, E.J.L. and Lilly, H.A. (1975) Gloved hands as applicator of antiseptic to operation sites. *Lancet* ii, 153.

Lowbury, E.J.L., Lilly, H.A. and Ayliffe, G.A.J. (1974) Preoperative disinfection of surgeons' hands: use of alcoholic solutions and effects of gloves on skin flora. *British Medical Journal* iv, 369.

Maki, D.G., Alvarado, C.J., Hassemer, C.A. *et al.* (1982) Relation of the inanimate environment to endemic nosocomial infections. *New England Journal of Medicine* 307, 1562.

Maurer, I.M. (1985) *Hospital hygiene*, 3rd edn. Bristol: Wright PSG.

Medical Devices Agency (1995) *Device bulletin. The reuse of medical devices supplied for single use only. MDA DB 9501.* London: Medical Devices Agency.

Medical Devices Agency (1996a) *Device bulletin. Decontamination of endoscopes. MDA DB 9607.* London: Medical Devices Agency.

Medical Devices Agency (1996b) *Device bulletin: The purchase, operation and maintenance of benchtop steam sterilizers. MDA DB 9605.* London: Medical Devices Agency.

Medical Devices Agency (1998) *Device bulletin: The validation and periodic testing of benchtop vacuum steam sterilizers. MDA DB 9804.* London: Medical Devices Agency.

Microbiology Advisory Committee to Department of Health Medical Devices Agency (1996) *Guidance on decontamination. Part 1. Principles. Part 2. Protocols. Part 3. Procedures* (in preparation). London: Medical Devices Agency.

Murray, S.M., Freiman, J.S., Vickery, K. *et al.* (1991) Duck hepatitis B virus: a model to assess efficacy of disinfectants against hepadnavirus infectivity. *Epidemiology and Infection* 106, 435.

Newsom, S.W.B. (1998) Special problems in hospital antisepsis. In Russell A.D., Hugo W.B. and Ayliffe G.A.J. (eds), *Principles and practice of disinfection, preservation and sterilization*, 3rd edn. Oxford: Blackwell Science. 416.

NHS Estates (1997) *Health Technical Memorandum HTM 2030. Washer disinfectors. Operational management, design considerations, validation and verification*, London: HMSO.

NHS Executive (1999) *Variant Creutzfeldt-Jacob disease: minimising the risk of transmission. Controls assurance in infection control: decontamination of medical devices.* London: Department of Health.

Rotter, M. (1984) Hygienic hand disinfection. *Infection Control* 5, 18.

Rotter, M. (1996) Hand washing and hand disinfection. *Hospital Epidemiology and Infection Control* 79, 1052.

Royal College of Obstetricians and Gynaecologists (1997) *HIV infection in maternity care and gynaecology.* Working Party Report. London: RCOG Press.

Rutala, W.A. (1990) APIC guidelines for selection and use of disinfectants. *American Journal of Infection Control* 18, 99.

Sattar, S.A., Springthorpe, V.S., Karim, Y. *et al.* (1989) Chemical disinfection of non-porous inanimate surfaces experimentally contaminated with four human pathogenic viruses. *Epidemiology and Infection* 102, 493.

Selkon, J.B., Babb, J.R. and Morris, R. (1999) Evaluation of the antimicrobial activity of a new superoxidised water, Sterilox, for the disinfection of endoscopes. *Journal of Hospital Infection* 41, 59.

Spach, D.H., Silverstein, F.E. and Stamm, W.E. (1993) Transmission of infection by gastrointestinal endoscopy and bronchoscopy. *Annals of Internal Medicine* 118, 117.

Taylor, D.M. (1992) Inactivation of unconventional agents of the transmissible degenerative encephalopathies. In Russell A.D., Hugo W.G. and Ayliffe G.A.J. (eds), *Disinfection, preservation and sterilization,* 3rd edn. Oxford: Blackwell Scientific Publications, 222.

Taylor, L.J. (1978) An evaluation of handwashing techniques. *Nursing Times* 74, 108.

Tyler, R., Ayliffe, G.A.J. and Bradley, C.R. (1990) Virucidal activity of disinfectants: studies with the poliovirus. *Journal of Hospital Infection* 15, 339.

Williams, J. D., Waltho, C. A., Ayliffe, G.A.J. and Lowbury E.J.L. (1967) Trials of five antibacterial creams in the control of nasal carriage of *Staphylococcus aureus. Lancet* 2, 390.

chapter 7

PREVENTION OF INFECTION IN WARDS. I. INCLUDING THE INFECTION CONTROL ELEMENTS OF ROUTINE NURSING CARE AND WOUND MANAGEMENT TECHNIQUES

INTRODUCTION

This chapter and the next deal with the methods by which patients in hospital wards can be protected against micro-organisms from various sources, in particular from other patients, and those transmitted by staff, by contaminated objects (fomites) and by air, with specific reference to the nurse's role together with other health-care workers in the prevention of transmission of micro organisms by the routes outlined in Chapters 1 and 8. Surgical patients are exposed to special hazards of infection during the relatively short period of the operation, and the prevention of these hazards is the subject of Chapter 11. Infection of wounds may also occur in the ward, where the period of exposure of some unhealed wounds may be prolonged. A clean, closed surgical wound is unlikely to become infected after 24 hours following the operation, and the duration of exposure for change of dressing is usually short, but the risk may be greater and more prolonged in some patients, especially those with drained or · open wounds and those with burns. Patients with chronic infected or colonized lesions and other infective conditions will often be nursed in the same ward as patients who are at increased risk of infection because of inadequate host defences. The largest reservoir of infective micro-organisms is among patients, and the most important mode of transfer is by the staff who have contact with them. It is therefore important to ensure that adequate infection control measures and protection are co-ordinated with routine elements of care.

Control of infection in wards, as in operating theatres, involves the application ⸴ of the principles of aseptic and infection control techniques in the numerous details of patient care (Glynn *et al.*, 1997; Ward *et al.*, 1997). It also involves the design, equipment and ventilation of the ward in such a way that patients may, when necessary, be placed in isolation to prevent infection passing either from or to them. Research and experience have shown that good buildings, although important, are less vital to the prevention of infection than good aseptic and infection control procedures, but patient isolation methods involve both structures and procedures. Isolation methods are discussed in Chapter 8. This chapter is concerned with the general principles of aseptic and infection control techniques which apply in all hospital wards. The requirements of special departments and some individual procedures are considered in Chapters 16 and 17. Examples of methods used for performing various aseptic procedures are presented in Appendix 7.1, at the end of this chapter.

NURSING CARE AND MANAGEMENT

The prevention of infection is the responsibility of all staff, but particularly of those responsible for direct patient care. The nurse's role is highlighted in the assessment, planning and implementation or delivery of the patient's care needs and evaluation of the success of the care delivered (commonly referred to as the nursing process). This problem-solving approach to individual patient care lends itself well to the prevention of primary infection and cross infection to others by encouraging assessment of risk of infection throughout the patient's stay, and allows reassessment as the patient's care needs change (Bowell, 1990).

ASSESSMENT

The patient may have a known transmissible infection (e.g. hepatitis B, MRSA, pulmonary tuberculosis) or be at high risk of acquiring an infection as a result of lowered host defences or severe disease process (e.g. leukaemia, high-dose steroid or cytotoxic therapy). This should be identified during the assessment process.

PLANNING

Requirements for preventing the spread of infection from the patient or for protecting the patient against infection should be incorporated in the care plan or patient profile (e.g. requirements for single-room isolation, if necessary).

IMPLEMENTATION

This should ensure that effective infection control methods, (e.g. handwashing, the wearing of protective clothing, etc.) are communicated to all staff and are applied to ensure that the goals can be attained. It should also include the psychological needs of patients, (e.g. patients in single-room isolation or patients with specific fears and concerns regarding transmission of their infection to others).

EVALUATION

The success of the plan and its outcome is assessed. This could be the absence of spread of infection to others, or the prevention of acquired infection in a patient identified as high risk on initial assessment. The possible reasons for any failures should be examined.

This systematic approach to patient care should enable problems to be identified more readily in the individual and effective control measures highlighted.

MODELS OF NURSING CARE

A nursing 'model' is a complete framework of all aspects of the care to be delivered to the individual patient, ensuring that nothing is missed or overlooked.

When using a nursing model, it must be flexible and take into account the disease process and any associated problems if control or prevention of infection is to be achieved in the ward setting. Infection control can be incorporated into all commonly used nursing models (Worsley *et al.*, 1990). Although each individual patient's needs remain paramount to good quality nursing care, the risks to other patients must also be considered. In some instances a compromise may have to be reached to ensure that cross-infection does not occur. For example, balancing the risks of psychological trauma in isolating a patient with a transmissible infection (e.g. MRSA) against the risk of infection spreading to other patients on a surgical ward may be achieved by increased nursing and other input and support to the isolated patient to ensure that all of the patients are protected from the organism.

WARD STRUCTURE AND FACILITIES

Spread of infection (particularly staphylococcal infection) is more likely to occur in large open wards. Wards should therefore be subdivided into units of four to six beds if possible, with complete separation from other areas and with adequate single rooms for isolation of infected patients. Although single rooms for 25% of patients have been recommended, a smaller number is probably sufficient (e.g. four single rooms for a 30-bedded adult ward), depending on whether a hospital isolation unit or ward with single rooms that can be used flexibly for a wide range of infections or conditions is available. To ensure that single rooms can be adapted adequately for isolation, wherever possible they should be equipped with *en-suite* facilities (e.g. shower, toilet and handwashing sink). Patients with communicable infections, including staphylococcal sepsis if caused by an epidemic or highly resistant strain, should be given priority for isolation if single-room accommodation is limited, but an isolation unit with designated experienced staff is preferred (see Chapter 9). To reduce risks of cross-infection further, bed centres should be at least 7 to 8 feet apart and overcrowding with extra beds should be avoided. A day room for ambulant patients will also reduce the number of patients in the clinical area. Toilet facilities should be adequate and provided with hand-washing basins. As patients are now allowed out of bed much earlier than formerly, washing facilities should be correspondingly increased. Separate toilet and handwashing facilities should be available for the staff. Showers should be provided whenever possible, in addition to or preferably instead of baths.

Handwashing basins for the staff should be readily available in the clinical area and supplied with paper towels of good quality. Hot-air hand dryers are slow, often noisy and should be avoided in clinical areas. Staff often do not completely dry their hands with these dryers, which results in sore hands. Sluice rooms should be adequate in size with suitable racking and storage space for bedpans, urinals and cupboards for urine testing and other equipment. Storage areas for domestic cleaning equipment should be provided. Wards should be kept in a good state of repair and provided with intact and readily cleanable surfaces.

ASEPTIC TECHNIQUES

The terms *asepsis* and *aseptic technique* are used to describe methods which have been developed to prevent contamination of wounds or other susceptible sites (e.g. the urinary tract) in the operating-theatre, the ward and other treatment areas, by ensuring that only sterile fluids or uncontaminated objects will make contact with these sites and that the risks of airborne contamination are minimized. When first introduced, the term *asepsis* was used to refer to the provision of heat-sterilized instruments and equipment in the operating-theatre, to supersede *antisepsis* by immersion of instruments in a phenolic solution as used by Lister. Today the word asepsis is not used in contrast with antisepsis, but includes antiseptic methods. Antiseptics are solutions used in skin disinfection (e.g. chlorhexidine, povidone iodine and alcohol). Any procedure which involves penetration of the skin, exposure of wounds or instrumentation (except non-operative endoscopies) should be performed with sterile instruments and materials supplied by an SSD, using a non-touch technique with forceps or gloves. The details of aseptic techniques vary to some extent from one hospital to another, but are similar in principle (Crow, 1989).

MASKS

The principal role of the mask is to protect the patient against organisms dispersed from the upper respiratory tract of the nurse or other attendant. Most of the bacteria that are dispersed during sneezing or talking come from the mouth and are normally harmless to wounds (although occasionally *Streptococcus pyogenes* and *Staphylococcus aureus* may be present in the mouth). *Staphylococcus aureus* is commonly present in the nose, but the nose disperses very few staphylococci directly into the air. *Staphylococcus aureus* is commonly shed into the environment on skin scales, so a mask will do little to reduce dissemination. Experimental studies and trials have indicated that masks contribute little or nothing to the protection of patients in wards against infection, and their routine use for aseptic ward procedures, including post-operative dressings, is therefore unnecessary (Taylor, 1980).

If a mask is thought to be necessary, most of the commercially available types will reduce the risk of impaction of bacteria from the mouth and may be considered satisfactory, but a 'filter'-type mask is preferred for barrier nursing if considered necessary to protect the nurse against respiratory pathogens such as TB (especially MDR strains). The mask should be close-fitting and filter particles larger than 5 μ in diameter.

PROTECTIVE CLOTHING

Clothing may be of some importance in the contact transfer of *Staphylococcus aureus* (Hambraeus, 1973). The front of the apron is the area most often contaminated. It is therefore wise for health-care workers to wear protective clothing while they are performing aseptic procedures, in order to prevent the transfer of bacteria from the uniform to the patients, and also to prevent contamination of their own uniform. It is unnecessary to change the apron between patients following routine procedures, except for procedures on infected patients or aseptic procedures, and in high-risk units (see also Chapter 8 for procedures on infected patients).

Wearing a gown or apron routinely (e.g. in the ITU) is unnecessary unless the staff member is handling the patient or associated items (e.g. charts).

Cotton is permeable to bacteria and moisture, and a water-repellent apron that is impermeable to bacteria is more appropriate. A single-use plastic apron worn during dressing and other aseptic procedures is cheap and convenient. There is little advantage to wearing a gown rather than a plastic apron because the shoulders and upper arms are unlikely to become contaminated in normal circumstances (Babb *et al.*, 1983). However, a gown may be preferred for lifting infected patients or for nursing neonates.

HANDS

The hands of nurses, doctors, physiotherapists and others who handle patients are probably the most important vehicles of cross-infection, and it is essential that effective methods are used to minimize this hazard. Handwashing with a good technique covering all surfaces of the hands at the right time is more important than the agent used or the length of time of handwashing. In tests of handwashing with a dye, it was found that over 50% of the nurses did not wash some part of the thumb, and many also missed areas of the finger tips and palm (Taylor, 1978). These are the areas most likely to come into contact with patients and equipment, and therefore to transfer infection. A standardized technique for handwashing should therefore be used (see Chapter 6; Ayliffe *et al.*, 1978). A satisfactory handwash or alcoholic rub can be completed by this method in 10–20 s. Studies have indicated that handwashing by both nurses and doctors is too infrequent. However, excessive handwashing will damage the skin and increase the likelihood of colonization of the hands with potential pathogens. Hands should be washed:

- on arrival for duty and on leaving the ward;
- after using the toilet and before handling food or medicines;

- after attending infected patients or patients in source isolation, and before attending patients in protective isolation;
- before and after aseptic procedures;
- after handling potentially contaminated materials;
- after removing gloves.

An unpublished study on hand contamination after various procedures showed that, from 1 to 10 in order of risk, procedures 1 to 5 listed below were least likely to be associated with significant hand contamination, whereas procedures 6 to 10 were most likely to be associated with contamination and required a handwash:

1 handling sterile or disinfected materials;
2 handling materials not handled by patients (e.g. charts, etc.);
3 handling items minimally handled by patients (e.g. furniture);
4 handling materials in close contact with bedding of non-infected patients;
5 minimal patient contact (e.g. taking pulse);
6 handling moist objects likely to be contaminated (e.g. cleaning materials);
7 handling bedding from infected patients, bed-bathing of any patient, handling of bedpans and urinals;
8 handling secretions or excretions or body fluids;
9 handling secretions, excretions or body fluids from infected patients;
10 direct contact with infected patients.

It is not possible to lay down absolute rules, and the requirement for handwashing must be assessed in each individual circumstance (e.g. following every contact with a patient colonized with MRSA). Disposable gloves may be used to prevent gross contamination of the hands, and they should also be used for handling highly contaminated objects and contaminated materials (e.g. drainage tubes, endotracheal tubes) or patients who are faecally incontinent. For aseptic procedures, sterile gloves or forceps should preferably be used. Handwashing/disinfection is also more important in high-risk wards and during epidemics.

Gloves are often recommended for the handling of all blood and body fluids ('universal infection control precautions') (see Chapter 8). Organisms are more readily removed from gloves than from hands by washing, but the value of repeatedly washing gloves rather than changing between patients remains controversial (Doebbeling et al., 1988; Newsom and Rowland, 1989) and depends on the purpose. Unless this is carefully carried out, organisms may remain on washed gloves (as on the hands), and gloves may be damaged on repeated washing. Hands should be washed when gloves are removed after handling an infected patient or potentially contaminated objects. However, it should be possible to remove gloves carefully without contaminating the hands. A further problem is that even unused gloves may have small defects and may thus allow penetration of organisms. For this reason, any cuts or lesions on the hands should be covered. It is therefore preferable to remove gloves after any relevant procedures, if supplies are adequate.

In the course of their work, nurses and doctors will touch many objects contaminated with staphylococci and other organisms capable of causing wound infection. They can easily transfer pathogenic organisms which have just been picked up from one infected or colonized patient to the next patient whom they visit in the ward. Such recently acquired contaminants are 'transient' bacteria which are not growing on the skin and which, unlike the 'resident' bacteria, can be greatly reduced in numbers by an effective handwash with soap and water or disinfection with 70% ethanol or isopropanol. Bacteria which remain on the skin may become 'residents'. For most purposes in the ward, a thorough wash with soap and water is adequate. Antimicrobial preparations (see Chapter 6) may be indicated for handwashing in special units such as intensive care, infectious diseases and special care baby units, and in general wards during an outbreak of infection. Some antimicrobial agents (e.g. chlorhexidine) have a persistent effect which may reduce transient organisms, but the value of this effect in prevention of the transfer of infection remains uncertain. More effective hand disinfection can be achieved if, following washing with soap and water, an alcohol handrub (e.g. 70% ethanol or isopropanol) is used (Ayliffe *et al.*, 1988; Rotter 1996). The use of 70% alcohol with an emollient, with or without an additional antimicrobial agent, is of particular value in wards that lack convenient handwashing facilities, or during medical staff rounds or dressing techniques. A suitable routine for a ward would be soap for general handwashing, with an alcoholic preparation available for special procedures (e.g. changing an IV infusion); alcoholic gels are particularly convenient. During an outbreak of a non-enveloped virus infection, washing with soap and water before the application of alcohol is advised as some viruses (e.g. some enteroviruses and other small round viruses) are resistant to isopropanol and relatively resistant to ethanol. Although 90% ethanol is preferred, 70% ethanol is effective against rotaviruses as well as enveloped viruses.

Soap containers used on wards may be a source of contamination (see Chapter 6). Containers for bar soap should be easy to clean and regularly cleaned. Liquid soap dispensers should be regularly cleaned and maintained, and antimicrobial liquid soap preparations should preferably be wall-mounted and operated by elbow, wrist or foot. A replaceable cartridge or equivalent will reduce risks of contamination compared to refilling the original container. Paper towels are advised for drying the hands, and should have good drying properties and be aesthetically acceptable. If hand taps are used, these can be turned off with a paper towel after the hands have been washed.

WOUND DRESSINGS

The place where wounds are dressed will be determined by the structure of the ward and the availability of single rooms, and also whether the hospital has central treatment rooms. If the design of the dressing room is poor and without mechanical ventilation, dressing all wounds in one small room increases the risk of infection by creating a high level of airborne contamination when the wounds are exposed. A single room, preferably with an extractor fan or other form of mechanical ventilation, should be used for source isolation of patients with wounds infected or colonized by multi-resistant strains of *Staphylococcus aureus* (e.g. MRSA) (see Chapter 8). These patients may then have their wounds dressed in their own rooms. Dressings of small wounds may reasonably be changed at the bedside in an open ward, if care is taken to avoid dispersal of bacteria from dressings that are being removed. Such procedures usually cause little increase in airborne contamination by wound pathogens. For large wounds and burns it may be desirable to change dressings in a mechanically ventilated dressing room or operating-theatre, if source isolation of the patient in a mechanically ventilated single room is not possible.

If a wound dressing or treatment room is considered to be necessary, it should be ventilated with 8 or more air changes per hour (a burns dressing station should have 20 air changes per hour). Adequate facilities should be available for laying up equipment and handwashing, and the doors should be large enough for a bed to pass through. At least 10 minutes should be allowed after use by an infected patient, and the cover on the surface of the couch should be intact and cleaned and/or a disposable paper cover should be changed after each patient. The ventilation system should be checked regularly by the engineers (e.g. at least every 3 to 6 months). Even if the room is adequate in all respects, it may be impracticable and time-consuming to move some patients in their beds to a dressing station (e.g. those in traction beds). In addition, where team nursing or patient allocation to individual nurses is practised, one dressing room may be inadequate.

As the cost of a correctly ventilated room is high and the evidence of its value (except for burns) is limited, it would rarely seem to be worthwhile incorporating a plenum-ventilated dressing room either in a new general ward or in an old, open general surgical ward. However, a small treatment room with a limited ventilation system (e.g. extractor fan) may be useful for preparing trolleys and for carrying out minor procedures on ambulatory patients. This system should be adequate if single rooms or an isolation unit are available for patients with wounds infected by organisms likely to be transmitted in the air (e.g. antibiotic-resistant *Staphylococcus aureus*).

Some hospitals have central treatment rooms. A suite of ventilated single rooms is available for dressings, and for aseptic and other procedures usually performed in the ward (e.g. lumbar puncture and laser procedures). It has the advantage of a controlled environment, adequate and appropriate supplies and experienced trained staff, and is available 24 hours a day for wards, out-patients and day cases. It is convenient to work in and removes the problem of not performing aseptic procedures while cleaning or bed-making is in progress. It has the disadvantage of fragmenting care, but patients do not perceive this to be a problem. There is also a potential risk of transfer of infection between wards, but if techniques are sound this should not occur.

DRESSING MATERIALS (Anon., 1991a,b)

The main functions of a dressing are as follows:
- to protect the wound from trauma or bacterial contamination;
- to promote healing;
- to prevent the transfer of organisms from an infected wound to other sites on the same or other patients.

It should absorb excess exudate, but maintain warm and moist conditions at the wound surface to improve healing, and it should allow gaseous exchange. It should be impermeable to bacteria. Gauze swabs are not the most suitable of dressing materials, as they tend to adhere to the wound and become soaked with exudate. The healing process is thus disturbed, and once 'strike through' of exudate has occurred there is no barrier to the passage of micro-organisms either to or from the environment.

Dressing materials vary in their properties and require selection appropriate to the nature of the wound (Leaper, 1995). Factors to be considered in the selection of dressings or topical agents are size of wound, site, depth and the presence of slough or infection. The progress of the wound should be accurately recorded. Clean, undrained surgical wounds seldom require dressing if they can be protected against contact and friction. Semi-permeable adhesive films are useful as they are permeable to water vapour but not to bacteria, and they allow the wound to be observed without the need to remove the dressing. They can be used for clean superficial wounds and are also useful for sealing infected lesions during surgery (e.g. for enclosing a pressure sore during a hip replacement operation). However, these films would not be appropriate on wounds with excessive exudate, although it is possible to aspirate exudate with a syringe and needle. A wide range of other dressing materials is available, including gel and colloid dressings. These are occlusive or semi-occlusive (Hutchinson and Lawrence, 1991), and they adhere to dry skin and form a gel with moisture on the wound surface. The evidence from rigorous controlled trials on the effectiveness of these dressings is limited, and it is difficult to make firm recommendations. These newer products tend to be expensive, but improved healing may reduce the time spent in hospital or off work.

Wounds can be conveniently classified as black (necrotic), yellow (infected or containing slough) or red (granulating).

The dressing required differs according to each of these categories. Hydrocolloid dressings are useful for necrotic, sloughing or granulating wounds, but not usually for infected wounds. They may also prevent infection. Hydrogels can be used on black necrotic or infected wounds and provide good healing conditions. Alginate dressings are used to remove exudate (e.g. in 'yellow' and infected wounds) and assist wound healing. Dextranomers (e.g. as beads) may be appropriate for sloughing wounds or infected wounds with exudate. Foam dressings (e.g. silicone foam) are slightly absorbent, and can be used on deep open granulating wounds.

CLEANING OF WOUNDS AND TOPICAL AGENTS

Clean operation wounds should not require routine cleaning, although the removal of blood or other exudate may reduce the presence of nutrients which may aid bacterial growth. Sterile normal saline is adequate for this purpose. The technique of cleaning is of doubtful relevance, and most methods only redistribute organisms present in the wound and on the adjacent skin.

The use of disinfectants is also of doubtful value, but some (e.g. 'Savlon') are effective cleaning agents for dirty wounds. Hypochlorite solutions (e.g. Eusol) are often used as debriding agents, but are toxic to cells and should preferably not be used at all, or at least only for a short period (Leaper, 1995). Some dressing materials (see previous section) are preferable for removing necrotic materials and slough, and do not impair healing. The disadvantages of hypochlorites also apply (but to a lesser extent) to hydrogen peroxide and iodophors. Chlorhexidine is less toxic to cells and has been shown to reduce the emergence of infection in minor burns. Silver sulphadiazine is commonly used to prevent infections in burns. There is some evidence that the wound exudate has antibacterial properties, and complete removal of all exudate may be undesirable. The role of bacteria in delaying the healing of pressure sores and ulcers is also uncertain, and it is generally unnecessary to apply antibacterial agents, although there is some evidence that healing may be delayed in the presence of large numbers of organisms (i.e. over 10^5/g or cm^2). Systemic antibiotics may be necessary in the presence of clinical sepsis, and the possibility of an anaerobic infection should be considered. Topical antibiotics, particularly those used for systemic treatment (e.g. gentamicin and fusidic acid), should be avoided as resistance is likely to emerge. However, if topical antibiotics are considered to be necessary, treatment should be limited to 5–7 days. Aminoglycosides (e.g. neomycin) may also be associated with hypersensitivity if they are used for long periods. The use of mupirocin should also be restricted, as resistance may emerge, and if it is used the time of application should be restricted as with other agents.

DRESSING TECHNIQUES

These are described in Appendix 7.1. They may require modification in the light of further studies or under special circumstances (Kelso, 1989). Some general principles are considered here. The evidence suggests that the recommended routine ward cleaning methods (see Chapter 6) do not significantly increase the numbers of airborne organisms. Certain other procedures may disperse much larger numbers of organisms into the air. These include bed-making, high dusting and changing curtains. It is often impracticable to stipulate that all of these activities must cease while dressings are in progress, particularly on wards where allocation of patients to individual nurses or team nursing is practised, as is now generally the case. Nevertheless, it is clearly desirable that cleaning activities should be avoided if possible during dressing sessions and, if unavoidable, reduced to a minimum. It is more practicable to ensure that these procedures do not take place in the immediate vicinity of the bed where the dressing is being done. To reduce opportunities for airborne contamination to a minimum, a wound should be exposed for the minimum time and dressings should be removed carefully and quickly placed in a bag and sealed. A large paper or clinical waste plastic bag should be available for disposal of large dressings.

Sterile Services Department (SSD) packs should be supplied in dispenser racks or boxes, stored in a preparation room and transferred to the dressing trolley when required. All instruments should be supplied by the SSD, and chemical disinfection before use should now be unnecessary. The dressing-trolley top should be thoroughly cleaned at the beginning of a dressing round with 70% alcohol, a chlorine-releasing product or a clear soluble phenolic disinfectant. The top of the trolley must be dry before the sterilized paper pack is placed on it. Repeated cleaning of the trolley top during a dressing round is unnecessary.

An aseptic or non-touch technique is important. Forceps are usually used, but disposable gloves (or a plastic bag, enclosing a hand) could with advantage be used more often, particularly for removing large, contaminated dressings. There is evidence to indicate that ungloved hands, if previously disinfected with an alcohol-based hand disinfectant, are more convenient than forceps and do not expose the patient to an increased infection risk (Thomlinson, 1987), but gloves are usually worn to protect the operator. Dispersal of organisms may be further reduced by inverting the glove (or plastic bag) over the dressing and discarding both together.

The dressing pack should be opened carefully with washed hands as instructed. The paper working surface should lie flat on the trolley top and should never be flattened with the fingers. Forceps used for removal of stitches or for inserting safety-pins in drains should be capable of holding the sutures or the pin firmly, otherwise gloved fingers should be used.

If dressings on clean and dry wounds without drainage are thought to be necessary, they should be left in place until the stitches are removed, unless there are signs of infection or leakage. These wounds are unlikely to become infected in the ward and, depending on surgical approval, may be left after the first 24–48 hours without a covering dressing. Drained wounds should be covered with a dressing until the drainage wound is healed and dry. This may not be necessary with very small drains with a closed drainage system (e.g. 'Redivac') until after removal. Drains should not be used unless absolutely necessary, and should be removed as quickly as possible. If required at all, drainage must be adequate. 'Redivac' and other small tube drains are less likely to be associated with acquired infection. Contaminated wounds (e.g. after colectomy, abdominoperineal excision of the rectum, and operations on pelvic abscess), although initially infected with the patient's own sensitive organisms, may acquire antibiotic-resistant hospital strains if care is not taken with aseptic techniques. All discharging wounds should be adequately covered, and dressings must be changed immediately if they are soaked, as micro-organisms readily penetrate wet dressings.

Septic wounds and contaminated wounds (e.g. colostomy) should be dressed at the end of the dressing list. Sutures should be removed at the beginning of the list. The use of absorbable sutures may allow a patient to be sent home earlier. Any procedure which reduces the patients time in hospital either pre- or post-operatively will reduce the hazards of infection.

INJECTIONS

Several studies have shown that the risk of infection is minimal following an injection without prior disinfection of the skin. Skin disinfection is often not recommended for insulin injection in diabetics, and some hospitals have given up the practice except before intravenous injections. Nevertheless, many hospital patients are particularly susceptible to infection, (e.g. elderly patients in whom heavy skin contamination with Gram-negative bacilli or *Staphylococcus aureus* is possible, particularly in the area of the upper thigh). As it is difficult to know which patients are at special risk until adequate trials on hospital patients of all age groups have been carried out, it is recommended that the skin of the injection site should be thoroughly cleaned by rubbing with 70% ethanol or isopropanol, and then allowed to dry. This is relatively inexpensive, and disinfection for some procedures and not others may cause confusion.

INTRAVENOUS INFUSIONS

The setting up of intravenous infusions should be carried out with strict aseptic precautions (Elliott *et al.*, 1994). The hands of the operator should be disinfected with an antiseptic detergent, or preferably with 70% ethanol or 60% isopropanol, for at least 30 s. The skin of the infusion site should also be thoroughly disinfected with 70% ethanol or isopropanol, preferably with added chlorhexidine, povidone-iodine or triclosan, and allowed to dry. The site should not be palpated after disinfection. Shaving of the skin should be avoided if possible. Disposable gloves should be worn by the operator and assistant if contamination of the skin with blood is likely. The wearing of a mask is unnecessary. For central venous catheterization, sterile gloves should be worn in addition to a sterile disposable gown, and the procedure should preferably be carried out in an operating-theatre with full surgical precautions, although another clean area may be adequate (Ward *et al.*, 1997). This is particularly desirable if tunnelling of the catheter under the skin is required.

The infusion container should be inspected for faults, leaks, cloudiness or particulate matter before connecting to the drip set, and if any of these are present it must be discarded. It should be recognized that the fluid can remain clear despite the presence of significant numbers of organisms. The rubber plug or diaphragm must be swabbed with 70% alcohol before the cannula is introduced on the infrequent occasions when a bottle rather than a bag is used. When a bottle is used, a single-use sterile air inlet is inserted. Check that the cotton-wool plug is present in the air inlet, and if it becomes wet at any time the plug should be changed. The insertion site should be covered with a sterile dressing. Either a non-woven or a transparent semi-permeable dressing can be used, which is changed every 3–7 days depending on the state of the dressing or the life of the catheter after dressing (Maki and Ringer, 1987). A semi-permeable dressing is usually preferred, and allows good observation of the site, but it can be associated with an increased growth of micro-organisms on the skin underneath the dressing. For this reason, a highly vapour-permeable membrane should preferably be used, and it should be changed if moisture accumulates under the dressing.

The insertion site must be inspected daily to detect phlebitis or infection. The value of treating the site at the time of a dressing change with an antibacterial agent is uncertain, although colonization of the cannula has been shown to be reduced by the use of a neomycin, bacitracin and polymyxin ointment (Maki and Band, 1981).

Spraying with povidone-iodine or chlorhexidine or applying a chlorhexidine or povidone-iodine solution is sometimes recommended. Ensure that the cannula is not damaged by alcohol if it is used. Reduction of colonization has also been reported with 2% mupirocin applied after skin disinfection and before insertion of the cannula, but selection of resistant organisms could be a problem, and the cannula may be damaged. The intravenous line should be securely anchored. The giving set should be changed at least every 72 hours and immediately after giving blood or lipids. The bags or bottles should be changed at least every 24 hours, and preferably every 12 hours. Peripheral cannulae should be re-sited every 48–72 hours if suitable alternative sites are available.

Peripheral cannulae should be removed when the earliest signs of infection or phlebitis are observed, and the catheter tip should be cultured. The skin around the catheter site should be disinfected with 70% alcohol before removal. Central venous catheters should not be routinely moved in the absence of infection. They should be removed if there are signs of infection, although in some instances they may be left *in situ* if no other suitable site is available, or they may even be replaced in the same site using a guide wire if appropriate antibiotics are given. Blood culture should be taken at another site.

The tip of the catheter should be placed in a sterile container for microbiological culture if considered necessary.

Although infection is usually caused by skin micro-organisms colonizing the outside of the cannula, it can arise from micro-organisms gaining entrance to the system. A closed system should be maintained as carefully as possible. Therapeutic substances should preferably be added to the infusate in the pharmacy in a laminar-flow cabinet or isolator. However, trained medical or nursing staff can often carry out this procedure more conveniently in the ward. Provided that the fluid is used immediately, the risk of infection is small. Most intravenous fluids will not support the growth of organisms that are normally present in the air. The risk of infection is increased by the use of three-way taps and injection ports, but the use of protective caps and cleaning with 70% alcohol before injection will reduce the hazard. Multilumen catheters are sometimes convenient, but the risk of infection may be slightly increased. However, the evidence for this is controversial. There is some evidence that an antiseptic-impregnated cuff or coating of catheter (e.g. with silver or benzalkonium chloride) may reduce the infection rate in central venous catheters, but further studies are needed (Maki *et al.*, 1988). If catheters are coated with an antiseptic, it should include the inside and outside and the whole length of the catheter.

In-line filters reduce the incidence of phlebothrombosis and prevent the access of bacteria. However, studies on the prevention of clinical infection have shown variable results (Spencer, 1990). Their use may be considered for patients who are particularly at risk.

Parenteral hyperalimentation therapy is now commonly used, and should be given through a dedicated line. The risk of infection is particularly high because of the possibility of bacterial or fungal growth in the fluid. Few organisms grow in saline or dextrose-saline, but Gram-negative bacilli, and especially yeasts, are able to grow in some of these solutions.

Prevention of infection depends on scrupulous aseptic techniques both when inserting the cannula and in subsequent daily care. Infection can be minimized if central catheters are inserted by an experienced operator and subsequently managed by a trained IV team. However, the advantages of a team over well-trained ward nurses are uncertain (Abi-Said *et al.*, 1999). The fluid should be used immediately, but if not should be kept at 4°C and should be administered within 24 hours.

URINARY CATHETERS

MANAGEMENT OF INDWELLING CATHETERS

Bacteria enter the bladder either through the lumen of the catheter or between the catheter and the wall of the urethra. The latter is more difficult to prevent (Falkiner, 1993). The likelihood of infection increases with the duration of catheterization, and catheters should be removed as soon as possible, preferably within a few days following urological surgery. Urethral catheterization may be avoided in some patients by suprapubic drainage, condom drainage systems, or by the use of absorbent pads to avoid the necessity for artificial drainage (Stickler and Zimakoff, 1994).

It has been demonstrated that, with closed drainage, infection can be prevented for several days. A continuous unbroken connection is required extending from the urethral catheter to the receptacle. However, even this system does not remain closed, as the bag must be drained at intervals, allowing possible entrance of bacteria. It is suggested that silicone catheters are preferable for long-term catheterization, as they are less irritant. Teflon and polyvinylchloride catheters can be used for intermediate periods (4–6 weeks), but latex catheters are adequate for short-term use (latex sensitivity should be excluded). Drainage bags with a tap are now most frequently used, but great care is needed in handling and emptying them. Most of the so-called 'non-return valves' allow bacteria to ascend into the bag and into the tubing above, particularly if the bag is tipped upside down or accidentally sat on by the patient. The bag should be kept below bladder level, but not on the floor, and drainage should not be obstructed. Bags vary in design, with non-return valves, drip chambers and different type of tap, etc., but design improvements may considerably increase the cost without necessarily reducing infection. The addition of a disinfectant to the bag remains of uncertain value, and cannot be recommended on the basis of the available evidence. An experimental study has shown that organisms deposited on the outside of the tap can reach the patient end of the catheter within several days (Bradley *et al.*, 1986). Hands should be washed prior to emptying a bag. When emptying the bag, the nurse's hands are often heavily contaminated with Gram-negative bacilli (over 10^6/mL) which may be incompletely removed by handwashing. The wearing of disposable gloves is recommended – one pair for each patient – and the use of alcohol for hand disinfection after emptying each bag. The bag should be emptied into a separate disinfected or disposable container for each patient. Some Gram-negative bacilli (e.g.

Klebsiella species) may survive better than others in a dry environment and on hands (Casewell and Phillips, 1977).

Specimens for culture should be collected using a syringe and needle after thoroughly cleaning the sample port with 70% alcohol. Care should be taken to avoid an inoculation injury. The closed system should not be broken to collect samples, and samples should not be collected from the bag.

Irrigation of the bladder should be avoided if possible. There is little evidence that irrigation with an antiseptic is of value in preventing or treating an infection. If irrigation is necessary to remove or prevent blood clots post-operatively, it should be performed as part of the closed drainage system using a three-way Foley catheter.

Infection in catheterized patients mainly occurs by the spread of micro-organisms along the outside of the catheter. The application of disinfectants or topical antibiotics to the catheter–material junction has had limited success in preventing infection via this route (Classen *et al.*, 1991). However, daily meatal-catheter care with sterile saline would seem to be a reasonable hygienic measure. The incorporation of an antimicrobial agent (e.g. silver compounds or antibiotics) into the catheter material would appear to be a promising approach as suggested for central venous catheters, but as yet a proven method that is suitable for routine use has not been commercially produced.

The use of systemic prophylactic antibiotics to cover the insertion of the catheter or the period of urological surgery remains controversial. However, patients with infected urine at the time of operation or catheterization should be treated with the appropriate antibiotic.

Urinary tract infection is the commonest cause of hospital-acquired infection, and is usually associated with catheterization. Although some patients with indwelling catheters remain free from bacteriuria for long periods, a catheter-care regime which will consistently prevent infection has not yet been defined. Nevertheless, the present recommendations should be carefully followed and the catheter removed as soon as possible (Ward *et al.*, 1997).

COLLECTION OF CLINICAL SPECIMENS FOR LABORATORY EXAMINATION

Hazards of infection, both to patients and to staff, occur during collection of specimens, during transport to the laboratory and during examination in the laboratory. The last of these hazards is discussed in Chapter 17 (see also Health Services Advisory Committee, 1991). The following notes are not intended as a guide to techniques for collecting laboratory specimens, but merely as a consideration of infection hazards in the collection and delivery of specimens, and ways in which they may be prevented.

Faulty technique during collection may result in inadequate, misleading or delayed laboratory reports which may affect a patient's treatment, including management of infection. During collection, especially of urine specimens, the patient may become infected. The nurse may be infected by contamination of the hands or clothing, or by inhalation of infected aerosol material during transfer to the containers. During transit, the person carrying the specimen may be infected by contaminants on the outside of the container, or through leakage or breakage of the container. In addition, the environment may become contaminated during these procedures and lead to an indirect spread of infection. Laboratory staff who receive unlabelled, potentially hazardous material (e.g. sputum from a patient with suspected pulmonary tuberculosis, or blood from a patient with suspected hepatitis) are also at risk. To ensure thorough and appropriate investigation, specimens should be correctly labelled and accompanying request forms should contain appropriate and adequate clinical details. Specimens should not be collected by inexperienced or untrained staff unless they are under close supervision. Specimens should routinely be transported in an upright position in dual-compartment plastic bags. Many laboratories advise that specimens should be labelled 'biohazard' if they are from known high-risk patients (e.g. with tuberculosis, HIV, HBV or enteric infections), although if all specimens are treated with the knowledge that the patient could be from a high-risk group (universal precautions), such labelling is probably unnecessary.

SWABS

Swabs collected from infected sites such as the throat, infected surgical wounds or vagina should be carefully transferred to the swab container and inserted slowly to avoid contamination of the rim with infected material. The container should be held as near to the infected site as possible to avoid shaking infected material in the air. If a spatula has been used, this should be discarded unbroken into the waste container, as the jerking movements involved in breaking a spatula may cause infected material to be released into the air. The swab should be sent to the laboratory as soon as possible. If there is a heavy discharge of pus from an infected wound or abscess, it is preferable to send a sample of pus in a sterile universal container, rather than sending a swab.

FAECAL SPECIMENS

These should be collected from a bedpan with a small applicator or scoop, and sent as soon as possible to the laboratory. A sterile container with an integral scoop is preferred. For bacteriological examination only, a small amount of faeces, approximately the size of a pea, is all that is necessary. There is no need to fill a container. A waterproof container with a wide mouth and a tight-fitting screw cap is essential, so that the specimen can easily be placed in the container and leakage does not occur. Samples of faeces collected on bacteriological swabs (especially rectal swabs) are usually unsuitable, although a sample of liquid faeces may be collected in hospital by this method. If a rectal swab is taken, ensure that the faeces are actually sampled; most anal specimens are useless.

URINE SPECIMENS

Apart from renal tuberculosis and typhoid fever, the organisms which are found in urinary tract infections are not usually infective for the person collecting the specimen. However, faulty collection technique may lead to contamination of the specimen and an erroneous diagnosis of urinary infection when this does not exist. Specimens should be collected with care, following the prescribed technique exactly, and sent as soon as possible to the laboratory. Examination of the urine is necessary before contaminating bacteria begin to multiply in it (i.e. within 2 hours). Alternatively, if delays are unavoidable, the specimen should be placed in a designated refrigerator soon after collection. A dip slide is useful if laboratory facilities are not immediately available, or boric acid can be added to the urine to prevent growth of organisms.

Infection can be transferred to a patient while a specimen is being collected from an indwelling catheter, and care must be taken to avoid this.

ASPIRATED FLUIDS (INCLUDING CEREBROSPINAL FLUID)

Equipment used to aspirate fluids from the thoracic cavity, joints, cerebrospinal space, facial sinuses, etc., must be supplied sterile from the SSD. An effective skin disinfectant (e.g. 70% ethyl alcohol) is used to prepare the site. Antibacterial agents with a strong residual effect (e.g. chlorhexidine) should preferably not be used if bacteriological examination of the aspirate is required. When cerebrospinal fluid (CSF) is aspirated from patients with certain infectious diseases (e.g. acute poliomyelitis or untreated meningococcal meningitis) a protective mask (see Chapter 9) is probably advisable. The organisms may be highly infectious, and some degree of aerosol production is almost unavoidable when screw caps and syringes are handled, although infection from this procedure is very rare. It may also be advisable on rare occasions to wear a protective mask when aspirating purulent fluids from other sites, although in general a mask is not essential for these procedures. The wearing of gloves is not essential, but is usually recommended to protect the wearer. Care must be taken to avoid contamination of the skin with pus. Having collected the fluid, the operator should disconnect the needle (if any) and expel the material gently into the container, avoiding spraying of droplets or release of aerosols.

SPUTUM SPECIMENS

It is often difficult to obtain a specimen of sputum without contamination of the rim and outside wall of the vessel, and contamination will occur even when wide-mouthed bottles are used. Some protection to porters and laboratory staff can be given if, after collection of the specimen, the rim and outside of the vessel are wiped with a paper tissue to remove any major contamination before replacing the lid of the container. The tissue should be discarded as clinical waste. If the patient is suspected of having tuberculosis, gloves should be issued for handling the container, which should be placed in a small plastic bag and sealed before transport to the laboratory.

BLOOD SPECIMENS

In addition to HBV, HCV and HIV infection (see Chapter 10), several other infections, including typhoid fever, can be acquired from blood specimens.

Blood specimens should therefore be regarded as potentially infected and gloves should be worn. Care should also be taken to avoid the dispersal of droplets which occurs when the blood is squirted vigorously into the container, although there is little evidence that aerosols are an infection hazard. Before discharging blood into a container, the needle should be separated from the syringe with care, using forceps or gloves. However, it is often recommended that the syringe and needle are discarded without separating into an approved sharps container (BS7320). Whichever method is used, the system should be designed to avoid a needle injury. In cases of known HBV, HCV or suspected HIV infection (UK Health Departments, 1998) needles should not be recapped unless a safe technique is available. Nozzles of syringes should not be broken before discarding, unless a safe method is available. Blood samples are frequently collected with an evacuated container system rather than a syringe and needle. Blood contamination may occur at the puncture site in the plug of the container on withdrawal of the needle, and should be removed with 70% ethanol. If the needle holder is contaminated with blood it should be discarded. The evacuated container should be safer than a syringe if used correctly. The hands should be thoroughly washed after taking a blood sample. Gloves should be worn when taking blood from high-risk patients, and are usually recommended for all blood-sampling. For protection of the patient during collection of blood specimens, only autoclaved or pre-sterilized disposable equipment should be used. When finger-prick specimens are taken, an individual single-use device is essential.

MISCELLANEOUS PROCEDURES

WARD EQUIPMENT

The cleaning and disinfection of many items of equipment, including nailbrushes, soap dishes, shaving equipment, thermometers, bedpans, urinals, suction, gastric aspiration and rectal equipment, beds, bedding and curtains are described in Chapter 6.

WASHING AND BATHING

Patients should use wash-basins in the washing areas whenever possible, and their own soap, hand and bath towels and other toilet requisites. Communal towels should not be available. Bathing or showering in the bathroom is preferred to bed-baths, but if bed-baths are necessary, patients should preferably have their own individual wash bowls. If this is not possible, bowls should be thoroughly cleaned between use by different patients (see Chapter 6). Water from the wash bowls should be emptied into a sink and bathing trolleys should not be used. Bathroom furniture should be simple, easily cleaned and reduced to a minimum, and the bathroom should not be used as a store room.

Communal bath mats should not be used. Instead, patients should use a towel unless disposable mats can be supplied. A routine of cleaning baths after each use should be instituted. Instructions on the correct method of cleaning the bath or wash-basins should be given to staff and also to patients if they are expected to clean their own bath. Cleaning is particularly important before and after a bath if the patient has an open wound; such patients should preferably not use a bath that has been used by pre-operative patients. Showers should overcome this problem to some extent. Salt is still occasionally added to the bathwater, but the practice has little if any value as an antimicrobial measure. If a disinfectant is required (e.g. during an outbreak or as part of the treatment of infected patients and carriers) the patient should apply an antiseptic detergent to the skin (see Chapter 6). This will also disinfect the bath water. Disinfection of the bath before or after use is still necessary, even if a disinfectant is used for bathing.

PRE-OPERATIVE PREPARATION (see Chapter 11)

Patients should preferably be admitted on the day of or the day before operation, and should have a shower if this is available, rather than a bath. If a bath is required, it should be disinfected before use. Pre-operative shaving should be avoided if possible to reduce the risk of infection from small cuts or abrasions (see Chapter 11; Cruse and Foord, 1980). If shaving is required, it should be done on the day of operation. Alternatively, hair may be removed by clippers, a depilatory cream or with an electric razor. The head of the electric razor (not the motor) should be disinfected by immersion in 70% alcohol for 5 minutes. Shaving brushes should not be used, and only experienced staff should shave patients, so that local trauma can be reduced to a minimum.

Preliminary disinfection of the operation site in the ward is not usually necessary (see also Chapter 6). The value of repeated bathing with chlorhexidine detergent before prosthetic hip or cardiac surgery is controversial, and is discussed in Chapter 11.

TREATMENT OF PRESSURE AREAS

Staff who perform these treatments should wash their hands between patients. Patients with bedsores should be treated as infected and may be nursed in isolation, if this is indicated from bacteriological examination (e.g. if multi-resistant organisms, particularly MRSA, are isolated). This should be balanced by considering the psychology and effect of isolation on the patient. All breaks in the skin should be treated as wounds. If these patients are bed-bathed, the water should be disposed of carefully without splashing, as it may be heavily contaminated. Nurses who carry out these procedures should wear disposable plastic aprons. *Staphylococcus aureus* is often dispersed in large numbers from healed as well as open pressure sores.

MOUTH-CLEANING AND DENTURES

Mouth care is required to keep the mouth clean, moist and free from infection. The most effective method is to brush the teeth, gums and tongue with a soft toothbrush. Alternatively, a sponge stick moistened in a sodium bicarbonate solution (1 in 60 dilution) may be used. A mouth pack can often be supplied by the

SSD, the contents of which should be discarded after use or returned for processing if appropriate. The use of an antiseptic mouthwash has a limited effect on the mouth organisms, and is not required as a routine. Rinsing with water is usually adequate. If glycerine and thymol are also used, they should be supplied in small containers and discarded daily, as contamination of the solution is frequent. Dentures may be stored in the patient's own preparation (e.g. 'Steradent'), but if this is unavailable a weak hypochlorite solution may be used (e.g. 'Milton', 1 in 80 dilution, or another chlorine-releasing agent containing 125 ppm available chlorine). Solutions should be changed daily. Paper bags should be supplied for the disposal of foam sticks, paper wipes, etc.

RESPIRATORY SUCTION TECHNIQUES (see Chapters 6 and 16)

A non-touch technique with closed suction, non-sterile gloves and a sterile catheter should be used for each suction procedure (Creamer and Smyth, 1996; Ward *et al.*, 1997). The saline solution should be discarded after each use. Suction tubing should be changed daily and between patients. Hands should be washed or disinfected before and after each procedure whether gloves are worn or not, and a plastic apron should be worn. In suspected cases of pulmonary or laryngeal tuberculosis, the operator should wear a mask to protect the wearer from direct contamination (see Chapters 8 and 16).

DISPOSAL OF SPUTUM

Sputum containers should be disposable and regularly discarded, and the responsibility for this task should be clearly defined. Used containers and paper wipes that have been used by patients should be placed in a plastic bag, sealed and disposed of as clinical waste (see also Chapter 8).

ENTERAL FEEDS

Enteral feeds using a nasogastric tube may be required in patients who are unable to tolerate a normal diet, and are an alternative to parental feeding. Feeds can be given either as a bolus or as a continuous drip monitored by a pump. There is a risk of contamination of feeds during preparation in the hospital or from inadequate refrigeration. Commercially prepared feeds are preferred (Bastow *et al.*, 1982; Casewell *et al.*, 1982). If special feeds are required, care must be taken to ensure that they are prepared using clean equipment and careful hygienic practices. If liquidizers are used, these must be thoroughly cleaned and dried after use.

Infection of the respiratory tract may occur from reflux of contaminated stomach contents, mouth secretions or contaminated feeds.

A non-touch technique should be used. Hands should be washed or disinfected before inserting the tube or handling and giving a feed. Non-sterile gloves and a plastic apron are worn for insertion of tubes, but are unnecessary for giving a feed. The nostrils should be cleaned and checks should be made that the tube is in the stomach before a feed is given. The patient should be kept in an upright position if possible. The tube should be flushed with sterile water from a sterile receptacle before and after feeding. The in-use feed should be discarded and the administration set changed at 24 hours or less. Opened feeds should be kept in the refrigerator and discarded after 24 hours. Nasogastric tubes should be changed weekly (or at longer intervals if indicated by the manufacturers). Nasogastric feeding should cease as soon as possible, and staff should be well trained in its use (Ward *et al.*, 1997).

EYES

The hands should be thoroughly washed before carrying out any procedures, and a non-touch technique or gloves should be used. Non-woven gauze, fluids or ointments should be sterilized (see Chapter 16).

DEAD BODIES

Most bodies are not infective, in which case no special care is necessary, and washing the body with soap and water is adequate. Bedding can be disposed of in the usual way, and mattresses and pillows may be cleaned by the recommended routine. Bed frames do not require routine cleaning. Disinfection of these or other items associated with the patient is not necessary unless death was due to or associated with a communicable disease (for details of disposal of infected dead bodies, see Chapter 9).

APPENDIX 7.1 USE OF PACKS IN SURGICAL PROCEDURES

PREPARATION OF TROLLEY AND PATIENT: GENERAL PRINCIPLES

The patient is made comfortable and the screen is drawn and the procedure explained. The nurse washes his or her hands or uses a 70% alcohol handrub and prepares the trolley. At the beginning of each dressing round the trolley top should be wiped with 70% alcohol and allowed to dry.

The requisite pack, supplementary packs, lotions and non-sterile items such as bandages, adhesive plaster and dressing scissors are placed on the lower shelf of the trolley. Lotions should be kept in small containers and replaced daily, or preferably supplied as single-use sachets.

The trolley is taken to the bedside and the patient prepared. Bedclothes and clothing are gently removed to expose the appropriate site, and the patient is placed in a suitable position.

The dressing pack is opened and the inner pack is placed in the centre of the trolley top. A bag of adequate size is fixed to the side of the trolley nearest to the patient for soiled dressings, and another bag is fixed to the opposite side for soiled and unused instruments. On completion of the procedure, instruments are placed in one bag (or directly into the used instrument container) and the unused dressings and disposables are rolled up in the paper towel covering the trolley top and placed in the soiled dressings bag.

ROUTINE DRESSING TECHNIQUE

The trolley and patient are prepared as described previously. The wound should not be cleaned unnecessarily. Some antiseptics have an adverse effect on wound healings, and there is evidence that the cleaning techniques traditionally used are ineffective in removing bacteria. The inner wrap is opened, handling the corners only, and forms the sterile field. Supplementary packs are opened and the contents are gently slid on to the sterile field.

The pack contents are arranged using handling forceps, and the handles of instruments are placed in a small defined handling area near the edge of the trolley. The lotion, if required, is poured into the gallipot.

The adhesive plaster is loosened and the dressing is removed with handling forceps, or a non-sterile glove or a plastic bag, and discarded into the soiled dressing bag. The forceps (if not disposable) are placed in the other bag. The wound can be more effectively cleaned with a gloved hand than with forceps. Clips or sutures are removed if necessary, and the dressing is completed using two pairs of sterile forceps or gloved hands (Thomlinson, 1987). After securing the dressing, instruments and unused or soiled materials are placed in bags as described above. If two nurses are available, the assistant prepares the patient, opens the outer bag of the pack and supplementary packs and pours the lotions. The dresser prepares the trolley and the sterile field and performs the dressing technique.

URINARY CATHETERIZATION

The patient, trolley and sterile field are prepared as described above. In male patients the penis is held with sterile gauze, the foreskin is retracted if necessary, and the glans and external meatus are thoroughly cleaned with sterile saline or aqueous povidone iodine or chlorhexidine (Falkiner, 1993). The local anaesthetic (sterile single use) is inserted into the urethra and left for 2–5 min). The nurse opens the catheter packet and the catheter is slid into a sterile receiver. A surgical drape is placed over the patient's thigh and the receiver with the catheter is placed between the patient's thighs. The penis is held with sterile gauze and the catheter is passed into the bladder. Catheters should only be handled with sterile gloves or forceps and should not be touched unless sterile gloves are worn. On removal, the catheter is discarded into the soiled dressing bag.

If two nurses are available, the assistant prepares the patient, opens the outer bag and supplementary packs and pours the lotion. The assistant also opens the catheter pack and slides the catheter carefully into the sterile receiver.

REFERENCES

Abi-Said, D., Raad, I., Umphrey, J. *et al.* (1999) Infusion therapy team and dressing changes of central venous catheters. *Infection Control and Hospital Epidemiology* **20**, 101.

Anon. (1991a) Local applications to wounds. 2. Dressings for wounds and burns. *Drugs and Therapeutics Bulletin* **29**, 27.

Anon. (1991b) Healing of cavity wounds. *Lancet* 1, 1010.

Ayliffe, G.A.J., Babb, J.R. and Quoraishi, A.H. (1978) A test for hygienic hand disinfection. *Journal of Clinical Pathology* 31, 923.

Ayliffe, G.A.J., Babb, J.R., Davies, J. *et al.* (1988) Hand disinfection and comparison of various agents in laboratory and ward studies. *Journal of Hospital Infection* 11, 226.

Babb, J.R., Davies, J.G. and Ayliffe, G.A.J. (1983) Contamination of protective clothing and nurses' uniforms in an isolation ward. *Journal of Hospital Infection* 4, 149.

Bastow, D., Greaves, P. and Allison, S.P. (1982) Microbial contamination of enteral feeds. *Human Nutrition: Applied Nutrition* 36a, 213.

Bowell, E. (1990) Infection control and the nursing process. In Worsley, M.A., Ward, K.A., Parker, L., Ayliffe, G.A.J. and Sedgwick, J.A. (eds), *Infection control. Guidelines for nursing care*. London: Infection Control Nurses Association, 1.

Bradley, C.R., Babb, J.R., Davies, J. *et al.* (1986) Taking precautions. *Nursing Times* 82, (Supplement), 70.

Casewell, M.W. (1982) Bacteriological hazards of contaminated enteral feeds. *Journal of Hospital Infection* 3, 329.

Casewell, M.W. and Phillips, I. (1977) Hands as a route of transmission of *Klebsiella* species. *British Medical Journal* ii, 1315.

Classen, D.C., Larsen, R.A., Burke, J.P. *et al.* (1991) Daily meatal care for prevention of catheter-associated bacteriuria. Results using frequent applications of polyantibiotic cream. *Infection Control and Hospital Epidemiology* 12, 157.

Creamer, E. and Smyth, E.G. (1996) Suction apparatus and the suctioning procedure: reducing the infection risks. *Journal of Hospital Infection* 34, 1.

Crow, S. (1989) *Asepsis: the right touch*. Bossier City, LA: Everett Co.

Cruse, P.J.E., and Foord, R. (1980) The epidemiology of wound infection. A ten-year prospective study of 62, 939 wounds. *Surgical Clinics of North America* 60, 27.

Doebbeling, B.N., Pfaller, M.A., Houston, A.C. *et al.* (1988) 'Removal of' noso-comial pathogens from the contaminated glove: implications for glove re-use and handwashing. *Annals of Internal Medicine* 109, 394.

Elliott, T.S.J., Faroqui, M.H., Armstrong, R.F. *et al.* (1994) Guidelines for good practice in central venous catheterization. *Journal of Hospital Infection* 28, 163.

Falkiner, F.R. (1993) The insertion of indwelling urethral catheters – minimizing the risk of infection. *Journal of Hospital Infection* 25, 79.

Glynn, A., Ward, V., Wilson, J. *et al.* (1997) *Hospital-acquired infection. Surveillance policies and practice*. London: Public Health Laboratory Service.

Hambraeus, A. (1973) Transfer of *Staphylococcus aureus* via nurses' uniforms. *Journal of Hygiene* 71, 799.

Health Services Advisory Committee (1991) *Safe working and the prevention of infection in clinical laboratories*. London: HMSO.

Hutchinson, J.J. and Lawrence, J.C. (1991) Wound infection under occlusive dressings. *Journal of Hospital Infection* **17**, 83.

Kelso, H. (1989) Alternative technique. *Nursing Times* **85**, 68.

Leaper, D.J. (1995) Risk factors for surgical infection. *Journal of Hospital Infection* **30 (Supplement)**, 127.

Maki, D.G. and Band, J.D. (1981) A comparative study of polyantibiotic and iodophor ointments in prevention of vascular catheter-related infection. *American Journal of Medicine* **70**, 739.

Maki, D.G. and Ringer, M. (1987) Evaluation of dressing regimes for the prevention of infection with peripheral intravenous catheters. *Journal of the American Medical Association* **258**, 239.

Maki, D.G, Cobb, L. and Garman, J.K. *et al.* (1988) An attachable silver-impregnated cuff for prevention of infection with central venous catheters: a prospective randomized multicentre study. *American Journal of Medicine* **85**, 307.

Newsom, S.W.B. and Rowland, C. (1989) Application of the hygienic hand disinfection to the gloved hand. *Journal of Hospital Infection* **14**, 245.

Rotter, M. (1996) Handwashing and hand disinfection. In Mayhall, C.G. (ed.), *Hospital epidemiology and infection control*. Baltimore, MD: Williams & Wilkins, 1052.

Spencer, R.C. (1990) Use of in-line filters for intravenous infusion. *Journal of Hospital Infection* **16**, 281.

Stickler, D.J. and Zimakoff, J. (1994) Complications of urinary tract infections associated with devices used for long-term bladder management. *Journal of Hospital Infection* **28**, 177.

Taylor, L.J. (1978) Evaluation of hand-washing techniques. Parts 1 and 2. *Nursing Times* **74**, 54, 108.

Taylor, L.J. (1980) Are masks necessary in operating-theatres and wards? *Journal of Hospital Infection* **1**, 173.

Thomlinson, D. (1987) To clean or not to clean. *Journal of Infection Control Nursing* **35**, 71.

UK Health Departments (1998) *Guidance for clinical healthcare workers: protection against infection with bloodborne viruses*. London: Department of Health.

Ward, V., Wilson, J., Taylor, L. *et al.* (1997) Preventing hospital-acquired infection. *Clinical guidelines,* London: Public Health Laboratory Service.

Worsley, M.A., Ward, K.A., Parker, L. *et al.* (eds) (1990) *Infection control: guidelines for nursing care*. London: ICNA.

chapter 8

PREVENTION OF INFECTION IN WARDS. II. ISOLATION OF PATIENTS, MANAGEMENT OF CONTACTS AND INFECTION PRECAUTIONS IN AMBULANCES

INTRODUCTION

The spread of infection to patients in hospital can be controlled by physical protection (isolation), and the extent of this control varies with the methods used (Bagshawe *et al.*, 1978; Garner, 1996). The emphasis on physical isolation in a single room has declined in recent years, and the risks of transmission of infection to staff, particularly with HIV, has led to the introduction of universal precautions, followed by body substance isolation (BSI). The new Centres for Disease Control (CDC) and Hospital Infection Control Practices Advisory Committee (HICPAC) guideline has combined these into 'standard' precautions which are designed to reduce the spread from unrecognized sources (Garner, 1996). These measures involve wearing clean non-sterile gloves when touching blood, body fluids, secretions, excretions and contaminated items, and handwashing after removal of gloves. Eye protection and gowns are worn if splashing of blood and body fluids is likely. Care is required when handling soiled equipment, linen and waste, particularly in the safe disposal of needles.

Also included in the HICPAC guidelines are airborne, droplet and contact isolation precautions. These are additional precautions to the 'standard' ones.

Many countries have adopted universal precautions, most of which are generally accepted as good routine infection control measures. However, the wearing of gloves for all of these purposes can be expensive, and there is little evidence that wearing of gloves is more effective than handwashing alone, which is still required after the removal of gloves. To avoid confusion we would recommend the use of the term 'universal infection control precautions' (UICP) (Wilson and Breedon, 1990), rather than 'standard' precautions, which is retained for basic isolation requirements in these recommendations.

RISK ASSESSMENT OF THE NEED FOR ISOLATION

The decision as to the type of isolation should where possible be tailored to the requirements of the individual patient (Ayliffe *et al.*, 1999). The following should be considered:
- the mode of transmission of the micro-organism;
- the level of risk of spread to other patients and staff;
- the potential severity of the infection and the availability of effective treatment;
- the mental state of the patient and their likely response to isolation (e.g. anxiety about possible neglect, loneliness, stigmatization) and the care required;
- hospital guidelines.

The possibility of rapid transfer of patients from hospital to the community may also influence decisions on the isolation of certain patients (e.g. MRSA colonization). The relative weighting of these factors is often difficult, and scoring systems have been suggested (e.g. Wilson and Dunn, 1996; Rao *et al.*, 1999).

METHODS OF PHYSICAL PROTECTION

The methods of physical protection are as follows:
- universal infection control precautions (UICP) (e.g. gloves and an apron, as described above) – these reduce the risks of contact spread between patients, as well as protecting the staff;
- segregation – in single rooms, cubicles or plastic isolators, which reduces airborne spread to and from patients. Cohort nursing may sometimes be useful, and consists of isolating patients with the same infection together in a separate ward or section of a ward;
- mechanical ventilation – which reduces the risks of airborne spread by removing bacteria from the patient's room and, in protective isolation, by excluding from the room bacteria that are present in the outside air.

The transfer of infection by the airborne route (e.g. respiratory infections) can only be controlled by confining the patient in a single room or isolator, whether for source or protective isolation. On the other hand, the control of diseases spread by contact (e.g. enteric fever) depends primarily on UICP.

The term 'isolation' is commonly used in the sense of segregation of the patient in a single room. It is used here to include all methods by which the patient may be physically protected. UICP is one of the basic components of patient isolation, and can be used on its own or together with other components.

MODES OF SPREAD OF INFECTION IN WARDS
(see Table 8.1)

Direct contact spread refers to the transfer of infection to the patient by direct contact with an infected person, or with a healthy carrier of a virulent organism.

Indirect contact spread refers to transfer of such organisms on needles, instruments, bedding and other 'fomites', in food, or on the hands of staff. This includes the transfer of dysentery and other intestinal infections through faecal contamination – the 'faecal–oral' route. Airborne spread refers to spread of infection through the air in small droplets (i.e. droplet nuclei – 5 μm or less in diameter) from the mouth (e.g. *Mycobacterium tuberculosis,* chicken-pox), or on skin scales, or in dust particles. Droplet transmission consists of the transmission of large droplets for short distances (i.e. 3 feet or less). It is often considered to be included in the category of contact transmission. Droplets are generated from coughs, sneezes and certain procedures such as tracheal or bronchial suction (and include the transmission of invasive influenza B, Neisserial meningitis, Gram-negative bacilli and most respiratory viruses). These are mainly deposited on the conjunctiva or mucous membranes of the respiratory tract of the host. Droplets are also produced by nebulizers, cooling towers and water-supply systems. These droplets may travel for longer distances and can transmit Gram-negative bacilli (e.g. *Legionella*), and should be included in a separate category.

Some infections are transmitted by more than one route (e.g. staphylococcal infections can be spread by direct and indirect contact and also by airborne transfer, and poliomyelitis may be acquired either by inhalation or by ingestion).

INFECTIONS THAT ARE UNLIKELY TO SPREAD FROM PERSON TO PERSON IN HOSPITAL

Actinomycosis, amoebiasis, aspergillosis, brucellosis, cat scratch fever, campylobacter enteritis, cryptococcosis, cryptosporidiosis, gas gangrene, histoplasmosis, infectious mononucleosis (glandular fever), legionellosis, leptospirosis, pneumonia, rabies, rheumatic fever, tetanus, toxocara infections, toxoplasmosis and worm infestations are unlikely to be transmitted in hospital. However, spread can occasionally occur with organisms causing some of these infections (e.g. *Campylobacter*, penicillin-resistant *Streptococcus pneumoniae*, Epstein-Barr virus), and special precautions are necessary for some of these diseases (see Chapter 9).

Table 8.1 Mode of person-to-person spread of transmissible diseases in hospital

Disease	Routes and possible routes of transfer			
	Airborne	Droplet	Faecal-oral route	Hands, personal and/or fomites
Anthrax	X (pulm.)			X
AIDS (see human immunodeficiency syndrome)				
Candidiasis				X
Chicken-pox	X			X
Cholera			X	X
Clostridium difficile infection			X	X
Cryptosporidiosis				X
Diphtheria (pharyngeal)		X		X
Fungal infections (skin)				X
Gastroenteritis in babies			X	X
Gonococcal ophthalmia neonatorum				X
Hepatitis A and E			X	X
Hepatitis B and C				X[a]
Herpes simplex				X
Herpes zoster	X			X
Human immunodeficiency syndrome				X[a]
Influenza		X		X
Measles	X	X		X
Meningitis				
(a) meningococcal		X		X
(b) viral		X	X	X
Mumps		X		X
Plague (pneumonia)	X	X		X
Pneumonia (viral and some bacterial, e.g. *Staphylococcus aureus*)		X		X
Poliomyelitis		X	X	X
Psittacosis		X		X
Q fever		X	X	X
Respiratory syncytial virus	[b]	X		X
Rubella		X		X
Salmonella and *Shigella* infections			X	X
Staphylococcal disease	X			X
Streptococcal disease		X		X
Syphilis (mucocutaneous)				X
Tuberculosis (open pulmonary)	X			X
Typhoid and paratyphoid			X	X
Vancomycin-resistant enterococcal infection			X	X
Viral haemorrhagic fevers		?	X	X[a]
Whooping cough	[b]	X		X
Wound infection				X

[a] Spread by blood/body fluid route usually percutaneously.
[b] Possibly airborne (Aintablian *et al.*, 1998).
Legionnaire's disease and aspergillosis are transmitted by airborne route, but not person to person.

VARIETIES OF ACCOMMODATION FOR ISOLATING PATIENTS

There are various types of isolation that offer different degrees of protection.

HIGH-SECURITY INFECTIOUS DISEASES ISOLATION UNITS

These are usually part of an infectious diseases unit, and have facilities for treating patients with highly communicable viral infections, having a high mortality rate and no or limited definitive treatment (e.g. Lassa, Marburg and Ebola fevers). Total environmental control is usually achieved by the use of negative-pressure plastic isolators, although a lesser degree of isolation is probably adequate.

INFECTIOUS DISEASES UNITS

At the present time these units are usually separate from other hospital buildings, but they may be situated in a general hospital. If so, separate ventilation and nursing staff should be provided. Facilities are available for the treatment of all infections, but not necessarily the African viral haemorrhagic fevers. Patients with untreated pulmonary tuberculosis, especially if caused by a highly resistant strain, should be treated in a cubicle with an extraction system. Patients are admitted both from the community and from other hospitals.

GENERAL HOSPITAL ISOLATION UNITS

These provide source isolation facilities for hospital-acquired infections and for most community-acquired infections. They can also provide facilities for protective isolation and for the screening of patients with suspected infections before admission to a general ward or transfer to a communicable diseases unit if necessary.

SINGLE ROOM OF A GENERAL WARD (WARD SIDE ROOMS)

These provide less secure source isolation than the above methods because of their close proximity to other patients and sharing of nursing and domestic staff with a general ward. Their value in protective isolation depends on the types of patient in the general ward, the thoroughness of barrier nursing, whether the room is self-contained (with WC), and the type of ventilation used.

OPEN WARD

Universal infection control precautions can be effective in controlling infections transferred by contact but not by air. An open ward can be used for nursing a number of patients with infections caused by the same organism (e.g. an MRSA ward).

ISOLATORS IN OPEN WARDS

Plastic enclosures ('isolators') for individual patients have been shown to be of value as a form of protective isolation for high-risk patients and of source isolation for infected patients, but are now rarely used.

ULTRA-CLEAN WARDS

Units have been set up in special centres for organ transplantation and treatment of leukaemia, choriocarcinoma and other diseases associated with extreme suscepti-bility to infection.

REQUIREMENTS FOR AN ISOLATION UNIT

At present very few general hospitals have satisfactory isolation units, often because of the high cost or even the lack of a sufficient number of single rooms for the treatment of patients who are suffering from or particularly susceptible to infection. The size of a general hospital isolation unit depends on a number of factors, such as the avail-ability of single-room accommodation in the general wards (which should have not less than two such rooms), the proximity of a major communicable diseases unit and the size of the hospital. The number of rooms in such a unit might vary from 10 to 20, depending on the above factors. A certain proportion of these rooms (about one-third) should have an appropriate form of mechanical ventilation for patients with severe infections which are likely to be spread by air. The number of beds required would be greater if paediatric patients are included. As these wards are likely to contain ill patients from all areas of the hospital, and as they are in individual rooms, a much higher nurse-patient ratio (e.g. two nurses to each patient over the 24-hour period) is required than in general wards. A specially trained team of domestic workers should be available for cleaning isolation rooms or units. Most hospitals are unlikely to be able to staff separate isolation wards for source and protective isolation (Rahman, 1985). A single unit for both would be appropriate, but requires particular care by the staff to prevent the spread of infection (Ayliffe *et al.*, 1979).

CATEGORIES OF ISOLATION

Various systems for categorizing patients have been proposed. A widely used method is to subdivide patients into categories according to the mode of spread of the organism (e.g. respiratory, enteric, wound, skin and blood), and includes strict isolation for highly transmissible and dangerous infections, and protective isolation for highly susceptible patients.

Coloured cards with nursing instructions can be attached to the door of the room. A more recently described system is disease-specific isolation, in which precautions are decided on the basis of the individual infection rather than the category. The advantages and disadvantages of these systems have been discussed by Haley *et al.* (1985). We propose a simplified system consisting of three main categories, namely standard, protective and strict. This has been successfully used for many years. Strict isolation (e.g. for viral haemorrhagic fevers and diphtheria) is rarely required and should only be undertaken in a Regional Infectious Disease Unit.

SUGGESTED LABELS FOR CATEGORIES OF ISOLATION

Adhesive labels are recommended for rooms occupied by patients in isolation. These should be attached to the door of the isolation room and will help to inform staff going into the room of the measures to be taken. Examples of colour codes are as follows:

- red – strict isolation;
- white – protective isolation;
- blue – standard isolation.

The requirement should be ticked where appropriate.

A brown card may be used for enteric precautions, although a single card for all source isolation may be preferred. An example of a card is shown in Figure 8.1. A special card is not necessary for blood precautions if universal precautions are routinely used. The visitor's line only should be translated into other languages as required. If the disease-specific system is used, requirements for gowns, masks, etc. are filled in separately for each patient, depending on the infection. Guidelines are provided to allow ward staff to make the appropriate decision.

In a general isolation unit, instructions for each patient are unnecessary, but an unmarked coloured card is still useful for the staff, particularly for domestic staff when cleaning cubicles in an agreed order. Protective isolation cubicles (white label) should be cleaned before source isolation cubicles (blue label). In single rooms in general wards, the instruction to visitors to report to the nurse in charge should be included on the isolation label or card.

STANDARD ISOLATION (see Appendix 8.1)

The main diseases requiring isolation in a general hospital are diarrhoeal infections (e.g. salmonella, shigella, rotavirus infection) and also untreated pulmonary tuberculosis and infections caused by highly resistant *Staphylococcus aureus* (e.g. MRSA) or vancomycin-resistant enterococci (VRE). Additional isolation facilities may be required for childhood communicable diseases (e.g. measles, chicken-pox, respiratory syncytial virus infection) or their contacts. Patients infected with antibiotic-resistant Gram-negative bacilli can be treated in an open ward with

VISITORS	PLEASE REPORT TO SISTER'S OFFICE BEFORE ENTERING ROOM
SINGLE ROOM	Necessary for all infections transferred by air and preferred, when available, for all communicable infections. Door must be kept closed
GOWNS OR PLASTIC APRONS	Must be worn when attending to patients
MASKS	Not necessary
HANDS	Must be washed before and after patient contact
GLOVES	Must be worn when handling blood, body fluids, secretions, excretions and contaminated materials
ARTICLES	Normal supplies. Linen and waste disposed of according to guidelines
COMMENTS	BLUE LABEL

Figure 8.1 Standard source isolation.

suitable precautions against contact spread, but single-room isolation may be preferred if available (Fryklund *et al.*, 1997).

Although it is recognized that special precautions may sometimes be necessary (e.g. for enteric infections), the following guidelines are applicable to most patients who require isolation, with some modifications. It is easier to maintain strict and minimal practices than to observe a list of rules without defining priorities. Discipline of the staff is of major importance, and the main requirements of standard isolation are as follows:

- keep the door of the room closed at all times when not in use;
- wash hands after handling the patient or his or her immediate surroundings (and before, if the patient is in protective isolation);
- wear disposable gloves (non-sterile) for handling blood, body fluids, secretions, excretions and contaminated materials. Wash hands after removing gloves;
- wear a disposable apron or gown when handling a patient or his or her immediate surroundings (this may be unnecessary for patients with airborne infections, but removes the need to make decisions on individual patients. Many infections that are spread by the airborne route are also spread by contact).

It is also necessary to ensure that the staff of an isolation unit are protected against tuberculosis, measles, rubella, poliomyelitis and hepatitis B. Evidence of a past infection with chicken-pox should be recorded and, if uncertain, antibody levels should be measured. Staff with inadequate levels and those who are chicken-pox contacts should be excluded from nursing susceptible patients who are in protective isolation.

ACCOMMODATION

This can vary from a ward side room to a fully equipped suite with an airlock. The minimal requirement is a side room of a main ward. It should have a handwash-basin and preferably also a toilet. A ventilation system (consisting of at least an extractor fan and providing 8–10 air changes per hour) is desirable for patients with a communicable respiratory or airborne infection, especially for chicken-pox and untreated pulmonary tuberculosis, and is preferred for heavy staphylococcal dispersers. An air extraction system is essential for untreated pulmonary tuberculosis caused by a highly resistant strain. A positive-pressure system (plenum) providing 8–10 air changes per hour is required for patients in protective isolation. If in a unit with mixed source and protective isolation facilities (Ayliffe *et al.*, 1979), a room with both systems for positive- and negative-pressure ventilation can be used for either source or protective isolation, but requires a decision on the direction of airflow required for individual patients. Although an airlock is generally unnecessary, an airlock with an extractor system can be similarly used for both types of patient isolation, and avoids the need to change the airflow depending on the type of patient. An airlock requires more space and may reduce contact between staff and patient. A plenum system filtering to a standard of 95% for 5 μm particles is generally adequate, but more efficient filtration may be needed in bone-marrow and liver transplantation units where *Aspergillus* infection is a potential hazard (see Chapter 9).

A ventilated room with toilet and shower or bathroom *en suite* and an airlock provides the highest standards of isolation, apart from a plastic isolator or the use of laminar-flow ventilation. However, if a toilet or bathroom is not present in the isolation suite, particular care is necessary to prevent contact between patients using the ward facilities, and to ensure adequate disinfection of the toilet and bath or shower after use.

The isolation room should not contain unnecessary furniture, and the surfaces should be washable. Good visibility of the patient is desirable, and glass panels in the walls and door are helpful. The room should have talk-through panels, or a good communication system and a television set to reduce the adverse psychological effects of isolation.

NURSING PROCEDURES FOR STANDARD ISOLATION

HANDS (see Chapter 7)

Handwashing before and after contact with the patient is the most important measure in preventing the spread of infection. Either a non-medicated soap or an antiseptic detergent is adequate for routine purposes, but 70% ethanol or isopropanol is more effective for killing transient flora, and should be used at least in high-risk situations. An alcohol rub is preferred by many during outbreaks (e.g. of MRSA). Prior washing is still necessary after handling patients with enterovirus infections.

Disposable gloves which need not be sterilized are used when directly handling contaminated materials, and for handling blood, body fluids, secretions and excretions. Hands should be washed after removing gloves.

GOWNS AND APRONS

Disposable plastic aprons are preferred. Aprons with a different colour on each side are more expensive, but can be reused with less potential risk of contamination to the wearer. Cotton gowns provide limited protection. Gowns may be required for lifting of patients. If aprons are used for this purpose, the arms should be kept bare to the elbows and should be washed after handling the patient. Gowns made of water-repellent materials (e.g. ventile or suitable non-woven materials) which have a low permeability to bacteria, give better protection than cotton gowns but, like disposable gowns, they can be expensive (see Chapter 11). The gown or apron should be left hanging inside the room and changed daily, although evidence exists that contamination does not increase if the gown is used over longer periods (Babb *et al.*, 1983).

MASK AND EYE PROTECTION

Masks are rarely necessary and are of doubtful value in protecting against organisms spread in the air. However, if they are used they should be of the filter type. Goggles, spectacles or a visor may sometimes be required (e.g. for procedures involving possible splashing of blood from patients). Masks may be recommended to be worn by staff for cases of untreated pulmonary tuberculosis. These should be close-fitting and of a filter type. Particulate respirators may be required in rooms occupied by patients with antibiotic-resistant pulmonary tuberculosis (see section on strict isolation). A positive tuberculin test is a requirement for staff handling patients with tuberculosis.

CAPS AND OVERSHOES

These are not required.

MEDICAL EQUIPMENT

Disposable or autoclavable equipment should be used whenever possible. Equipment such as stethoscopes, sphygmomanometers and thermometers should preferably be left in the room and terminally disinfected on discharge of the patient.

OTHER EQUIPMENT

A bedpan washer and dishwashing machine that heat to 80°C for 1 or more minutes or an equivalent time-temperature relationship should be available in the isolation ward. The temperature profile of the cycle should be monitored regularly. Disposable crockery and cutlery should be used for enteric infections and untreated pulmonary tuberculosis if a suitable washing machine is not available.

LAUNDRY

Linen from patients with open pulmonary tuberculosis, salmonella and shigella infections, HBV and HIV (if bloodstained) and others specified by the infection control doctor should be sealed in water-soluble bags and enclosed in a red outer bag (Chapter 12). Linen from other patients can be treated routinely as 'used' linen.

WASTE

Waste contaminated with body fluids or secretions from patients listed above should be disposed of as clinical waste for incineration in a UN-approved (UN3291) container or bag. If fluids are present, then a 'gel' should be used to reduce the fluid content. If fluids are disposed of in the sluice, protective clothing should be worn. Prior disinfection before disposal is rarely necessary.

CHARTS

Patients' charts should be kept outside the contaminated areas, if only to discourage frequent visits to the room. The infective hazard of contamination from charts is small.

TRANSPORTING PATIENTS

Patients should be sent to other departments only if this is absolutely essential. The department in question should be notified in advance, so that it may make arrangements to prevent possible spread of infection. It may be advisable for the order in which patients visit other departments to be arranged in advance.

SECRETION, EXCRETION, EXUDATE AND BLOOD PRECAUTIONS

These are precautions against infected oral or other secretions, or against pus and other infected exudates. They will usually be part of routine universal infection control precautions. The hands should be washed/disinfected after these procedures.

Oral secretions

Patients should be encouraged to cough or spit into a paper tissue and then discard this into a plastic container which, when sealed, must be disposed of as clinical waste.

Exudate

A 'non-touch' technique using forceps or disposable gloves should be employed and contaminated material should be placed in sealed paper or plastic bags. These should be disposed of as clinical waste.

Excretion

For patients with enteric fever, dysentery, cholera and other infections spread by urine or faeces, disposable gloves should be worn to take the bedpan from the patient to the disposal area. It is necessary for the nurse to put on a plastic gown to prevent contamination of their uniform. The pan should be covered with a disposable paper bag before transport. Gloves and aprons should be disposed of as clinical waste. Disposable gloves and a plastic apron or gown should be worn when handling contaminated equipment or linen, and when cleaning the perineal areas (see Chapter 7 for details of disinfection of bedpans, etc.)

Blood

See Chapter 10 (UK Health Departments, 1998).

DISPOSAL OF PERSONAL CLOTHING

Used clothing requires no special treatment unless it is from patients with an infection that is potentially hazardous to staff. Infected clothing should be transferred to the hospital laundry in a sealed water-soluble or alginate-stitched bag and treated by the routine method used for this category of linen (see Chapter 12). Rarely, other methods of disinfection (chemical or low-temperature steam) or incineration may be necessary for heat-sensitive materials. Articles from patients with anthrax should be autoclaved. Articles from patients with viral haemorrhagic fevers should be treated as 'infected' linen and must not be sorted. Autoclaving before transport to the laundry may be preferred.

DISPOSAL OF THE DEAD

When death of a person suffering from a Notifiable Disease occurs in a hospital, provision is made under the Public Health Act (1936. S. 163 164) to prohibit the removal of the body from the hospital except for the purpose of being taken direct to a mortuary or being forthwith buried or cremated. Under the Act, every person having charge or control of premises where such a body may be lying must take such steps as may be practicable to prevent individuals from coming into unnecessary contact with or proximity to it. Wakes over such bodies are prohibited. Furthermore, a Justice of the Peace has the power to order the removal or burial of such a body subject to a medical certificate issued by the Consultant in Communicable Disease Control (CCDC) (or other registered practitioner on his or her staff) stating that the body constitutes a risk of spread of infection. In practice, the above powers are not generally enforced today. Cremation is perhaps the safest method of disposal of the infected dead, and relatives should be encouraged to agree to this method, but it cannot be legally enforced.

Death may occur from infectious diseases which are not notifiable, and the corpse may remain infectious to those who handle it. The precautions described above for handling infected patients do not become unnecessary with the patient's death. The isolation category should be stated on a card attached to the body. Porters, mortuary attendants, pathologists and funeral undertakers must be informed of the possible danger in order that appropriate precautions may be taken. The bodies of patients with infections that are potentially transmissible to personnel (e.g. typhoid and other enteric infections, open tuberculosis, HBV, HCV or HIV infections) should be sealed in a leak-proof cadaver plastic bag, labelled as above. However, it should be possible to arrange for the face of such a patient to be seen by relatives if required, provided that suitable precautions are taken against spread.

TERMINAL DISINFECTION OF ISOLATION ROOMS

All surfaces, including beds, other furniture, wash-basins, etc. and the floor, should be washed. The need to use a disinfectant is doubtful, but may be advisable if there is visible contamination, or following the presence of infections transferred by contact (e.g. MRSA, VRE, *Clostridium difficile*) which survive well in the environment, or are hazardous to personnel (e.g. untreated tuberculosis) (see Chapters 5 and 6). It is unnecessary to wash walls and ceilings unless they are visibly contaminated. The room may be occupied when the surfaces are dry. If disinfectants are used, every consideration must be given to comply with COSHH guidelines.

STRICT ISOLATION TECHNIQUES (IN ADDITION TO THE STANDARD)

If the infection is likely to be airborne and the personnel are non-immune, masks that are protective to the wearer (of a recommended filter type stored outside the room) or particulate respirators should be put on before entering the room and discarded into a pedal bin before leaving. Disposable water-impermeable gowns, with a low permeability to bacteria are preferred to aprons. Clean gowns should be stored outside the room and discarded into a pedal bin on leaving. Patients with a suspected or confirmed viral haemorrhagic fever must be transferred between hospitals in specially equipped ambulances with crews wearing protective clothing. Disposable gloves should be worn when handling such patients or their immediate surroundings (see also p. 198–201).

PROTECTIVE ISOLATION

This is required for diseases, lesions or therapy associated with an increased susceptibility to infection and in which patients need special protection from the hospital environment. The type of infection (bacterial, viral and fungal) and the risks of infection vary with the condition and procedure. Precautions are required to prevent the acquisition of exogenous organisms which may be more hazardous to immunosuppressed than to healthy individuals. Isolation requirements vary with the degree of immunodeficiency, but these are ill-defined. These requirements are usually minimal, but more intensive measures are included here as they may be preferred in some hospitals. Isolation measures are usually maximal for liver and bone-marrow transplantation and minimal for kidney transplantation patients. Most infections acquired by immunosuppressed patients are endogenous, and isolation in a single room is of doubtful value (Nausef and Maki, 1981; Fenelon, 1995). However, cross-infection can be a hazard, and single rooms, preferably in a self-contained unit (with shower and toilet) and a positive-pressure ventilation system (8–10 air changes per hour) are preferred at the present time for highly immunosuppressed patients (e.g. those with very low neutrophil counts). High standards of hygiene to prevent contact spread of infection (e.g. by hand-washing and wearing plastic aprons) are probably of greater importance (see standard isolation techniques). Masks are rarely required. No special precautions are required for the disposal of waste and linen, and terminal disinfection is not necessary. Filtration of air with HEPA filters to reduce airborne aspergilli is also advisable when nursing highly susceptible patients, particularly in liver and bone-marrow transplant units. The cost of a laminar-flow air system would appear to be unwarranted, and a failure in filtration of the recirculated air could represent a greater hazard. Positive-pressure plastic isolators are sometimes used for bone-marrow and cardiac transplant patients, but their use is now rare. Other measures may sometimes be recommended (e.g. sterile linen, sterile food and other supplies, decontamination of the mouth or other orifices, gut and skin, and prophylactic systemic antimicrobial agents such as co-trimoxazole). The evidence for the effectiveness of these procedures is conflicting, and they are not routinely recommended, although some measures may be of value (e.g. prophylactic co-trimoxazole in the prevention of pneumocystis infection in bone-marrow or liver transplant patients). Uncooked food, particularly salads, may be contaminated with Gram-negative bacilli or listeria, and should generally be avoided in highly immunosuppressed patients. Similarly, routine screening of the nose, throat, faeces and skin of immunosuppressed patients, although frequently recommended, is of uncertain predictive value.

MANAGEMENT OF CONTACTS OF INFECTED PATIENTS IN HOSPITAL

See Brewer and Jeffries (1990) for viral infections.

CHICKEN-POX

If indicated, an injection of human-specific zoster immunoglobulin (ZIG) may be given to patients who are suffering from or contacts of chicken-pox and who are on steroid therapy or receiving cytotoxic or immunosuppressive drugs (e.g. patients with leukaemia). Non-immune contacts should be sent home or isolated from 8 days after contact.

CYTOMEGALOVIRUS INFECTION

Children who are excreting cytomegalovirus are not normally a hazard to pregnant women, provided that the usual hygienic precautions are taken, especially handwashing.

DIPHTHERIA

Throat and nasal swabs should be taken from all close contacts of patients who develop diphtheria while in hospital. They should be given prophylactic erythromycin (1 g daily for 7 days) and swabs should be taken from carriers on completion of treatment. The Consultant in Communicable Disease Control (CCDC) should be informed. Active immunization of contacts, if they are not known to be immune, should be started (see Chapter 13). All contacts should be kept under surveillance, and if any individuals develop sore throat or nasal discharge, antitoxin should be given.

INFANTILE GASTROENTERITIS

If an outbreak of gastroenteritis due to enteropathogenic or toxigenic *E.coli* occurs, stools should be cultured from all contacts, and admissions to the ward must be suspended. Children who are well enough to go home should be discharged as soon as possible. The isolation of a gastroenteritis serotype of *E.coli* in the laboratory from a child without symptoms should not cause alarm, but is an indication that this child should be kept away from any susceptible children (i.e. under 2 years old) in the ward. Nurses working in a ward where cases of gastroenteritis are present should not be transferred to other wards. Infantile gastroenteritis is also commonly caused by viruses, especially rotaviruses.

INTESTINAL INFECTIONS (including typhoid fever, other salmonellosis, cholera and bacillary dysentery)

Other patients and staff in the ward should be kept under surveillance, and stool samples should be obtained from those who develop signs of the disease. Under certain circumstances it may be necessary to close a ward or unit. When typhoid contacts, in whom the incubation period may be prolonged to 3 weeks, are discharged from hospital the general practitioner should be made aware of the contact so that cases are not missed. The Occupational Health Department should be informed of contacts among members of staff.

MEASLES

Contacts under 2 years of age and other children in whom measles might be particularly dangerous (eg. those suffering from chronic or debilitating diseases such as leukaemia, or receiving corticosteroid drugs) should be given an injection of human normal immunoglobulin as soon as possible after contact. It may be necessary to close a children's surgical ward because operations on children with measles can be dangerous. Admissions should be limited to children who have had a definite attack of measles or who have been immunized.

MENINGOCOCCAEMIA

Household contacts should be kept under surveillance and throat swabs should be taken. A prophylactic course of rifampicin or a single dose of ciprofloxacin (see Chapter 15) should be given to close family contacts, or to staff contacts if they have given mouth-to-mouth respiration.

POLIOMYELITIS

All contacts, both staff and patients, should be offered oral poliomyelitis vaccine.

HAEMOPHILUS MENINGITIS

A prophylactic course of rifampicin should be given for close family contacts (children only).

RUBELLA

Rubella is generally a benign disease, but infection during the first 4 months of pregnancy is associated with fetal abnormality. Estimation of the antibody titres in the blood of contacts in early pregnancy can be helpful and should be done without delay. Immunoglobulin is not recommended. Rubella vaccine should be considered for women of child-bearing age who are found to be non-immune to rubella.

SCABIES

When scabies is diagnosed in a patient admitted to hospital, arrangements must be made for all home contacts to be treated.

TUBERCULOSIS (OPEN PULMONARY)

The names of all close patient contacts of a case of sputum-positive tuberculosis should be notified to the appropriate Consultant in Communicable Disease

Control (CCDC) and to the general practitioner. Staff contacts are reported to the hospital occupational health departments and their immune status is checked. Tuberculin tests and chest X-rays may be indicated on close contacts in long-stay wards or at 6 weeks depending on the time of contact, and also in neonatal, paediatric (under 3 months) or immunocompromised close contacts.

VIRAL HEPATITIS

Human normal immunoglobulin gives protection against hepatitis A but not against hepatitis B. A 500-mg dose should be given to debilitated contacts and pregnant women. Hepatitis A vaccine may be given in certain situations (see Chapter 14). Human-specific immunoglobulin, which confers protection against HBV, is available for those at risk due to accidental exposure to infection, and hepatitis B vaccine should be given (see Chapter 10).

VISITING OF PATIENTS IN ISOLATION HOSPITALS

INFECTED PATIENTS

In general, patients in hospital who are suffering from infection should be allowed visitors in the normal way, and daily visiting of small children by their parents is encouraged. However, under certain circumstances some restrictions may have to be imposed for the protection of visitors, or to prevent the spread of disease. It is sometimes necessary for the visitor to wear a gown or plastic apron (e.g. if handling a child with an intestinal infection), and instructions must be given on handwashing. Language and cultural difficulties may have to be considered in some cases. Visitors must not visit patients other than those whom they have come to see. It is unwise to allow children to visit patients in isolation or communicable disease units, and adults who are not considered to be immune to a particular infection should be excluded from contact with that disease. Pregnant women who are non-immune must not visit patients with rubella.

PATIENTS IN PROTECTIVE ISOLATION

Parents may visit children, but contacts should be restricted, especially when visiting immunosuppressed patients. If the intending visitor has an infection of the respiratory or intestinal tract, boils or other septic lesions, the visit should be postponed.

AMBULANCE SERVICES – GENERAL PROCEDURES FOR CONTROL OF INFECTION

Many diseases are infectious before symptoms appear, and contact with a sick person before a final diagnosis is made will always carry some risks of infection. Most infections (e.g. bronchitis, pneumonia, abscesses and urinary tract infections) will not be transferred to normal healthy staff, and the risk of acquiring infection is minimal. The inanimate environment within the ambulance is unlikely to be an infection hazard, and the risk of transfer of infection from one occupant to the next is remote.

The minimal measures required are as follows:

- immunization of ambulance staff (if not already immune) against poliomyelitis, tuberculosis, hepatitis B and tetanus;
- handwashing after a patient and his or her belongings have been removed from the ambulance. Bedding (blankets, sheets and bedcovers) should be sealed in a plastic bag and laundered after use by a patient with a notifiable or other communicable disease, or if soiled with blood, secretions or excreta, whether the patient has a known infection or not. Spillage should be removed with disposable wipes, which should be sealed in plastic bags for incineration;
- the use of an alcoholic rub is more convenient than washing, and will usually be preferred.

Disposable plastic aprons and gloves should be available for handling contaminated patients (e.g. those with diarrhoea and vomiting) and cleaning up contaminated surfaces. A chlorine-releasing agent (1000 ppm available chlorine) may be used for cleaning contaminated surfaces.

ADDITIONAL PROCEDURES FOR SPECIAL INFECTIONS

A few infections are potentially dangerous to staff as well as to patients and require special care. These include typhoid, dysentery, HBV, HCV and HIV infections, diphtheria and open tuberculosis. For a discussion of potentially dangerous infections (e.g. Lassa and other haemorrhagic fevers and rabies), see Chapter 9.

SUGGESTED PROCEDURES

Typhoid, dysentery and other gastrointestinal infections
Bedpans, urinals, vomit bowls, etc., should be either washed in a bedpan washer with a steam disinfection cycle or washed in a chlorine-releasing agent or a phenolic disinfectant. Disposable cups should be used. If the surfaces are extensively contaminated, the ambulance should be taken out of service and all surfaces cleaned with a chlorine-releasing agent or a phenolic disinfectant. All surfaces should be dry before the ambulance is reused. Fumigation of the ambulance interior with formaldehyde is unnecessary.

HBV, HCV and HIV infections
As above, but disinfect with a chlorine-releasing agent. Rinse to reduce corrosion of fixtures and fittings after a short exposure (e.g. 1 min) to a chlorine-releasing agent.

Tuberculosis (open untreated pulmonary)
As above. Sputum containers and wipes used for removing secretions from patients should be sealed in a plastic bag and incinerated. Disinfect contaminated surfaces with a phenolic solution or 70% ethanol after cleaning.

Diphtheria

As for typhoid, dysentery, etc., above. Prophylactic antibiotics for contacts may be recommended by the CCDC.

Methicillin-resistant *Staphylococcus aureus*

Infection caused by these organisms is no special hazard to personnel or their relatives. Lesions should be sealed if possible (see Chapter 9).

To reduce the risks of transfer to another patient, ambulance staff should use an alcoholic handrub after contact with a patient with MRSA.

Surfaces in contact with the patient should be cleaned with 70% alcohol or, for larger areas, with a chlorine-releasing agent. If a chlorine-releasing agent is used, it should be rinsed off after 1–2 min.

Nasal carriers of MRSA and those with enclosed lesions can be transported with other patients unless they are at high risk of infection. If further measures are required, the ICT should inform the ambulance service (Working Party Report, 1998).

AMBULANCE

If an ambulance is specially designated for transport of infected patients, it is advisable:

1 to remove any equipment not considered to be necessary (e.g. spare stretcher);
2 to seal the equipment locker with adhesive tape (terminal cleaning of the inside will not then be necessary);
3 to seal clean blankets and bedding in a plastic bag and carry them in the bag, and to seal the box containing resuscitation equipment so that only the outside of the box will require cleaning or disinfection.

Respiratory resuscitation equipment should be returned to a hospital SSD or equipment cleaning and disinfection department for processing.

APPENDIX 8.1 ISOLATION METHODS FOR INDIVIDUAL DISEASES

IF UNIVERSAL INFECTION CONTROL PRECAUTIONS ARE IN USE, EXCRETION, SECRETION, EXUDATE AND BLOOD PRECAUTIONS WILL ROUTINELY BE INCLUDED.
STANDARD ISOLATION REQUIRES A SINGLE ROOM OR SPECIAL ROOM

Isolation for infections

This section lists diseases in alphabetical order, with the category of isolation and special nursing procedure, if any, required. The following abbreviations are used:

HIU	hospital isolation unit
HSIU	high security isolation unit
IDH	infectious diseases hospital
SR	single-bedded side room
CCDC	Consultant in Communicable Disease control

Actinomycosis	Isolation unnecessary
	Exudate precautions
Acquired immunodeficiency syndrome (AIDS)	See human immunodeficiency virus syndrome infection
Amoebiasis	Isolation unnecessary
	Excretion precautions

Anthrax

Category of isolation	Strict (pulmonary or systemic); standard (cutaneous)
Period of isolation	Length of illness (e.g. until completion of successful chemotherapy)
Place of isolation	HIU, IDH or SR for cutaneous infection.
	HSIU, or IDH for pulmonary infection.
	Laboratory must be warned of any specimens sent for examination.
	Notify CCDC

Aspergillosis	No special precautions (see Chapter 9)
Brucellosis	Exudate precautions only if a draining lesion

Campylobacter enteritis

Category of isolation	Standard
Period of isolation	Until diarrhoea stops
	Excretion precautions without single-room isolation usually adequate

Candidiasis (moniliasis, thrush)	Exudate precautions
Category of isolation	Standard isolation in neonatal wards
Cat scratch fever	No special precautions

Chicken-pox

Category of isolation	Standard (in room with extractor fan)
Period of isolation	7 days from start of eruption
Place of isolation	HIU or IDH

Comments	Take precautions with secretions. Isolate non-immune contacts from 7–8 days after exposure. Staff who have not had the disease must be excluded. Visitors who have not had the disease must be warned of the risks

Cholera

Category of isolation	Standard
Period of isolation	Length of illness
Place of isolation	IDH
Comments	Excretion precautions. Notify CCDC

Clostridium difficile infection

Category of isolation	Standard
Period of isolation	Duration of illness
Place of isolation	SR or HIU
Comments	Excretion precautions

Common cold	See influenza
Conjunctivitis (gonococcal)	See ophthalmia neonatorum and venereal diseases
Cryptosporidiosis	Excretion precautions

Diarrhoeal disease of unknown origin

Category of isolation	Standard
Period of isolation	Duration of illness
Place of isolation	SR or HIU
Comments	Excretion precautions

Diphtheria

Category of isolation	Strict
Period of isolation	Until bacteriologically negative
Place of isolation	IDH
Comments	See section on contacts
	Notify CCDC

Dysentery, bacillary (Shigellosis)

Category of isolation	Standard
Period of isolation	Until three consecutive negative stools after acute phase, whenever possible
Place of isolation	SR, HIU or IDH
Comments	Notify CCDC
	Excretion precautions

Dysentery, amoebic	Isolation unnecessary
	Excretion precautions for stools
Comment	Notify CCDC
Ebola virus disease	See viral haemorrhagic fevers
Enterococcal infection	See vancomycin-resistant enterococci

Food poisoning
Staphylococcal and clostridial   No special precautions
                                  Notify CCDC

Salmonella   See p. 176

Fungal infections
Systemic, e.g.   No special precautions
    cryptococcosis,
    histoplasmosis
Ringworm   Precautions against contact transfer
                                  Isolation in a cubicle may be advisable, especially in children's wards

Gastroenteritis in babies
Category of isolation   Standard
Period of isolation   Length of illness or until stools are negative
Place of isolation   HIU, or IDH, or SR
Comments   Excretion precautions are important
                                  Notify CCDC in Northern Ireland only

Gas gangrene   No special precautions

Gonorrhoea   See venereal diseases

Herpes simplex
Category of isolation   Standard (children's wards only)
Period of isolation   Length of illness
Place of isolation   SR or HIU
Comments   Staff with infection should be excluded from neonatal, maternity or
                                      children's wards, and should cover cuts or abrasions on fingers if
                                      in contact with an infected child

Herpes zoster
Category of isolation   Standard
Period of isolation   Length of acute illness (when lesions stop discharging)
Place of isolation   SR or HIU
Comments   Staff who have not had chicken-pox must be excluded. Visitors who
                                      have not had the infection should be warned of the risk

Hepatitis A and E
Category of isolation   Standard
Period of isolation   Isolation probably not required once jaundice has developed.
                                      However, patients are infectious in the early febrile phase of the
                                      illness
Place of isolation   SR or HIU
Comments   Excretion precautions
                                  Notify CCDC

Hepatitis B, C and E   Isolation not required
                                  Blood and body fluid precautions

Human immunodeficiency virus   Isolation only required in special circumstances (e.g. superadded
  infections   TB or salmonellosis)
                                  Blood and body fluid precautions

Infectious mononucleosis   Oral secretion precautions

Influenza
Category of isolation   Standard (if admitted with disease)
Period of isolation   Length of illness
Comments   Isolation of doubtful value if acquired in hospital or if other patients
                                             with the disease are in the ward

Lassa fever   See viral haemorrhagic fevers

Legionnaire's disease   Isolation unnecessary
                                             Oral secretion precautions

Leprosy
Category of isolation   Standard
Period of isolation   Length of hospital stay
Place of isolation   HIU or IDH
Comments   Not infectious following adequate treatment

Leptospirosis   Isolation unnecessary
                                             Notify CCDC
                                             Excretion precautions (urine)

Listeriosis   Person-to-person spread rare: isolation unnecessary apart from
                                             neonates
                                             No special precautions

Malaria   Isolation unnecessary
                                             Contact CCDC

Marburg disease   See viral haemorrhagic fever

Measles
Category of isolation   Standard (preferably in room with extractor fan)
Period of isolation   5 days from onset of rash
Place of isolation   SR, HIU or IDH
Comments   Secretion precautions
                                             Notify CCDC
                                             If outbreak in paediatric ward, do not admit children who are not
                                             immune until 14 days after the last contact has gone home (see
                                             section on contacts)

Meningitis (meningococcal)
Category of isolation   Standard
Period of isolation   48 hours after onset of treatment
Place of isolation   SR, HIU or IDH
Comments   Secretion precautions. See section on contacts
                                             Notify CCDC

Meningitis (tuberculous)   See tuberculosis, p. 178

Meningitis (viral) and meningo-encephalitis
Category of isolation   Standard

Period of isolation	Length of acute illness
Place of isolation	SR, HIU or IDH
Comments	Excretion precautions
	Notify CCDC

Meningitis (pneumococcal, haemophilus, coliform and other causes
No isolation required
Notify CCDC

Mumps

Category of isolation	Standard
Period of isolation	9 days after onset of parotid swelling
Place of isolation	SR, HIU or IDH
Comments	Secretion precautions
	Exclude staff who are not immune
	Warn visitors who are not immune

Nocardiosis
No isolation required unless immunosuppressed patients are in the ward
Exudate and secretion precautions

Ophthalmia neonatorum (see also venereal diseases)

Category of isolation	Standard
Period of isolation	Length of illness (24 hours after start of chemotherapy)
Place of isolation	SR
Comments	Secretion precautions
	Notify CCDC

Orf
No isolation required
Exudate precautions

Paratyphoid fever
See typhoid and paratyphoid

Plague

Category of isolation	Strict
Period of isolation	Until bacteriologically negative
Place of isolation	IDH or HSIU
Comments	Secretion and exudate precautions
	No visitors if pneumonic
	Notify CCDC

Pneumonia
No isolation or special precautions required for lobar (unless due to antibiotic-resistant strains of *Streptococcus pneumoniae*) or evidence of transmissible strain or primary atypical (mycoplasma) pneumonia. For other causes see staphylococcal infection, plague and psittacosis, Legionnaire's disease

Poliomyelitis

Category of isolation	Standard
Period of isolation	Until stools are negative for poliovirus (or 7 days from onset)
Place of isolation	IDH

Comments	Excretion precautions. Visitors and staff should be immunized
	Notify CCDC

Psittacosis

Category of isolation	Standard
Period of isolation	For 7 days after onset
Place of isolation	SR, HIU or IDH
Comments	Secretion precautions
	Notify CCDC

Puerperal sepsis

Category of isolation	Standard
Period of isolation	Until bacteriologically negative (48 hours or longer)
Place of isolation	SR or HIU
Comments	Exudate precautions
	Notify CCDC

Q fever — As for psittacosis

Rabies

Category of isolation	Standard (person-to-person transfer is unlikely) (see Chapter 9)
Period of isolation	Length of illness
Place of isolation	IDH or SR in intensive-care unit
Comments	Secretion precautions
	Immunize staff in close contact
	Notify CCDC

Rheumatic fever — No isolation or special precautions required

Ringworm — See fungal infections

Rubella

Category of isolation	Standard
Period of isolation	5 days from onset of rash
Place of isolation	SR or HIU
Comments	Exclude young women staff or visitors who may be pregnant, unless they are immune. The congenital rubella syndrome is highly infectious

Salmonella infections (food poisoning)

Category of isolation	Standard
Period of isolation	Until three stools negative, whenever possible, or cessation of symptoms
Place of isolation	SR, HIU or IDH
Comments	Excretion precautions
	Visitors avoid close contact with patients
	Notify CCDC
	Carriers – send home and inform CCDC

Scabies

Category of isolation	Standard until successfully treated

Comments	See sections on contacts, and on human infestation
Scarlet fever	See streptococcal infections
Schistosomiasis	No isolation or special precautions
Shigellosis	See dysentery

Staphylococcal infection (epidemic, e.g. MRSA or other highly resistant strains), including pneumonia

Category of isolation	Standard
Period of isolation	Until the organism is no longer isolated from the lesion
Place of isolation	SR or HIU
Comments	Exudate and secretion precautions (see Chapter 9)

Staphylococcal infection (sensitive, or resistant only to penicillin)

	No isolation needed, unless in maternity and neonatal wards or evidence of epidemic strain

Streptococcal infection (including scarlet fever and erysipelas)

Category of isolation	Standard
Period of isolation	Until organism no longer isolated, following chemotherapy (or not less than 3 days)
Place of isolation	SR or HIU
Comments	Exudate and secretion precautions (see Chapter 9)

Syphilis	See venereal diseases
Tapeworm	No isolation needed
	Excretion precautions
Tetanus	No special source isolation precautions, but patient should be in SR for medical reasons
Threadworms	No isolation needed
	Excretion precautions
Tonsillitis	See streptococcal infection
Toxocara	No isolation needed
	Excretion precautions
Toxoplasmosis	No isolation or special precautions
Trichomoniasis	No isolation needed
	Exudate precautions

Tuberculosis (open, including pulmonary, urinary or draining lesions)

Category of isolation	Standard (respiratory – air extraction)
Period of isolation	2 weeks after beginning effective treatment (or 4 weeks in neonatal and paediatric wards or if immunosuppressed patients are present)
Place of isolation	SR, IDH (or special hospital) or HIU
Comments	Secretion and exudate precautions
	Staff and visitors who are not immune should be warned of risk and given suitable protection

| | See section on contacts |
| | Notify CCDC |

Tuberculosis (closed) — Isolation and special precautions not needed
Notify CCDC

Typhoid and paratyphoid fever (and carriers)

Category of isolation	Standard
Period of isolation	Until six negative stools, and urine samples if applicable
Place of isolation	IDH, HIU
Comments	Excretion precautions
	Notify CCDC
	It is not necessary to keep the patient in hospital until he or she is no longer excreting typhoid bacilli

Vancomycin-resistant enterococcal infection

Category of isolation	Standard
Period of isolation	Duration of illness
Place of isolation	SR or HIU
Comments	Exudate and secretion precautions

Venereal diseases (syphilis [mucocutaneous] and gonorrhoea)

Category of isolation	Standard
Period of isolation	Until bacteriologically negative; this will occur after 48 hours in syphilis and after 24 hours in gonorrhoea unless the strain is resistant to the antibiotic
Place of isolation	SR or HIU
Comments	Use of gloves for handling secretions or infected sites

Varicose ulcers (with sepsis) — See wounds

Viral haemorrhagic fevers

Category of isolation	Strict
Period of isolation	Until virus is no longer isolated
Place of isolation	HSIU
Comments	See Chapter 9
	Secretion, excretion and blood precautions
	Notify CCDC

Whooping cough

Category of isolation	Standard
Period of isolation	3 weeks after onset of paroxysmal cough, or 7 days after appropriate chemotherapy (e.g. erythromycin or amoxycillin)
Comments	Secretion precautions
	Notify CCDC

Wounds
Extensive wounds (with sepsis caused by epidemic or highly antibiotic-resistant *Staphylococcus aureus* or Gram-negative bacilli)

| Category of isolation | Standard |
| Period of isolation | Until wound is healed or organism is eliminated |

Place of isolation	SR or HIU
Comments	Exudate precautions

Worm infestations (see also tapeworm, threadworm and toxocara)	Isolation not necessary Excretion precautions only

Isolation for susceptible patients

Neutropenic, leukaemic and immunosuppressed patients

Category of isolation	Protective
Period of isolation	Duration of illness or period of immunosuppression
Place of isolation	SR, HIU
Comments	See p. 165

Burns

Category of isolation	Combined protective and standard source
Period of isolation	Duration of hospital stay for larger burns (see p. 194)

REFERENCES

Aintablian, N., Walpita, P. and Sawyer, M.H. (1998) Detection of *Bordetella pertussis* and respiratory syncytial virus in air samples from hospital rooms. *Infection Control and Hospital Epidemiology* 19, 918.

Ayliffe, G.A.J., Babb, J.R., Taylor, L.J. *et al.* (1979) A unit for source and protective isolation in a general hospital. *British Medical Journal* 2, 461.

Ayliffe, G.A.J., Babb, J.R. and Taylor, L.J. (1999) *Hospital-acquired infection. Principles and practice,* 3rd edn. Oxford: Butterworth and Heinemann.

Babb, J.R., Davies, J.G. and Ayliffe, G.A.J. (1983) Contamination of protective clothing and nurses' uniforms in an isolation ward. *Journal of Hospital Infection* 4, 149.

Bagshawe, K.D., Blowers, R. and Lidwell, O.M. (1978) Isolating patients in hospital to control infection. *British Medical Journal* ii, 609, 684, 744, 808, 879.

Brewer, J. and Jeffries, D.J. (1990) Control of viral infections in hospitals. *Journal of Hospital Infection* 16, 191.

British Society of Antimicrobial Chemotherapy, Hospital Infection Society and Infection Control Nurses Association (1998) Working Party Report. Revised guidelines for the control of methicillin-resistant *Staphylococcus aureus*. *Journal of Hospital Infection* 39, 253.

Fenelon, L.E. (1995) Protective isolation: who needs it? *Journal of Hospital Infection* 30 (Supplement), 218.

Fryklund, B., Haeggman, S. and Burman, L.G. (1997) Transmission of urinary bacterial strains between patients with indwelling catheters – nursing in the same room and in separate rooms. *Journal of Hospital Infection* 36, 147.

Garner, J.S. (1996) The Hospital Infection Control Practices Advisory Committee. Guideline for isolation precautions in hospitals. *Infection Control and Hospital Epidemiology* 178, 53.

Haley, R.W., Garner, J.S. and Simmons, B.P. (1985) A new approach to the isolation of hospitalized patients with infectious disease: alternative systems. *Journal of Hospital Infection* 6, 128.

Nausef, W.M. and Maki, D.E. (1981) A study of simple protective isolation in patients with granulocytopenia. *New England Journal of Medicine* 304, 448.

Rahman, M. (1985) Commissioning a new hospital isolation unit and assessment of its use over five years. *Journal of Hospital Infection* 6, 65.

Rao, G Gopal and Jeanes, A. (1999) A pragmatic approach to the use of isolation facilities. *Bugs and Drugs* 5, 4.

UK Health Departments (1998) Guidance for clinical health care workers: protection against infection with bloodborne viruses. London: Department of Health.

Wilson, J. and Breedon, P. (1990) Universal precautions. *Nursing Times* 86, 67.

Wilson, P. and Dunn, L.J. (1996) Using an MRSA isolation scoring system to decide whether patients should be nursed in isolation. *Hygiene Medicine* 21, 465.

chapter 9

SPECIAL PROBLEMS OF MISCELLANEOUS INFECTIONS AND HUMAN INFESTATION

OUTBREAKS OF *STAPHYLOCOCCUS AUREUS* INFECTIONS IN GENERAL HOSPITAL WARDS

Staphylococcus aureus is one of the commonest causes of wound infection. Many infections are endogenous, and major outbreaks due to methicillin-sensitive strains are now uncommon in UK hospitals. However, methicillin-resistant strains (MRSA) are a major problem in some hospitals in the UK, and are endemic in hospitals in many countries.

Strains of *Staphylococcus aureus* which have a propensity for spreading and causing sepsis in a ward are known as 'epidemic strains'. In the UK there are three predominant epidemic strains (designated EMRSA3, EMRSA15 and EMRSA16) (British Society of Antimicrobial Chemotherapy, Hospital Infection Society and Infection Control Nurses Association, 1998). These are usually resistant to two or more antibiotics. However, not all multiple-resistant strains spread readily to other patients. Antibiotic-sensitive strains (or strains resistant to penicillin only) rarely spread in wards (apart from neonatal units), but may be responsible for infection in the operating-theatre, or for self-infection of the patient (Ayliffe *et al.*, 1999). People are the most important source of infection, as staphylococci multiply in noses, on the skin (e.g. the perineum) and in lesions, but not in the inanimate environment. Nevertheless, staphylococci, which can survive for some time outside the body, especially in dry conditions, may spread from the inanimate environment (e.g. bedding and baths are sometimes important reservoirs). Some infected patients, and occasionally healthy individuals who may be carriers, are responsible for heavy environmental contamination, mainly on contaminated skin scales. They are known as 'dispersers' and are a special hazard in a ward or operating-theatre (Solberg, 1965).

Staphylococci may be transferred by direct (i.e. personal) or indirect (i.e. fomite-borne) contact, or through the air. Transfer of organisms from an infected patient on the hands of members of staff is an important mode of transmission. Strains carried in the noses of staff are rarely responsible for wound infection acquired in the ward, but nasal carriers of epidemic strains of MRSA are potentially more hazardous as sources in high-risk units. Individuals with concealed lesions (e.g. a boil in the axilla or on the buttock) may be an important source of infection.

CONTROL OF INFECTION

Control of infection is based on a good reporting system, high standards of aseptic technique and immediate isolation or removal from the open ward of any patient with a potentially epidemic strain (Wenzel *et al.*, 1991; Ayliffe *et al.*, 1995, British Society of Antimicrobial Chemotherapy, Hospital Infection Society and Infection Control Nurses Association, 1998).

In addition, the following infection control measures should be in use throughout the hospital and must be regularly monitored:

- gloves for handling body fluids and contaminated materials (including bedding of patients with epidemic methicillin-resistant *Staphylococcus aureus* [EMRSA] or during outbreaks); handwashing/disinfection after removal of gloves;
- a disposable apron or gown for handling the patient and their immediate surroundings;
- high standards of cleaning;
- careful handling of used linen and clinical waste;
- avoiding overcrowding and minimizing inter-ward transfers;
- maintaining adequate levels of trained ward staff;
- an antibiotic policy.

The effort required to control infection due to *Staphylococcus aureus* depends on the type of environment and the risk to the patient. Areas considered to be high risk might include intensive care units, high-dependency units and certain surgical units (e.g. orthopaedic wards and vascular surgical units). Infection control measures in these high-risk units may need to be quite draconian, particularly in the case of demonstrated cross-infection due to MRSA.

At the other end of the spectrum are minimal-risk areas such as long-stay geriatric wards, geriatric day hospitals and nursing homes (see p. 189). Significant infection, as opposed to colonization, is rare in these settings, and eradication efforts, including isolation of colonized patients, is less justified (Working Party of the British Society of Antimicrobial Chemotherapy, and the Hospital Infection Society, 1995).

ISOLATION

All patients with an infection due to a highly resistant strain, especially if multi-resistant as well as methicillin-resistant, should if possible be transferred to a hospital isolation unit or to a single room (preferably equipped with appropriate mechanical ventilation) or, if clinically feasible, sent home. The doors of cubicles or side wards should be kept closed. Isolation should include precautions against contact transfer as well as against airborne transfer.

Priority of isolation

Since isolation facilities are limited in most hospitals, priorities may have to be considered. These depend on the type of ward, the susceptibility of the other patients, the infection and the virulence and transmissibility of the organism (see also Chapter 8). Infections that are likely to spread in the air should have a priority. Priority for isolation should also be considered for patients with the following lesions: major open staphylococcal sepsis (e.g. generalized eczema, chest infection, urinary tract infection, profusely discharging wounds, generalized furunculosis or skin sepsis, burns, bedsores) due to multiply-resistant epidemic strains, particularly strains resistant to methicillin, clindamycin, fusidic acid, gentamicin or mupirocin. Priority of single rooms is not always given to infected patients; often they are needed for difficult patients, or for social or compassionate reasons, although this should not mean that infected patients are nursed in open wards. Patients with major open sepsis caused by a highly resistant or epidemic resistant strain should be isolated in single rooms, as barrier nursing measures in an open ward are of limited value in reducing the spread of infection (especially staphylococcal infection) from such patients. Although side wards on general wards are preferable to open wards, the isolated patients are still nursed by the same staff, and an isolation unit with designated staff is preferable. In many hospitals the number of patients who require isolation due to colonization with MRSA exceeds the availability of isolation beds. In this situation cohort nursing is the most appropriate means of controlling the spread of these organisms. Ideally the cohort bay or ward should have dedicated nursing staff as well as appropriate facilities for hand hygiene. A scoring system may help to determine isolation priorities (e.g. Wilson and Dunn, 1996).

OTHER MEASURES

If no isolation facilities are available, and single-bed wards are already occupied with high-priority patients, some measures may help to limit the spread of infection. Topical chemoprophylaxis of burns with an effective agent contributes much more to the exclusion of hospital infection in a burns unit than isolation methods (see Chapter 16). In the absence of an outbreak (i.e. more than two or three infections due to the same phage or molecular type), a good aseptic technique and adequate covering of a wound may be sufficient to prevent the spread of infection from patients with minor sepsis. Infection can be spread from a patient with a small septic lesion (e.g. a bedsore), and even a healed lesion, or a healthy nasal or skin carrier of a multiply-resistant strain, can sometimes disperse large numbers of staphylococci. Additional measures which can be used when treating patients with sepsis or dispersing epidemic strains in the open ward (or in isolation) are as follows.

Treatment of nasal carriers

Apply a cream containing 2% mupirocin three times a day for 5 days. Although 2% mupirocin (Bactroban) has been shown to be more effective in eradicating nasal carriage of MRSA than other agents, there have been reports of mupirocin resistance emerging on treatment. Mupirocin resistance can be low level, in which case treatment with this agent is still effective, or high level, in which case an alternative agent must be chosen (e.g. neomycin and chlorhexidine – 'Naseptin' or another agent of equal effectiveness) to the anterior nares four times a day for 2 weeks or until the staphylococcus is no longer present (Hudson, 1994; Cookson, 1998).

Skin treatment
An effective antiseptic detergent preparation (e.g. 2% triclosan detergent solution or 4% chlorhexidine detergent) should be used for bathing and washing. This should be applied directly to the skin and rinsed off. 28.5mL 7.5 g of 2% triclosan concentrate added to bath water reduces the risk of transfer of infection via contamination of the bath, but is not effective as a treatment for colonization. Patients who are perineal carriers should wash the perineum and 'bathing-trunk area' daily with an effective detergent antiseptic preparation such as chlorhexidine detergent.

Open wounds and lesions (excluding burns)
Open and drained wounds, ulcers of the skin and pressure sores may be dusted with chlorhexidine (1%) powder or covered with dressings impregnated with chlorhexidine. These may be effective against *Staphylococcus aureus* but not against many Gram-negative rods. (It should be noted that hexachlorophane and chlorhexidine 'Hibitane' are different compounds. Hexachlorophane has toxic properties and must not be applied to open wounds.) An iodophor spray or dressing impregnated with povidone-iodine may also be used. Mupirocin (2%) may be applied to small wounds, but the treatment period should be limited to 7 days. Open or drained wounds and lesions should be covered with bacteria-proof dressings.

General measures
Disposable gloves and an apron and gown should be used when handling any infected patient or his or her immediate surroundings. Careful handling and disposal of bedding and dressings are important.

Bedding and clothing should be changed daily if possible, or every 2 days. Bedding should be carefully removed and transferred at the bedside to a container or bag which is immediately closed and sealed.

Contaminated dressings must not be handled with fingers but should immediately be placed, with forceps or gloves, into a bag and sealed. Large dressings are best handled with disposable gloves. Contaminated instruments should be placed into a sealed bag or container immediately after use and returned to the SSD.

Urine bottles used by patients with staphylococcal urinary infection should be handled carefully with gloves and the bottles should be disinfected after use, preferably by heat. Wash-bowls, bedpans, baths and the barber's razor should be disinfected after use by an infected patient (see Chapter 7). The infected patient should preferably retain his or her own wash-bowl which is terminally disinfected on discharge from hospital.

Special prophylactic measures
Patients. In the presence of a severe outbreak of staphylococcal infection, prophylactic treatment of the noses of all patients in the ward twice daily with a special

antibiotic cream or ointment such as mupirocin (see above) could be considered. All patients should also use antiseptic soap or detergent and take antiseptic baths. Hexachlorophane powder may be applied daily to the groins, trunk, buttocks and upper thighs of bed-ridden or long-stay patients, but hexachlorophane must not be applied to open lesions. Lesions and open wounds, whether infected or not, should be treated as described in the previous section.

Staff handwashing. All staff working in the ward (including physiotherapists, radiographers and laboratory technicians) should wash their hands with a chlorhexidine-detergent solution, or povidone-iodine detergent, or disinfect with a solution of 70% ethanol or 60% isopropanol rubbed on until the hands are dry, before and after handling any patient or his or her immediate environment (see Chapters 6 and 7).

SEPSIS AND NASAL CARRIERS IN HOSPITAL STAFF

Members of staff who are carrying an epidemic strain of *Staphylococcus aureus* in the nose or on the skin, especially if they are dispersers, or with a septic lesion caused by any strain of *Staphylococcus aureus*, require treatment. This should be controlled by the occupational health department and the microbiologist. It is not necessary to treat a nasal carrier of a strain which has not caused an infection or is not responsible for an outbreak of MRSA colonization or infection. Any member of staff with a septic lesion should be excluded from the wards until this has healed. Minor cuts and abrasions should be covered with a waterproof dressing. Prophylactic nasal treatment of staff is rarely required. Nasal carriers who require treatment should be treated with nasal cream (usually mupirocin) and antiseptic soap or antiseptic detergent (see above section on treatment of nasal carriers). If there is evidence of skin carriage of an epidemic strain or repeated septic lesions, daily baths with triclosan-detergent solution or another recommended antiseptic-detergent preparation should be taken for 1 week, and the hair should be washed twice weekly with triclosan detergent, or with povidone-iodine or cetrimide shampoo, in addition to the routine skin treatment. If the staphylococci are not removed after 1 week, a further course of nasal treatment should be given and bathing with triclosan or other antiseptic detergent solution should be continued. If eradication proves difficult, it may be necessary to continue skin treatment for long periods (e.g. 3–6 months). Changing to a different antiseptic-detergent preparation may sometimes be effective. Nasal treatment with mupirocin should not be given for more than 2 weeks.

CLOSURE OF WARDS

If there are increasing numbers of infections and carriers of an epidemic strain in a ward, and if measures have failed to control their spread, it may be necessary to close that ward. This entails stopping new admissions and limiting transfers to other wards. Patients who are on the ward should remain there, but patients may still be discharged home or to a long-term care establishment if this is clinically indicated. Once all colonized or infected patients, or patients who have been exposed to colonized or infected individuals, have been discharged or transferred to an isolation facility (i.e. an isolation ward, side ward or cohort ward), the ward can be reopened after a thorough clean. When it is reopened, all patients should be screened for the presence of the epidemic strain before they are admitted to the clean ward. Screening is particularly important if patients are transferred to the clean ward from another hospital or from another ward in the same hospital. Unless required for aesthetic reasons, cleaning of walls and ceilings is unnecessary. The use of a disinfectant for cleaning is controversial, but although thorough cleaning is most important, a phenolic or a chlorine-releasing agent is often used for surfaces, particularly if an epidemic strain was involved.

NEONATAL UNITS

Staphylococci are particularly likely to be transferred on the hands of staff. If an outbreak occurs, all babies should be treated with hexachlorophane powder (e.g. 'Ster-Zac') at each napkin change or twice daily (if this is not already routine procedure). The buttocks, groins, lower abdomen, umbilicus and axilla should be powdered. Infected babies should be bathed daily with chlorhexidine-detergent solution. A 4% chlorhexidine-detergent solution, or 70% alcohol solution rubbed to dryness, should be used for all handwashing by the staff. Staff should wear gloves and a gown or apron when handling babies during an outbreak. Routine screening of staff for *Staphylococcus aureus* is not necessary, but in an outbreak carriers of the epidemic strains should be treated. General control methods should be applied, especially isolation of infected babies.

EPIDEMIC METHICILLIN-RESISTANT *STAPHYLOCOCCUS AUREUS* (EMRSA)

Methicillin-resistant *Staphylococcus aureus* strains are not more virulent than sensitive strains, and only require different treatment because of their resistance and transmissibility. They do not differ in other respects from hospital strains isolated in the 1950s and 1960s. An increase in the number of outbreaks of methicillin-resistant staphylococcal infection has been reported in Australia, the USA, Eire, South Africa, the UK and many other countries (Wenzel *et al.*, 1991; Ayliffe *et al.*, 1995). The strains that cause these infections are often resistant to penicillin, tetracycline, erythromycin, clindamycin and trimethoprim, and possibly to gentamicin and sometimes to other antibiotics such as neomycin, chloramphenicol, fusidic acid and ciprofloxacin. Some epidemic strains are only resistant to two agents. Strains with low resistance to vancomycin have been described in Japan, the USA and France (Johnson, 1998). Many methicillin-resistant *Staphylococcus aureus* (MRSA) are not epidemic strains, but there is no laboratory test available to differentiate them rapidly from epidemic strains. However, experimental phages which can differentiate between strains of known epidemicity as well as other techniques are available for use in specialist centres (Marples *et al.*, 1986; Mulligan and Arbeit, 1991). More recently, various molecular methods have been described for typing strains of MRSA. PCR-based methods using random primers are rapid and relatively simple to perform. A more complex method involves analysis of the total genome by pulsed-field electrophoresis after restriction-enzyme digestion (Streulens, 1996). This method is highly discriminatory, but is still in the early stages of evaluation for routine epidemiological purposes. Some precautions must therefore be taken with all MRSA. Infections with EMRSA are often severe and the outbreaks are difficult to control. Most of the measures already described for prevention of spread of *Staphylococcus aureus* are appropriate, but additional measures to prevent inter-ward and inter-hospital spread are required (Wenzel *et al* 1998; Working Party Report, 1998). However, circumstances vary in different hospitals, and decisions should be based on the local situation.

A known or previously infected patient or carrier of EMRSA, or a patient admitted from a hospital or unit in which the strain is endemic or transferred from hospitals abroad, should be admitted directly to an isolation room and screened. The transferring hospital should inform the receiving hospital, and this is the responsibility of the infection control team. On discharge, infected or colonized patients should be identified by marking their medical records, or should be given cards so that the necessary action can be taken if they are admitted to another hospital. Staff transferred from wards or hospitals with this strain should also be screened. Particular care is required with agency staff, who should preferably not work in wards containing epidemic MRSA-infected or -colonized patients.

If a strain is first identified when the patient is in a ward, particularly if it is a surgical or intensive-care ward, or if immunocompromised patients are present, the patient should be immediately isolated, preferably in a special unit. Isolation in side wards is often ineffective. If more than one patient is found to be carrying the strain, all patients should be screened and appropriate action taken. Staff should also be screened if there is evidence of further spread.

Routine screening should include the nose, perineum/groin and any lesions. The role of throat carriers in transmission of staphylococci remains uncertain, but the taking of throat swabs should be considered if an epidemic continues despite maximal precautions, particularly in a high-risk ward, or if the usual nasal treatment fails. It should be agreed before sampling that if throat carriers are detected, they should be treated. Groin swabs are less sensitive than perineal swabs in detecting carriers, but are easier to collect when screening all patients in a ward. In elderly bedridden patients, the buttocks and other pressure areas should also be sampled irrespective of the presence of an actual lesion. EMRSA may also be found in the sputum, faeces and urine, and in association with indwelling lines, catheters and tracheostomies when present. Contact or sweep-plates from bedding are useful for identifying new infections or colonized patients, and can reduce the number of screening samples required. Contact plates taken from the floor are also helpful in determining whether a ward is clear of the organism, but will not necessarily detect the presence of non-dispersers.

Due to the higher incidence of infection in certain areas (e.g. intensive-care units and orthopaedic wards), it may be appropriate to screen all patients admitted to these units to allow rapid identification of carriers of EMRSA.

Eradication of the strain from a carrier is often difficult, but if the individual is a nasal carrier, mupirocin (2% in a paraffin base) applied three times daily for 5 days is usually effective, or if applied in a polyethylene glycol base it may also remove the organisms from superficial lesions, but treatment should be limited to 2 weeks (i.e. two courses) because of the possible emergence of resistance. Nasal carriers on the staff can be returned to duty on treatment before a negative swab is obtained, and after 2 days of treatment with mupirocin on a high-risk ward, but not if other topical agents are used. As already discussed, nasal treatment should be associated with bathing, washing and shampooing with antiseptic detergents such as 4% chlorhexidine, povidone-iodine or 2% triclosan, and similar agents or an alcohol rub should be used by staff for handwashing. Systemic agents for a short period, such as a combination of fusidic acid, ciprofloxacin or trimethoprim and rifampicin (for not more than 7 days) have been used to treat nasal or throat carriers, but this should not be a routine treatment as resistance to these agents can emerge rapidly and side-effects to rifampicin can occur.

Transferring infected or colonized patients to an isolation unit may abort an epidemic, but if such a unit is not available it may be necessary to convert an existing ward to an isolation ward and provide it with its own nursing staff. This can be very expensive.

Many hospitals are now finding that MRSA is endemic in some units or even in the entire hospital. At this point it becomes futile to try to eradicate the organism from these areas. It is more appropriate to accept the endemicity of the strain and to attempt to protect patients as much as possible. A combination of surveillance of clinical specimens for MRSA, improved hygienic measures (e.g. alcoholic hand disinfection, gloves for handling patients and their surroundings), isolation of positive patients and screening of patients and staff where there is evidence of cross-infection, depending on the type of ward and facilities, is probably the most cost-effective way of managing the problem in this type of situation. Attempts to eradicate MRSA from an entire acute hospital become particularly futile if the local community, including nursing homes, has a high incidence of colonization with these strains (Fraise et al., 1997). However, it may be useful to categorize patients for treatment priorities. Good hygienic standards are essential in all wards. The Working Party recommends the categorizing of patients (or wards) into infection-risk categories (British Society of Antimicrobial Chemotherapy, Hospital Infection Society and Infection Control Nurses Association, 1998) (see Table 9.1).

The intensity of control measures will vary with the category, particularly if endemic conditions exist throughout a hospital. However, each hospital should decide on its own category system depending on the local situation (e.g. a surgical ward or a medical ward or a tertiary referral unit may be classified as high risk and a burns unit as moderate or low risk).

Although some MRSA strains do not have epidemic potential, it may be advisable to treat patients colonized with any strain, epidemic or not, with a nasal ointment and skin antiseptics, and to isolate them, particularly if they are in a surgical or high-risk unit.

Table 9.1 Priorities for control of MRSA (Spicer, 1984; Ayliffe *et al.*, 1995; British Society of Antimicrobial Chemotherapy, Hospital Infection Society and Infection Control Nurses Association, 1998

High-risk areas	(e.g. intensive care, cardiothoracic, burns, transplantation, orthopaedic and trauma)
After one case	Screen all patients and staff
	Isolate and treat[a] carriers and infected patients
	Treat staff nasal carriers; consider screening admissions
Intermediate risk	(e.g. general surgery, urology, neonatal)
After one case	Isolate and treat[a] patient
After more than one case	Screen all patients, isolate and treat[a] carriers and infected patients
Low risk	(e.g. non-surgical wards)
	Isolate and treat[a] index and subsequent patients
Minimal risk	(e.g. long stay, care of the elderly, psychiatry)
	Basic control measures

[a] nose and skin

Three successive negative swabs from the nose and any other colonized sites are necessary before a patient is considered to be clear of MRSA, but even then late recurrences up to 12 months can occur.

Systemic treatment of infections

Glycopeptides (vancomycin and teicoplanin), either alone or in combination with other agents, are the choice of treatment for severe infections (Fraise, 1998). Vancomycin resistance has been described, but at present it is rare. Other anti-staphylococcal agents (e.g. rifampicin, erythromycin, ciprofloxacin, clindamycin, trimethoprim, minocycline or an aminoglycoside) may be used in combination for treating infections with vancomycin-resistant strains or less serious infections (British Society of Antimicrobial Chemotherapy, Hospital Infection Society and Infection Control Nurses Association, 1998, Anon., 1999). The strain should be sensitive to both agents in the combination.

Communication and staff education

These are important, and they apply to various departments (e.g. radiotherapy, physiotherapy and ambulance staff).

INFECTIONS DUE TO GRAM-NEGATIVE BACILLI (OTHER THAN INTESTINAL PATHOGENS)

Gram-negative infection is often due to self-infection from the patient's own bowel flora, but cross-infection is also common (including infections first acquired by the patient's intestinal flora from hospital food). Gram-negative bacilli are usually transferred by contact; airborne spread is rare. Transfer on the hands of staff is probably the main route of spread, although contaminated solutions or equipment are sometimes responsible for infection. Precautions against contact transfer should be taken for all infections, but for patients infected with Gram-negative bacilli (with the exception of some severe *Pseudomonas aeruginosa* infections and highly resistant strains) isolation in a single room should be given a lower priority than for patients with epidemic staphylococcal infection. Combined infection of wounds with staphylococci and Gram-negative bacilli is common, but *Pseudomonas aeruginosa* is less likely to spread by air then *Staphylococcus aureus*. Patients infected with highly resistant Gram-negative bacilli in special units – such as neonatal or intensive care units (especially in the presence of patients on mechanical ventilation), ophthalmic and neurosurgical units – or areas where patients are treated with immunosuppressive drugs should be isolated in single rooms because of the difficulty of preventing the spread of infection and the high susceptibility of the patients. If infection occurs in a ward where patients are particularly susceptible, staff should use povidone-iodine, chlorhexidine detergent or a 70% ethanol preparation for hand disinfection, and if it is necessary to bathe patients with discharging wounds, povidone-iodine detergent should be used for bathing. Since many of these hospital strains are resistant to several antibiotics, the rational use of antibiotics is important (Goldmann *et al.*, 1996).

INFECTIONS DUE TO LANCEFIELD GROUP A, β-HAEMOLYTIC STREPTOCOCCI (*STREPTOCOCCUS PYOGENES*)

These organisms can spread both by contact and through the air. All patients with infections in maternity units should be isolated in a hospital isolation unit or in single rooms, and treated with an appropriate antibiotic (e.g. benzylpenicillin or penicillin V for 7 days for mild infections), except for those with burns (see below). In an outbreak (two or more cases), staff and patients should be screened (nose, throat and lesion swabs) and staff carriers should be excluded from duty and treated. Other sources in patients may also be sought (e.g. vaginal and rectal lesions, and umbilical lesions in neonates). Staff carriers should be kept off duty for at least 3 days after commencing treatment. If the outbreak is not controlled, repeat swabbing is required and prophylactic treatment of all patients and staff should be considered. Patients in other wards, particularly surgical wards, with profusely discharging wounds or extensive skin sepsis due to this organism should be given a high priority for isolation. Failures of treatment with penicillin should be treated with a β-lactamase-stable antibiotic such as flucloxacillin or cefuroxime, and patients with colonized burns should initially be treated with flucloxacillin or erythromycin. All colonized burns patients (throat and burn) should be isolated and treated.

INFECTIONS DUE TO LANCEFIELD GROUP B STREPTOCOCCI

Outbreaks occasionally occur in neonatal wards. Early-onset infections are usually acquired from the mother, whereas late-onset infections may be acquired by cross-infection. In an outbreak, infected babies are isolated and treated with benzylpenicillin for 7 days. Swabs are taken from the throat and umbilicus of all babies, and carriers are treated with penicillin. The umbilici of all babies are treated with alcoholic chlorhexidine, and the babies are bathed with chlorhexidine detergent.

OUTBREAKS OF DIARRHOEA AND/OR VOMITING (see also Chapter 10)

Such outbreaks are commonly due to bacterial infection or intoxication, viral infection or, rarely, to chemical intoxication. One of the commonest causes of outbreaks of diarrhoea and vomiting in hospitals is the Norwalk virus, one of a group of viruses known as small round structured virus (SRSV). This infection has an acute onset and lasts 24–48 hours. It can spread by the airborne route as well as by contact and, although mild, can have serious consequences in debilitated patients. Closing the ward to new admissions and limiting transfers to other wards as soon as infection due to this agent is suspected is the most effective way of controlling an outbreak. Reinfection can occur, and staff are often affected. Infectivity lasts for approximately 48 hours after cessation of symptoms.

Occasionally, outbreaks may be traced to food. If a food source is suspected, a case-control study should be performed to implicate a particular food item. Consultants for Communicable Disease Control and environmental health officers may need to be involved at this stage.

INCUBATION PERIODS OF INTESTINAL INFECTIONS

Table 9.2 Incubation periods

Food poisoning	
Staphylococcus aureus	2–6 hours
Bacillus cereus	1–5 hours or 10–16 hours
Vibrio parahaemolyticus	8–16 hours
Clostridium perfringens	8–24 hours
Salmonella species	12–48 hours
Campylobacter species	2–5 days
Other organisms	
Shigella species	3–5 days
Enteropathogenic *E.coli*	1–3 days
Rotaviruses	1–2 days

Salmonella infections are particularly hazardous in neonatal, geriatric and psychiatric units. Campylobacter infections are now more common than salmonella, but infrequently cause hospital outbreaks. Rotavirus infections are the commonest cause of intestinal infection in neonatal nurseries, but also occur in paediatric and geriatric wards. Enteropathogenic or enterotoxic *E.coli* infections also occur in infant nurseries, but are now infrequent. Small outbreaks, probably of viral origin, are common in geriatric and psychiatric wards.

INVESTIGATION

1 Arrangements should be made to ensure that ward staff immediately report possible outbreaks to the infection control team and send specimens of faeces and/or vomit to the laboratory.
2 Infection control staff should visit wards and collect epidemiological data on onset of infection (e.g. whether one or more wards are involved, whether staff are affected and what food was eaten by infected patients). If food poisoning is suspected, a dietary history of infected patients and staff, and of non-infected controls, should also be investigated.
3 Arrangements should be made for isolation of infected patients (salmonella) or closure of the ward. Staff should be instructed in hygienic techniques.
4 If food poisoning is suspected, samples of suspect food should be collected from the kitchen. Catering staff should be questioned about symptoms, and samples of faeces should be collected if necessary. Hygienic practices in the kitchens should be investigated. A case–control study may be helpful in establishing the cause.
5 The Consultant in Communicable Disease Control (CCDC) should be notified if a notifiable disease or food poisoning is involved, and the environmental health officer if food poisoning is suspected.

Procedures for infection control in hospital have been outlined in a Department of Health document (Department of Health, 1995). Most outbreaks in hospitals will be small and can be managed by the infection control team without additional resources. Often no causative organism will be isolated and no further case will occur. If the outbreak is large or particularly severe (e.g. responsible for deaths in patients), the outbreak committee should be assembled and the procedures outlined on p. 22 should be adopted where applicable. It is particularly important to appoint a spokesperson to keep the media informed. A daily meeting of the outbreak committee may be necessary in the early stages of the outbreak.

A particular problem may occur if staff are also infected. If no cause has been found for an outbreak of diarrhoea, nursing staff can be allowed to return to work when they have been symptom-free for 48 hours. Instructions on hygienic precautions should be given. Catering staff who have been infected should not handle food until three negative faecal samples have been obtained. In the event of prolonged carriage, a discussion between occupational health, infection control departments and the manager involved may be necessary to determine the future of the individual.

ANTIBIOTIC-ASSOCIATED COLITIS/ PSEUDOMEMBRANOUS COLITIS

This is an infection caused by *Clostridium difficile*, which is a toxin-producing organism carried in the intestinal tract. It is usually associated with antibiotic therapy. Although clindamycin is thought to be a major risk factor, cephalosporins may represent a greater risk. Infection occurs most frequently in neonates or in the elderly. The spores survive well in the environment and have been isolated from floors, bedpans and the hands of staff. The infection usually occurs sporadically, but outbreaks have been reported (Cartmill et al., 1994; Department of Health/PHLS Working Group, 1994). Transfer on instruments such as sigmoidoscopes has been suggested. Infected patients should be treated with metronidazole or vancomycin and nursed with excretion precautions (e.g. gloves and disposable aprons). Handwashing by staff before and after handling patients and their environment is the most important control measure. Vancomycin is no longer recommended as a first-line treatment because it is a risk factor for the development of outbreaks due to vancomycin-resistant enterococci. During a possible outbreak, infected patients should be isolated if possible. Thorough cleaning of the ward with a detergent is recommended before reopening. Clostridium difficile is resistant to most disinfectants, but is killed by 2% glutaraldehyde in 10 min (see p. 84). However, single-use or autoclaved instruments should preferably be used on infected patients.

ENTEROCOCCAL INFECTIONS

Outbreaks of enterococcal infections have been increasingly reported in recent years (Wade, 1995). Some strains show increased resistance to glycopeptides, such as vancomycin, and may occasionally produce β-lactamase. There have been outbreaks of infection due to vancomycin-resistant enterococci, predominantly in renal units and in other tertiary centres, but they are becoming increasingly widespread. These strains are of particular concern, as there are few currently available antibiotics which can be used to treat them. Strains are often resistant to high levels of aminoglycoside, which reduces the effectiveness of combined β-lactam and aminoglycoside therapy. Enterococci are part of the normal flora of the gastrointestinal tract and may be selected by the use of third-generation cephalosporins or quinolones. Infection with resistant strains tends to occur in longstanding intra-abdominal or urinary tract infections and neurological diseases in severely ill or immunosuppressed patients, after repeated courses of antibiotics. Rapid identification of an epidemic strain and surveillance of faecal cultures is important (Hospital Infection Control Practices Advisory Committee, 1994). Spread is believed to be mainly via the hands of staff, but adequate decontamination of bedpans and urine bottles and effective care of indwelling catheters are also important. Enterococci are relatively resistant to heat, and therefore thermal disinfection may not always be adequate unless it is combined with effective cleaning (Bradley and Fraise, 1996). Patients who are infected or colonized with resistant strains should preferably be isolated, and excessive use of vancomycin, aminoglycosides, third-generation cephalosporins, vancomycin and quinolones should be avoided (Goldmann et al., 1996). If there are a number of cases, a cohort ward with dedicated nursing staff and equipment is recommended (Jochimsen et al., 1999).

INFECTIONS DUE TO *CLOSTRIDIUM PERFRINGENS* AND OTHER GAS-GANGRENE BACILLI

Hospital-acquired infection with *Clostridium perfringens* is almost always post-operative and derived from the patient's own bowel flora. Gas gangrene is rare, but it occasionally follows orthopaedic operations on the leg (especially above the knee) when the arterial blood supply is defective, and may occur after certain abdominal operations.

Because gas-gangrene bacilli which are no different to those that cause infection are carried in abundance by most healthy individuals in their bowel flora, and are also commonly found in the environmental air and dust, there is no reason to close a theatre after operations on patients with clostridial infection. All that is needed is a thorough routine cleaning of the theatre after the operation. Although, for the same reason, isolation to prevent cross-infection with *Clostridium perfringens* is unnecessary, a patient with gas gangrene should preferably be nursed in an isolation room because he or she is dangerously ill and requires special nursing care.

ISOLATION OF PATIENTS WITH BURNS
(Ayliffe and Lawrence, 1985)

Patients with burns are commonly thought to require protective isolation before the burns become infected, and to require source isolation if they do become infected. In practice, the burns are infected for at least 24 hours before this state can be recognized by bacterial cultures. Moreover, a patient may be infected with one pathogen (e.g. *Staphylococcus aureus*) but for the time being be free from other pathogens (e.g. *Pseudomonas aeruginosa*) from which he or she should be protected. For these reasons it is logical to use combined source and protective isolation for extensive burns.

Many burns, especially those of small or moderate extent, can be kept free from bacterial colonization for long periods by topical chemoprophylaxis (e.g. with 0.5% silver nitrate solution or silver sulphadiazine cream) (see Chapter 16). Segregation in cubicles, even with mechanical ventilation, has been shown to have little protective value for burned patients in a burns unit. Good barrier nursing techniques (especially the use of gloves for handling the patient) and topical chemoprophylaxis are of particular importance for such patients. Isolation in single bedrooms facilitates the aseptic handling of extensively burned patients and should be instituted. Such single bedrooms should ideally have plenum ventilation and an exhaust ventilated airlock. If no airlock is provided, the extracted air should not be discharged into the ward. For smaller burns, given effective local chemoprophylaxis, barrier nursing in an open ward with exudate precautions is acceptable, provided that the dressings can be changed in a mechanically ventilated dressing-room.

If a patient with burns (whether small or extensive) is in a general surgical ward, it is of the utmost importance that he or she should be source-isolated in a single bedroom. If a patient is nursed in such a room, it should be remembered that although staphylococci are commonly transferred by air, Gram-negative infections of burns, when not acquired from the patient's faecal flora, are more often acquired by contact. Barrier nursing techniques are more effective in preventing cross-infection of the patient than physical segregation by the walls that surround him or her, although this will facilitate barrier nursing and reduce the risk of cross-infection by discouraging unnecessary visits.

LEGIONNAIRE'S DISEASE (LEGIONELLA PNEUMONIA)

This is a potentially severe respiratory infection which was first recognized in 1976. It is caused by a Gram-negative bacillus, *Legionella pneumophila,* and several other related species. The organism is widely distributed in nature and is commonly found in soil and surface waters. It multiplies over a temperature range varying from 20°C to over 40°C. Colonization of static water is likely, and the organism may commonly be found in the hot-water systems of large buildings such as hospitals, hotels and offices, usually without any evidence of infection among staff or patients. Outbreaks have originated from air-conditioning systems, particularly their associated cooling towers. Hot-water systems and showers have also been recognized as sources of infection (Bartlett *et al.*, 1986; Fallon, 1994). However, the exact source of the outbreak is often far from easy to establish. Outbreaks in the UK have been reported in hospitals, usually new ones, and occasionally in hotels and other large buildings with cooling towers. Sporadic cases also occur in the community, with no recognizable source. Although some aspects of the epidemiology of the disease remain obscure, there is no evidence of person-to-person spread, nor is infection thought to be acquired by ingestion. It is believed that the pneumonia is acquired by inhaling fine aerosols consisting of *Legionella*-containing particles about 5 μ in diameter which are able to find their way into the lung alveoli. From this it also follows that some mechanism for generating a fine spray of *Legionella*-contaminated water should be sought as a possible source of any outbreak (e.g. cooling-tower drift, showers, 'whirlpools', etc.). The elderly, especially those with pre-existing chronic respiratory tract disease, and the immunosuppressed are particularly susceptible, but the disease can occur at any age. The organism has probably been one of the causes of pneumonia, particularly in the elderly, for many years, and the risk of acquiring legionella, as distinct from other pneumonias (e.g. pneumococcal pneumonia) has been exaggerated. Legionella has been reported to be responsible for 2–7% of community-acquired pneumonia.

Early detection of cases of infection is of major importance, and is usually based initially on clinical suspicion by the clinician or microbiologist. Sputum, if obtainable, is usually mucoid and shows scanty neutrophils and no predominant organism. Legionella can sometimes be identified by direct immunofluorescence and by culture of sputum, but usually additional techniques such as trans-tracheal or bronchial aspiration or lung biopsy are required. Antibody levels in the acutely ill are often of little help, but diagnosis can be made at a later stage if a fourfold increase is obtained, or a single high titre (>128), particularly if specific IgM is detected. Serotyping of the legionella strain may be useful if an epidemiological investigation is required. Isolation of the patient is unnecessary for infection control purposes, but may be indicated because of the severity of the established disease and the untoward publicity associated with it.

If the patient has been in hospital for 10 days or more, it is likely that infection was acquired in hospital, and enquiries may reveal other possible cases, which can be confirmed by antibody tests. However, further investigation is not usually warranted following a sporadic case, as legionellas are commonly found in hospital water supplies. These are rarely associated with infection, and control measures could be excessive and unnecessarily expensive.

Two or more cases warrant further investigation, which would include case–control studies, antibody testing and sampling of possible environmental sources. If there is evidence of a community-acquired outbreak, or if an extensive investigation is likely, the Public Health Laboratory Service should be asked for assistance as soon as possible. The outbreak committee should be convened and the hospital engineer should be co-opted.

If environmental sampling is required, this should be done before any control measures are instituted.

Five-litre samples of water should be collected from all known potential sources (e.g. hot and cold water systems and cooling towers). Samples should be taken from the mains supplies, holding tanks, calorifiers, hot and cold taps and showers. Temperatures should be recorded at hot-water taps both at the time of sampling and 3 minutes later. If a cooling tower is a possible source, samples should be taken from various points in the pipework, the cooling water return at the top and from the pond.

Routine sampling of the water supplies is not recommended, except possibly in wards for immunosuppressed patients, but a follow-up for a limited period is advisable after measures have been introduced to control an outbreak.

The elimination of legionellas from a water supply depends on chlorination or raising the temperature.

Chlorination of a cooling tower may be achieved by addition of a hypochlorite solution or tablets to give a level of available chlorine of 5 mg/L (ppm) for a period of several hours followed by cleaning and rechlorination. Higher levels of available chlorine (e.g. up to 50 mg/L) have been recommended. Levels of 50 mg/L are also suggested in header tanks for disinfection of hot or cold water supply systems. Continuous chlorination to give levels of 1–2 mg/L available chlorine is an expensive alternative. Moreover, metal corrosion may be a long-term consequence of continuous or repeated chlorination.

It is also recommended that hot water should be stored in tanks (calorifiers at 60°C and distributed to taps at 52°C ± 2°C). These temperatures are not always easy to achieve in practice, nor can they be relied upon to destroy the organism. In addition, patients, particularly the elderly and confused, must be protected from accidental scalding.

Good maintenance of equipment is the main preventative measure (Department of Health and Social Security, 1989; Health and Safety Executive, 1995).

Hospital engineers should ensure that water systems are correctly designed and adequately maintained. For example, storage tanks should have an adequate flow rate and have well-fitted covers, calorifiers should have facilities for easy drainage and cleaning and stratification should be minimized, 'dead legs' should be avoided, water pipes should be lagged to prevent incidental heating of cold-water pipes and loss of temperature from hot-water pipes, and washers should be replaced as necessary with approved types which do not support the growth of legionella. Cooling towers should be cleaned at least twice yearly and treated with appropriate biocides and corrosion inhibitors. Cold-water supplies should be maintained at 20°C or less.

Legionnaire's disease can also be transmitted by whirlpools, humidifiers and nebulizers. This equipment should be treated with hypochlorites, or if nebulizers are used for respiratory therapy they can either be disposable or disinfected by heat (e.g. low-temperature steam), although occasionally chemical disinfection may be required. Legionella is widely distributed, and it is not known why infection occurs on some occasions and not others. In the absence of infection it is not recommended that expensive additional measures are introduced. However, careful surveillance of patients to detect cases is necessary in hospitals, particularly in units for immunosuppressed patients.

ASPERGILLUS INFECTIONS

Invasive aspergillus infections occur mainly in highly immunocompromised patients, and particularly in liver and bone-marrow transplant patients. Prolonged neutropenia and use of high-dose steroids are important risk factors (Manuel and Kibbler, 1998).

Aspergilli (*Aspergillus fumigatus, Aspergillus niger* and *Aspergillus flavus*) are always present in air, dust, soil, etc., and infection mainly occurs through inhalation of airborne spores. Most outbreaks have been associated with demolition and renovation of adjacent buildings, presumably associated with the release of an unusually large number of spores. Occasional outbreaks have been associated with the release of spores within the hospital (e.g. from service ducts and contaminated filters in ventilation systems).

PREVENTION OF ASPERGILLI INFECTION

High-risk units (e.g. liver and bone-marrow transplantation units) should be provided with filtered air (Rhame, 1991). The filters should be capable of removing spores (diameter 2–3 μ). High-efficiency particulate air (HEPA) filters are commonly recommended, and these remove 99.97% of particles 0.3 μ in diameter (Tablan *et al.*, 1994). Laminar flow is not required.

The effectiveness of conventional filters of operating-room type removing 90% of particles 5 μ in diameter is uncertain, but these are probably adequate for most leukaemia units. If adjacent building operations are in progress, it is important to ensure that all windows are sealed. Service ducts passing through high-risk wards should be sealed. If an outbreak has occurred, the ward surfaces should be thoroughly cleaned with a solution of a chlorine-releasing agent (1000 ppm available chlorine), service ducts and windows should be sealed and a portable HEPA filtering unit should be introduced. A window unit introducing some external filtered air (e.g. 20%), in addition to recirculated filtered air, has the advantage of providing a positive pressure in the room. During an outbreak, prophylaxis with an antifungal agent (e.g. amphotericin B or itraconazole) may also be considered.

CRYPTOSPORIDIOSIS

Cryptosporidiosis is a diarrhoeal disease caused by protozoa that are species of *Cryptosporidium*. Infection is commonly acquired from water supplies, and is a common complication of HIV infection. Spread of infection in hospital has been rarely reported (Lettau, 1991a). *Cryptosporidium* oocysts are resistant to 70% ethanol, iodophors, chlorine-releasing agents, quaternary ammonium compounds and aldehydes over practicable exposure times. High concentrations of chlorine dioxide, ozone, hydrogen peroxide, peracetic acid and ammonia may be effective, but further tests are necessary under practical conditions (Department of the Environment and Health, 1990). There is no effective treatment for clinical infections, but thorough cleaning of contaminated equipment should minimize the likelihood of spread.

VIRAL HAEMORRHAGIC FEVERS (VHF)

These virus infections (Lassa fever, Marburg disease and Ebola virus and Crimean/Congo haemorrhagic fever) are endemic in West and Central Africa, parts of South America and some rural parts of the Middle East and Eastern Europe. All of them have a significant mortality, and there is no vaccine available. Treatment with tribavirin is effective in Lassa fever, which is the commonest of these infections. Lassa fever is contracted by humans from a rodent, *Mastomys natalensis,* which is widely distributed in Africa but not in Europe. Human-to-human transmission of infection is probably uncommon, and the risk of epidemic spread in the UK population is negligible. The incubation period of these infections is usually 7–10 days, with a range of 3–17 days. For control purposes, if no infection has occurred within a period of up to 21 days from exposure, a contact is usually considered to be free from infection (for more information, see *Management and Control of Viral Haemorrhagic Fevers*; Advisory Committee on Dangerous Pathogens, 1996). Hantaviruses can cause a haemorrhagic fever, but person-to-person spread has not been reported.

EARLY IDENTIFICATION OF KNOWN OR SUSPECTED CASES

A medical practitioner who suspects that a patient might be suffering from a viral haemorrhagic fever (on the basis of pyrexial illness, occupation or residence in an endemic area) should not refer the patient to hospital but should immediately seek the advice of a consultant in communicable or tropical diseases. If the patient is already in hospital, he or she should be confined in a single room until he or she has been seen by the consultant. If a suspected case arrives in a casualty department, the infection control doctor should be informed, and the patient should be placed in a room specially designated for this purpose, where a box containing special protective clothing is available. There is considerable urgency about making contact with the appropriate expert not only for epidemiological purposes, but also to exclude *Plasmodium falciparum* malaria, which can be rapidly fatal, as a cause of the illness. Typhoid fever should also be excluded.

In practical terms, the above advice applies to any patient with a pyrexia of unknown origin that arises during a period of 21 days after arrival from West or Central Africa. It is the duty of the medical practitioner who first sees the patient and/or the second opinion to notify the CCDC at the earliest possible opportunity.

The memorandum on *Management and Control of Viral Haemorrhagic Fevers* (Advisory Committee on Dangerous Pathogens, 1996) recommends that suspect patients should be graded according to the degree of suspicion (high, moderate or minimal risk). Recent evidence suggests that spread will not occur if adequate blood and body fluid precautions are taken. In countries without a high-security infectious diseases unit, patients may be isolated in a single room with blood and body fluid precautions (Holmes *et al.*, 1990).

RISK CATEGORIES

High risk
- A febrile patient from a known endemic area (usually viral) during the 3 weeks before illness who lived or stayed for more than 4 hours in a house where there were ill, feverish individuals known or strongly suspected to have a VHF.
- An individual who took part in nursing or caring for a person strongly suspected of having VHF or contact with body fluids, tissues or the dead body of such a patient.
- A laboratory, health or other worker who is likely to have come into contact with the body fluids or tissues of such a patient.
- An individual who has been in contact with such a patient or body fluids, but who has not been in an endemic area.

Moderate risk
- A febrile patient from an endemic area (usually viral) during the past 3 weeks, but with no other risk factors.
- A febrile patient who is not from a known endemic area, but who has suspicious symptoms.

Minimal risk

- A febrile patient who has not been in a known endemic area (e.g. who has been in a major city where the risk is negligible).
- A febrile patient from an endemic area (or in contact with a known or suspected source), more than 21 days after their first contact with a source.

A history of malaria prophylaxis should also be considered when grading the degree of suspicion.

ACTION

High risk

Admit the patient to a high-security infectious diseases unit. The CCDC should be informed so that they can carry out surveillance of close contacts for 21 days.

Moderate suspicion

Admit the patient to a regional infectious diseases unit for strict isolation. Review the level of suspicion if the illness proves to be more consistent with VHF, and if malaria and other infections have been excluded. The CCDC should be notified. Contacts should be identified, but need not be kept under surveillance unless the patient is re-categorized as high risk.

Minimal suspicion

Admit the patient to a regional infectious diseases unit or a district general hospital isolation unit with blood/body fluid precautions. A consultant in infectious diseases should review the case. If there is no immediate threat to life, the patient may remain at home.

With high and moderate risk categories, patients must be transported using specific ambulance precautions and laboratory specimens should be examined in a high-security (Category 4) laboratory. If the level of suspicion is high, and the patient is seen in the Accident and Emergency department or has been admitted to a ward, the hospital outbreaks committee should be convened to decide on the action required.

The names and addresses of close contacts of known infected patients should be obtained and surveillance should be continued for 21 days. If the patient is in a ward he or she should be transferred to a side room of the same ward and strict isolation precautions instituted involving a minimal number of staff (e.g. the doctor making the diagnosis and one nurse present).

NOTES

1 Protective clothing (cap, gown, mask, gloves and overshoes) and a disposable urinal and bedpan should be available in a box in the emergency department. This box can be taken to a ward if necessary or provided for the ambulance service.
2 Particular care is required in the disposal of blood, urine and faeces. The viruses are susceptible to the usual antiviral disinfectants. Autoclaving in the laboratory is preferable, but a hypochlorite solution would be appropriate, prior to incineration.

The CCDC is responsible for surveillance of contacts and for terminal disinfection of wards, departments or ambulances, but advice on disinfection should be obtained from the infection control doctor, who will usually be responsible for these procedures within the hospital.

3   Although all laboratory samples should be examined in a secure containment laboratory, films for malaria, after they have been rendered microbiologically safe (e.g. with formaldehyde), can be examined in the routine hospital laboratory as this is an urgent investigation.

More detailed information on surveillance of contacts, terminal disinfection and disposal of corpses, etc., can be found in the guidelines of the Advisory Committee on Dangerous Pathogens (1996).

RABIES

Human-to-human transmission of rabies has never been reported, and the strict precautions recommended for the prevention of transmission are therefore unnecessary in terms of risk assessment. However, the disease has emotive connotations for hospital staff, while the intensive medical and nursing care which is essential if the patient is to have any chance of survival increases the likelihood of exposure to infection.

The following precautions are recommended.

1   The patient should be isolated in a single room, preferably in an intensive therapy unit.
2   Attendant staff and other close contacts (e.g. anaesthetists) should be offered immunization with human diploid cell vaccine (4 intradermal injections of 0.1 mL given on the same day).
3   Staff should wear protective clothing, including goggles, mask and gloves.
4   Mouth-to-mouth resuscitation should not be used.
5   Pregnant female staff should not attend the patient.
6   Specimens from the patient should not be sent to routine diagnostic laboratories but only to a laboratory equipped for handling hazard group 3 pathogens. Prior notice is essential.
7   Equipment soiled by secretions or excretions must be destroyed or autoclaved. Further information is contained in the *Memorandum on Rabies* (Department of Health and Social Security, 1977).

HUMAN INFESTATION

Biting insects and burrowing mites may cause irritation, and scratching may lead to infections such as impetigo. Although insects and mites are unlikely to be a major source of infection in hospitals in the UK, the problem of infestation is often referred to infection control staff (Lettau, 1991b).

Lists of insecticides and acaricides suitable for treatment of the skin can be found in the *British Pharmacopoeia* or the *British National Formulary*. These include dosages, methods of application and contraindications. Most health authorities operate a rotating policy for the treatment of head lice to suppress the emergence of resistant strains. Details of the drugs currently recommended should be available from a pharmaceutical officer.

LICE

All three species of human lice are bloodsucking insects which are host-specific. The head and crab (pubic) lice are usually found in specific areas (e.g. scalp and pubic hair), but can also occur in the axillae, chest, legs, beard and eyebrows. The nits (eggs) are firmly attached to hair and not easily removed. Body lice are found mainly in clothing, but also on the body surface, especially in the axillae and around the waist. Superficial skin infection due to scratching is common.

Control measures
1 Carefully remove all clothing of patients with body or pubic lice and seal it in a bag. Disposable gloves and a plastic apron should be worn.
2 Process linen in the laundry in a washing-machine using conventional heat treatment.
3 In infestation with head or crab lice, treat the specific hairy areas of the host with an appropriate insecticidal lotion, such as 0.5% carbaryl or malathion or permethrin (1%), and repeat within 7–10 days. Patients with body lice do not require specific treatment but should be bathed.
4 No special treatment of the environment is required, as spread is by personal contact. However, body lice are capable of surviving for a limited time in stored clothing, but head and pubic lice rapidly die when detached from their host.

SCABIES (ITCH MITES)

Scabies is an allergic reaction to the presence of a small mite (0.3–0.4 mm in length) which burrows into the top layer of the skin. Symptoms consist of intense itching which may persist for some time after effective treatment, and the appearance of a hypersensitive rash. Burrows may occur anywhere, but are mainly on the hands and arms, and particularly the finger-webs. The associated rash is usually on the groin, elbows, inside thighs and around the wrists and waist. Transmission is by person-to person contact, and is usually assumed to require fairly prolonged and intimate contact. Hand-holding or patient support for long periods is probably responsible for most hospital-acquired scabies. Spread from bedding, clothing or fomites is unlikely. However, in elderly or immunosuppressed patients the mites multiply rapidly and large numbers of the parasites are present. This form of scabies is often known as 'crusty' or 'Norwegian' scabies, and is far more readily transmissible.

Control measures
1 Apply a suitable ascaricide, such as 0.5% malathion or 1% permethrin, to all areas of the body. A bath is not necessary prior to treatment, but if a bath is

given the skin must be thoroughly dry before applying the ascaricide, and it should not be washed off for 24 hours. If this is done effectively a second treatment should be unnecessary.

2 Treat bedding and clothing as described for lice.

3 No special environmental control measures are necessary.

4 Refer members of the patient's family and those in close physical contact to their general practitioner so that they can be treated if necessary.

FLEAS

Infestation is usually with dog, cat or bird fleas, which will bite humans in the absence of the preferred host. The human flea is more likely to be introduced from outside the hospital, but is now fortunately rare. Fleas are able to survive for several months in the environment without feeding. Elimination of the host or treatment of pets and the use of suitable insecticides on environmental surfaces is therefore essential if control is to be effective.

Control measures (patient admitted with fleas)

1 Remove all clothing and bedding and seal them in a bag. Whenever possible, process linen in the laundry in a washing-machine using conventional heat treatment. A hot-water-soluble plastic bag will allow transfer to the machine without handling. Clothing that is not suitable for washing may be sealed in a laundry bag and treated with low-temperature steam or a suitable insecticide.

2 Use aerosol dispensers containing insecticide to kill fleas and arrange with your pest control operative to treat surfaces in the environment concerned.

Control measures (infestation in a hospital ward)

1 Identify the flea and, if possible, treat or remove the host. If it is a cat flea, take steps to exclude feral cats from the site.

2 Heat treat clothing and bedding as described above.

3 Vacuum-clean floors, carpets, upholstery, fabrics, etc.

4 Contact your pest control operative to treat the environment (e.g. ducting, hard surfaces, and under fixtures) with a residual insecticide.

For further advice on control management of lice, scabies and human infestations, contact the Medical Entomology Centre at the University of Cambridge, Department of Applied Biology, Pembroke Street, Cambridge. (For details of Pharaoh's ants, see p. 252).

REFERENCES

Advisory Committee on Dangerous Pathogens (1996) *Management and control of viral haemorrhagic fevers* London: HMSO.

Anon. (1999) Tackling antimicrobial resistance. *Drug and Therapeutics Bulletin* 37, 9.

Ayliffe, G.A.J. and Lawrence, J.C. (1985) *Symposium on infection control in burns. Journal of Hospital Infection* 6 (**Supplement B**).

Ayliffe, G.A.J., Cookson, B.D., Ducel, G. *et al.* (1995) World Health Working Group on the global control of MRSA. Geneva: World Health Organization.

Ayliffe, G.A.J., Babb, J.R. and Taylor, L. (1999) *Hospital-acquired infection. Principles and prevention,* 3rd edn. London: Butterworth Heinemann (1995).

Bartlett, C.L.R., Macrae, A.D. and Macfarlane, J.D. (1986) *Legionella infections.* London: Edward Arnold.

Bradley, C.R. and Fraise, A.P. (1996) Heat and chemical resistance of enterococci. *Journal of Hospital Infection* 16, 191.

British Society of Antimicrobial Chemotherapy, Hospital Infection Society and Infection Control Nurses Association (1998) Report of a combined working party. Revised guidelines for the control of epidemic methicillin-resistant *Staphylococcus aureus* in hospitals. *Journal of Hospital Infection* 39, 253.

Cartmill, T.D.I., Panigraphi, H., Worsley, M.A. *et al.* (1994) Management and control of large outbreaks of diarrhoea due to *Clostridium difficile. Journal of Hospital Infection* 27, 1.

Cookson, B.D. (1998) The emergence of mupirocin resistance: a challenge to infection control and antibiotic-prescribing practice. *Journal of Antimicrobial Chemotherapy* 41, 11.

Department of the Environment and Health (1990) *Report of the Group of Experts on* Cryptosporidium *in water supplies.* London: HMSO.

Department of Health (1995) *Hospital infection control. Guidance on the control of infection in hospitals. Report of the Hospital Infection Working Group of the Department of Health and Public Health Laboratory Service.* London: Department of Health.

Department of Health/PHLS Working Group (1994) *The prevention and management of* Clostridium difficile *infections.* London: Department of Health.

Department of Health and Social Security (1977) *Memorandum on rabies.* London: HMSO.

Department of Health and Social Security (1989) *Report of the Expert Advisory Committee on Biocides.* London: HMSO.

Fallon, R.J. (1994) How to prevent an outbreak of Legionnaire's disease. *Journal of Hospital Infection* 27, 247.

Fraise, A.P. (1998) Guidelines for the control of methicillin-resistant *Staphylococcus aureus. Journal of Antimicrobial Chemotherapy* 42, 287.

Fraise, A.P., Mitchell, K., O'Brien, S.J.O. *et al.* (1997) Methicillin-resistant *Staphylococcus aureus* (MRSA) in nursing homes in a major UK city: an anonymised point prevalence survey. *Epidemiology and Infection* 118, 1.

Goldmann, D.A., Weinstein, R.A., Wenzel, R.P. *et al.* (1996) Strategies to prevent and control the emergence and spread of antimicrobial-resistant micro-organisms in hospital: a challenge to hospital leadership. *Journal of the American Medical Association* 275, 234.

Health and Safety Executive (1995) *The prevention and control of legionellosis.* Sudbury: HSE books.

Holmes, G.P., McCormick, J.B., Trock, C.C. *et al.* (1990) Lassa fever in the United States. Investigations of a case and new guidelines for management. *New England Journal of Medicine* 323, 1120.

Hospital Infection Control Practices Advisory Committee (1994) Recommendations for preventing the spread of vancomycin resistance. Recommendations of the Hospital Infection Control Practices Advisory Committee (HICPAC). *Morbidity and Mortality Weekly Report* **44 (Supplement RR-12)**, 1.

Hudson, I.R. (1994) The efficacy of intranasal mupirocin in the prevention of Staphylococcus infections. A review of recent experience. *Journal of Hospital Infection* **27**, 81.

Jochimsen, E.M., Fish, L., Manning, K. *et al.* (1999) Control of vancomycin-resistant enterococci in a community hospital. *Infection Control and Hospital Epidemiology* **20**, 106.

Johnson, A.P. (1998) Intermediate vancomycin resistance in *Staphylococcus aureus:* a major threat or a minor inconvenience? *Journal of Antimicrobial Chemotherapy* **42**, 289.

Lettau, L.A. (1991a) Nosocomial transmission and infection control aspects of parasitic and ectoparasitic disease. Part 1. *Infection Control and Hospital Epidemiology* **12**, 59.

Lettau, L.A. (1991b) Nosocomial transmission and infection control aspects of parasitic and ectoparasitic diseases. Part 3. *Infection Control and Hospital Epidemiology* **12**, 179.

Manuel, R.J. and Kibbler, C.C. (1998) The epidemiology and prevention of invasive aspergillosis. *Journal of Hospital Infection*, **39**, 95.

Marples, R.R., Richardson, J.F. and de Saxe, M.J. (1986) Bacteriological characters of strains of *Staphylococcus aureus* submitted to a reference laboratory related to methicillin resistance. *Journal of Hygiene* **96**, 217.

Mulligan, M.F. and Arbeit, R.D. (1991) Epidemiologic and clinical utility of typing systems for differentiating among strains of methicillin-resistant *Staphylococcus aureus*. *Infection Control and Hospital Epidemiology* **12**, 20.

Rhame, F.S. (1991) Prevention of nosocomial aspergillosis. *Journal of Hospital Infection* **18 (Supplement)**, 466.

Solberg, C.O. (1965) A study of carriers of *Staphylococcus aureus*. *Acta Medica Scandinavia*, **178 (Supplement 463)**.

Spicer, W.J. (1984) Three strategies in the control of staphylococci, including methicillin-resistant *Staphylococcus aureus*. *Journal of Hospital Infection* **5 (Supplement A)**, 466.

Streulens, M.J. (1996) Laboratory methods in the investigation of outbreaks of hospital-acquired infection. In Emmerson, A.M. and Ayliffe, G.A.J. (eds) *Surveillance of nosocomial infections. Clinical infectious diseases.* Vol. 3. London: Baillière Tindall.

Tablan, O.C., Anderson, L.J., Arden, N.H. *et al.* and the Hospital Infection Control Practices Committee (1994) Guidelines for the prevention of nosocomial pneumonia. *Infection Control and Hospital Epidemiology* **15**, 587.

Wade, J.J. (1995) The emergence of *Enterococcus faecium* resistant to glycopeptides and other standard agents – a preliminary report. *Journal of Hospital Infection* **30 (Supplement)**, 483.

Wenzel, R.P., Nettleman, M.D. and Pfaller, M.A. (1991) Methicillin-resistant *Staphylococcus aureus:* implications for the 1990s and effective control measures. *American Journal of Medicine* **91,** (Supplement 3B), 2215.

Wenzel, R.P., Reagan, D.R., Bertino, J.S. *et al.* (1998) Methicillin-resistant *Staphylococcus* outbreak: a consensus panel's definition and management guidelines. *American Journal of Hospital Control* **26,** 102.

Wilson, P. and Dunn, L.J. (1996) Using an MRSA isolation scoring system to decide whether patients should be nursed in isolation. *Hygiene Medicine* **21,** 465.

Working Party of the British Society of Antimicrobial Chemotherapy and the Hospital Infection Society (1995). Guidelines on the control of methicillin-resistant *Staphylococcus aureus* in the community. *Journal of Hospital Infection* **31,** 1.

chapter 10

CONTROL OF VIRAL HEPATITIS AND HUMAN IMMUNODEFICIENCY VIRUS (HIV) INFECTION

Deenan Pillay

Bloodborne viral infections represent a significant infection control problem in health-care settings. At present, the major concern rests with the hepatitis viruses B and C, and HIV 1 and 2. The infection control risks associated with hepatitis G virus are commensurate with the seemingly negligible clinical impact of this virus. The hepatitis viruses also include hepatitis A and E, both spread by the faecal–oral route, and hepatitis D, which requires the presence of hepatitis B in order to replicate. Thus all of the infection control implications of hepatitis B are relevant to hepatitis D virus (HDV).

VIRAL HEPATITIS

These viruses are traditionally grouped together purely because they infect the same organ. However, with respect to natural history and epidemiology they differ from each other. The bloodborne viruses will be discussed first.

HEPATITIS B

This disease has an incubation period of about 40–160 days, often about 90 days. The serum concentration of virus may approach 10^8–10^9 viral genome copies/mL, and virus can also be detected in saliva, semen and vaginal secretions. The commonest mode of acquisition of the infection world-wide is from mother to neonate, and these infants have a high risk of becoming lifelong carriers of the virus (defined as the presence of HB surface antigen [HBSAg] in serum for more than 6 months). Such individuals are also at a higher risk of developing the severe hepatic sequelae of HBV infection. Adults who acquire infection may be asymptomatic or suffer an acute hepatitis. However, they are likely to clear the virus (95% of cases) and become naturally immune.

Three different components of the virus may be detected in the serum of infected individuals. The presence of HBSAg defines an infection. HBSAg-positive individuals may also have 'e' antigen, which is associated with a highly infectious state. In contrast, the absence of 'e' and the presence of antibody to 'e' suggests low infectivity. Finally, serum HBV DNA can be detected and quantitated. These sensitive assays are used to predict and assess the response to drug therapy. As HB e Ag/Ab status can sometimes be a misleading surrogate of infectivity (due in part to the presence of viral variants which do not code for the e protein) it is likely that these markers will be replaced by HBV DNA quantitation (viral load) in future. Antibodies to core antigen (HB c Ab) develop soon after infection and persist, whether the infection is cleared or a carrier state develops. The presence of core antigen-specific IgM indicates recent acquisition of infection. By contrast, antibodies to S Ag only develop with clearance of surface antigen, and therefore signify immunity. Since HBV vaccine is composed of surface antigen alone, vaccine response is also assessed by the presence of these antibodies (Table 10.1).

The incidence of HBV infection ranges from 0.1 – 1.0% in the UK, USA and Northern Europe (low) to 4–5% in Southern Europe (medium) and more than 10% in the Far East and some areas of Africa (high). Screening of donated blood for HBSAg has minimized the risk of transfusion-associated HBV infection. Groups at higher risk of acquiring the infection include intravenous drug users and homosexual men and, where infection control procedures are suboptimal, renal dialysis patients and health-care workers (HCW).

Following a needlestick injury with blood from an 'e' Ag-positive HBV-infected patient, the risk of infection for a susceptible individual is estimated to be up to 40% (Table 10.2). HCW most at risk from such infection are those involved in invasive procedures, such as gynaecologists who often perform 'blind' deep pelvic surgery in which small innocuous cuts on their hands with suture needles are common, although non-apparent infection through mucous membranes may also occur. Of course, HBV infections in HCW may be due to risk activity outside work. As stated above, virus can be detected in saliva, albeit at 1000 to 10 000-fold lower concentration than in serum. Certainly transmission of HBV via bites has been documented, although mucosal contact with saliva poses little if any risk. In the UK, it is recommended that HCW who are e Ag-positive HBV carriers must not perform procedures where there is a risk that injury to themselves will result in their blood contaminating a patient's open tissues. This follows previous evidence that transmission of HBV from HCW to

Table 10.1 The meaning of HBV markers

	HBS Ag	HB core IgM	HB core Ab (total)	HB 'e' Ag	HB 'e' Ab	HBS Ab
Acute hepatitis	+/–	+	+	+/–	+/–	–
Chronic hepatitis	+	–	+	+/–	+/–	–
Natural immunity	–	–	+	–	–	+
Post-vaccine immunity	–	–	–	–	–	+

Table 10.2 Risks from occupational exposure to HBV, HCV and HIV[a]

Virus	Risk of infection from percutaneous contact (%)
HBV	2–40
HCV	3–10
HIV	0.2–0.5

[a] Adapted from Centers for Disease Control (1995).

patient was limited to such e Ag-positive staff. However, transmission from e Ag-negative surgeons has recently been documented, and a review of current guidance is being undertaken within the UK (Anon., 1997) (see below).

Treatment of chronic HBV with interferon has some benefit in producing loss of 'e' antigen. This is pertinent to 'e' Ag-positive HCW who have been prevented from continuing work, as long-term seroconversion to e Ag-negative status may allow a return to normal working. A number of newer nucleoside analogue drugs (e.g. lamivudine) demonstrate powerful anti-HBV activity, and these are now becoming available. Vaccination against HBV is by far the most important tool for eradication of this virus. The vaccine does not contain any genetic material of the virus, and is safe and effective. Passive immunization with hyperimmune globulin may be useful as an adjunct to active vaccination in the post-exposure prophylaxis setting (see below).

HBV VACCINATION OF HEALTH-CARE WORKERS

Immunization should be offered to those HCWs who have potential contact with blood or bloodstained body fluids, or with patients' tissues, including medical, dental, nursing, ancillary and technical staff. Current UK Department of Health guidelines stipulate that any HCW (including locum staff) involved in exposure-prone procedures must demonstrate evidence of an HBV vaccine response, or otherwise, that they are not infected with HBV, before starting work (see Figure 10.1). Such testing must be undertaken via an Occupational Health Department or, for instance, a general practitioner to ensure that the correct sample is tested (HCW who are aware of their HBV infection have been known to substitute a different sample to send to the laboratory) and that appropriate counselling can be instituted if necessary. Some medical schools now also require such evidence before acccepting students on to a medical course.

A full course of a recombinant HBV vaccine consists of 3 injections into the deltoid at 0, 1 and 6 months. In a low-prevalence region, such as the UK, pre-vaccine screening for evidence of prior infection or immunity to HBV is not cost-effective. Two months after the last dose, a blood sample should be tested for antibodies to HBSAg, reflecting the level of response to vaccine. A level of 10–50 mIU/ml is thought to be protective against infection, and 100 mIU/mL is therefore used as a safe cut-off value for determining a good vaccine response (see Table 10.3).

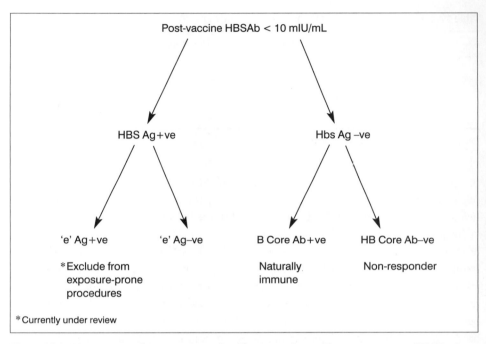

Figure 10.1 Management of exposure-prone health-care workers with non-response to HBV Vaccine.

It is expected that 90% of HCW will respond to vaccine. One reason for non-response is existing chronic HBV infection, and this should be checked for in non-responders. In such cases it is prudent first to check the post-vaccine blood sample for HB core antibodies. If a positive result is obtained, consent should be obtained before proceeding to HBSAg testing. However, most non-responders will be Hb Ab-negative, and therefore not infected (see Figure 10.1). A number of new HBV vaccines, incorporating additional immunogenic epitopes, are currently being evaluated, and should soon be available for those who do not respond to existing vaccines.

HEPATITIS D

This virus can only infect individuals in association with HBV. It is also spread parenterally. However, it is particularly prevalent among intravenous drug users, and in Southern Italy and parts of Eastern Europe. Prevention of HDV infection within a health-care setting is the same as for control of hepatitis B.

Table 10.3 Follow-up of HBV vaccines

Post-vaccine HBS Ab level (mIU/mL)	Action
< 10	Non-response
10–100	Booster 1 year
> 100	Booster 5 years

HEPATITIS C

Hepatitis C was identified in 1989 as the major cause of what had previously been known as post-transfusion non-A, non-B hepatitis. We now recognize that infection is commonly followed by long-term carriage, with up to 60–70% of infected individuals developing chronic liver disease after 20–30 years. Acute infection is often asymptomatic, and infection is therefore unlikely to be identified at this stage. It is estimated that there are 100 million HCV carriers world-wide, with a prevalence within Europe of 0.5 – 2% among the general population. Very high rates of infection are observed in intravenous drug users and haemophiliacs and, to a lesser extent, in haemodialysis patients. Transmission is therefore parenteral, although sexual and perinatal transmission has also been documented, albeit with far less frequency than hepatitis B (see Table 10.2). Of particular interest, around 40–50% of diagnosed HCV infections are of unknown source. Unlike HBV, the prevalence of HCV infection in HCW appears to be no greater than that in the general population, although needlestick transmission from patient to HCW has been described, and must therefore be seen as a potential risk.

Infection is diagnosed by the detection of antibodies to HCV. Infection diagnosed in this way should always be confirmed by further tests, as some antibody assays have less than optimal specificity. Increasingly, confirmation is undertaken by detection of the HCV viral genome in serum by the polymerase chain reaction (PCR), and the presence of virus in blood infers a potential infectious risk to others.

Combinations of interferon and ribavirin have good efficacy in clearing HCV virus from the circulation, although there is a significant rate of recurrence following cessation of treatment (Liang, 1998). The success of antiviral therapy can be predicted to some extent by the HCV genotype. This proven benefit of treatment may be seen by some as a rationale for actively following HCW who may have been infected by HCV. No vaccine is currently available, and there is no efficacy data for post-exposure prophylaxis.

HIV

This virus preferentially infects CD4+ T-lymphocytes, and leads to an inexorable immunodeficiency due primarily to a depletion of this class of T-cells. Primary infection is associated with a short-lived glandular fever-type 'seroconversion illness', which may include a widespread rash, flu-like symptoms and diarrhoea, as well as a generalized lymphadenopathy. This is then followed in the untreated individual by a long but variable asymptomatic period during which the total CD4 cell count declines. Quantitative plasma HIV RNA assays demonstrate a very large viral burden during this period, representing a rapid turnover of infected cells. The 'steady-state' viral load established following primary infection is predictive of the rapidity of progression of HIV disease. The data generated by these new assays also infers that HIV-infected patients are infectious to others throughout their infection. Although it is still the case that HIV infection inevitably leads to AIDS, the natural history of infection is changing, due to effective prophylactic therapies that reduce the risk of opportunistic infections such as pneumocystis and tuberculosis and the use of a range of antiretroviral drugs. These reverse transcriptase and protease inhibitors, when used in combination, can lead to dramatic reductions in the circulating viral load, which correlates with long-term clinical benefit. The net effect of these interventions is that individuals infected with HIV are living longer and with an improved quality of life.

The major routes of transmission of HIV include sexual intercourse, vertical spread and bloodborne spread. Widespread screening of blood donors has reduced the impact of transfusion-acquired infection, although such screening is by no means universal throughout the world. The prevalence of HIV infection is very variable, not only between countries but also within them. Figures of up to 10% of blood donors in some central African countries have been reported, and similar figures have also been cited for prostitutes in Bombay. Homosexual men still constitute the largest HIV-positive group within the UK, although the incidence of heterosexually acquired infection is growing rapidly. Data culled from a number of prospective studies of occupational exposure events suggests that the risk to HCW from percutaneous incidents involving blood from HIV-infected patients is approximately 0.32% (Table 10.2). Factors which independently predicted transmission of virus included deep injuries, visible blood on the device before injury, devices which were used on an artery or vein before injury, and exposure to a patient with AIDS (Beckmann et al., 1994). If we also consider that the risk of viral transmission from mother to infant is increased with a higher maternal plasma viral load, it becomes evident that transmission is a function of the inoculum of virus as well as the route of entry.

The presence of HIV-specific antibodies indicates infection. It may take 3–6 months for these to become detectable following infection, although during this 'window period' HIV antigen and RNA will be detectable in blood. As stated above, HIV RNA quantitation is routinely used for monitoring of infected individuals, and in part determines when initiation of antiretroviral drugs should occur, and when drug therapy is failing.

HIV-2 is prevalent in West Africa, and few cases have been diagnosed in the UK. Most of these cases have a clear geographical or personal link with this area of the world. HIV-2 infection also progresses to AIDS, although the speed of progression may be slower. The infection control implications of HIV-2 are similar to those for HIV-1, although the viruses show some differences in antiretroviral drug susceptibilities which will have a bearing on post-exposure prophylaxis regimes.

PREVENTION OF SPREAD OF BLOODBORNE VIRAL INFECTIONS IN HOSPITALS

One of the key issues in this area is whether to view all patients as potential sources of infection, or whether to use a two-tier level of protection based on the knowledge of which patients are infected with these agents. The former approach, known as 'universal precautions', is based on the premise that risk is associated with a particular procedure (e.g. venepuncture, lumbar puncture, laboratory testing, etc.), whereas implicit in the two-tier approach is that risk is associated with a particular patient. There is no doubt that a universal precautions approach involving routine use of gloves, double-gloving for invasive operations, and a low threshold for the wearing of masks, gowns and eye protection has major resource implications. However, the arguments in favour of this approach are powerful. First, by no means all patients infected with HBV, HCV or HIV will be aware of their infection (these infections are asymptomatic for long periods, during which infected individuals will present to health-care settings because of a range of related and unrelated conditions), and a two-tier system of infection control means that such individuals will be treated as 'safe'. Secondly, there are no doubt new bloodborne infections which have yet to be identified, for which spread to HCW will be reduced by the implementation of universal precautions. Thirdly, a two-tier approach may introduce differences in the quality of clinical care offered to patients (e.g. in the array of laboratory tests offered, or in the threshold for undertaking invasive procedures).

Nevertheless, the prevalence of HBV, HCV and HIV differs widely between different areas of the country, and the overall benefit of universal precautions when implemented in a large, urban hospital setting is likely to be greater than when this approach is introduced to a small rural hospital. The implementation of such a programme at one of the major clinical research facilities of the US National Institutes of Health, involving intensive training of all staff by means of videos and interactive sessions over a 2-year period, led to a progressive reduction in percutaneous injuries and adherence to universal precautions methods.

MANAGEMENT OF NEEDLESTICK AND OTHER HIGH RISK INJURIES AMONG HCW

GENERAL

Each hospital should have a clear and coherent needlestick policy, co-ordinated by named individuals. This should be widely advertised in order to maximize the reporting of such incidents, and would clearly be appropriate for incidents involving all staff and *any* patient, whatever their infection status. There should be 24-hour access to advice. Ideally, the co-ordinators should have full access to staff health records, including HBV vaccine status.

This policy should include advice on the following:

1 immediate care of injury (e.g. washing with soap and water);
2 responsibility for taking blood from the HCW and the patient, together with any relevant counselling. It is mandatory that blood should be obtained in all cases;
3 period of storage of blood samples (at least 2 years);
4 responsibility for compiling an accident report;
5 clear actions with regard to post-exposure prophylaxis and follow-up concerning HBV-, HCV- or HIV-risk incidents. This will incorporate

information on the particular risks of acquiring infection through different modes of incident (i.e. needlestick, mucous membrane contact, intact skin contact);

6 immediate access to antiretroviral drugs for HIV post-exposure prophylaxis;

7 maintaining the confidentiality of the HCW concerned.

HBV-RISK INCIDENTS – SPECIFIC MANAGEMENT

All incidents should be used to check HBV vaccine history opportunistically. The patient source of any incident should be tested for HB surface antigen. If previously vaccinated, the HCW can be checked for HBV S Ab levels. The recommended protocol is shown in Table 10.3.

HCV-RISK INCIDENTS – SPECIFIC MANAGEMENT

Where the source of a needlestick injury is known to be HCV infected, the HCW should be tested at 3 and 6 months for evidence of infection. As the risk of infection is very small, there is no need for a limitation of clinical activity during this period. There is currently no consensus on whether patients of unknown HCV status should be routinely tested following a needlestick injury. In view of the efficacy of antiviral treatment for HCV infection, and the fact that infection may be asymptomatic, it is this author's view that patients should be tested in these circumstances (with appropriate counselling). Thus, if found positive, there is an opportunity to monitor the HCW as above, and therefore to identify infection at an early stage.

HIV-RISK INCIDENTS – SPECIFIC MANAGEMENT

Until recently, there was no clear evidence that post-exposure prophylaxis following a needlestick injury from an HIV-infected individual was beneficial. Indeed, clear failures of zidovudine post-exposure prophylaxis (PEP) have been well documented. However, more recently a case–control study of HCW exposed to HIV has demonstrated that a failure to take zidovudine was associated with an increased risk of acquisition, with an odds ratio of 5.9 (Centers for Disease Control, 1995). This therefore provides the rationale for a more active policy of encouraging PEP in appropriate cases (see above).

Since this report in 1995, the Center for Disease Control in Atlanta, USA, has updated its recommendations for HIV PEP in the light of new potent antiretroviral drugs. These recommendations are as follows (Centers for Disease Control, 1998).

1 PEP should be recommended to exposed HCW after exposures associated with the highest risk (see above). They also categorize exposures with a lower risk (e.g. mucous membrane contact with blood and percutaneous exposure to bodily fluids containing visible blood), for which PEP should be offered, and with a negligible risk (non-blood fluids), for which PEP is not recommended.

2 Highly active antiretroviral therapy should be initiated within 4 hours of the risk incident. The precise combination used should be considered in the light of possible drug resistance variants, but comprises a minimum of three drugs.

3 PEP should be initiated promptly, preferably within 1–2 hours of the incident. Starting treatment after a prolonged period (1–2 weeks) may be considered in high-risk incidents. PEP should be continued for 4 weeks.

4 Initiation of PEP should be accompanied by relevant counselling (including a discussion of potential drug toxicity and sexual spread of infection), checks for seroconversion (up to 6 months if necessary) and laboratory monitoring for drug toxicity.

We believe that HIV PEP should be limited to high-risk exposures involving blood from known infected patients. It is incumbent on the co-ordinators of a hospital needlestick policy to highlight the minimal risk where the HIV status of the patient is unknown.

MANAGEMENT OF HEALTH-CARE WORKERS INFECTED WITH BLOODBORNE VIRUSES

HEPATITIS B

The infectivity of an HBV-infected individual is determined by the concentration of virus in the blood. The presence of 'e' antigen is associated with a higher level of virus, which in turn reflects a higher risk of transmission to others. Until recently, such transmission of HBV from HCW to patients has been limited to 'e' antigen-positive HBV-infected HCW leading the UK Department of Health to stipulate that such individuals should not perform exposure-prone procedures (NHS Executive, 1996; UK Department of Health, 1998). There is no restriction on carriers of the virus who are 'e' antigen-negative, unless they have been shown to be associated with transmission of the virus to a patient, in which case practice should be restricted. In this context, high-risk procedures encompass situations where the worker's gloved hands may be in contact with sharp instruments, needle tips or sharp tissues (e.g. bone spicules) inside the patient's open body cavity, wound or confined anatomical space where the hands or fingertips may not be completely visible at all times. Thus internal examinations or procedures that do not require the use of sharp instruments are not considered to be in this category, nor is normal vaginal delivery. By contrast, suturing or infiltration of local anaesthetic during and after delivery are high risk, as the fingers may not be continually visible.

More recently, the transmission of HBV to patients by four separate surgeons without 'e' antigen in their circulation has been reported. All four had an alteration in the viral genome which prevented production of this antigen (Anon., 1997). These cases have major implications for the policy on infected HCW, and UK recommendations are currently being reconsidered in the light of these data.

The identification of an HBV-infected HCW, either through routine post-vaccine follow-up or by screening, must be dealt with in a sensitive manner. An 'e' antigen-positive surgeon is threatened with a potential loss of livelihood. The possible role of interferon and/or lamivudine therapy in leading to a loss of 'e' antigen and reduction in HBV serum DNA (Hoofnagle and Di Bisceglia, 1997) could then be considered. Although 'e' antigen-negative surgeons may still practise invasive procedures, the identification of such individuals at an early stage of their training may provide an opportunity for a career change to a more appropriate clinical specialty. Occupational Health Departments should play an important role in these areas.

Once identification of a highly infectious surgeon has occurred, a team that includes public health experts should be convened to put in place a 'look-back' to assess the spread of infection to patients at risk. It is evident that patients have to be given detailed information in order for them to understand the purpose of retesting. The scope of this look-back exercise should be decided on the basis of local circumstances, such as the nature of the invasive procedures performed.

HIV

Transmission of HIV from an HCW to patients has been reported for both a dentist and a surgeon (Geberding, 1995). However, the risk is undoubtedly very small. Provided that general infection control measures are followed, the circumstances in which HIV could be transmitted to a patient are restricted to exposure-prone procedures, as outlined above. As is the case for HBV, the initial identification of an HIV-infected HCW involved in such procedures should lead to the establishment of an incident panel, including public health specialists, who will determine the precise nature of a look-back exercise.

It is important that an atmosphere is generated in which a HCW infected with HIV, or who feel themselves to be at risk, can present themselves to medical services with confidence that their case will be dealt with in an understanding manner. If not, then we run the risk of such individuals continuing to work in an exposure-prone specialty. However, if it is clear that such procedures have been performed, it remains the responsibility of the HCW to inform their local Director of Public Health (or equivalent) either directly or through their physician, on a strictly confidential basis. Subsequent medical management of the infected individual should be undertaken in close association with a specialist occupational health physician, who will be able to advise on subsequent occupationally related matters.

At present in the UK it is not recommended to test HCW routinely for evidence of HIV infection (Expert Advisory Panel on AIDS, 1994).

HCV

At the time of writing, no cases of transmission of HCV from HCW to patients have been clearly demonstrated. Nevertheless, as transmission of HCV can occur via needlestick injuries, it is naive to assume that such an incident will never occur. Therefore, in the case of the identification of an HCV-infected HCW who is involved with exposure-prone procedures (see above), it seems prudent to set in motion a look-back investigation as outlined previously. In addition, the HCW concerned should seek medical and occupational health guidance (Crawshaw *et al.*, 1994; Anon., 1996).

INVESTIGATION OF HBV, HIV OR HCV INFECTIONS POSSIBLY ACQUIRED IN HOSPITAL

Routine investigation of a sporadic case of HBV, HIV and HCV may identify a medical procedure as one possible risk factor (e.g. recent invasive gynaecological surgery). There should be a low threshold for initiating an investigation in such circumstances, especially in the absence of other clear risk activity. This should involve the relevant infection control team, clinical virologists, public health specialists and the physicians involved in the case. Among other factors, this investigation will consider the validity of further testing of hospital staff and other patients. If more than one infected individual is identified by such a procedure, molecular analysis of the isolates may be undertaken to identify a specific epidemiological link between them. Virological advice should be sought in order to access such testing.

NON BLOODBORNE HEPATITIS VIRUSES

HEPATITIS A VIRUS (HAV) INFECTION

Hepatitis A virus can lead to asymptomatic or symptomatic illness. The former is more common in children. The incubation period is 15–50 days, and the illness is usually short-lived, with symptoms including fever, malaise, dark urine and jaundice of acute onset. A small proportion of infected adults experience symptoms for up to 6 months. Very rarely, HAV can lead to a fulminant hepatitis. Virus is excreted in the stool, with peak levels shed in the 2 weeks preceding onset of the disease. The levels of virus decline after this time, although children can shed virus for longer periods of time.

Definitive diagnosis of HAV infection is made by the detection of HAV-specific IgM in serum. Long-lasting immunity is conferred by specific IgG. The virus is spread by the faecal-oral route and is thus highly prevalent in areas of poor sanitation and where water quality is low. Paradoxically, most individuals in such areas have acquired asymptomatic infection during childhood.

As patients admitted to hospital with acute HAV show minimal viral shedding at this time, there is little risk to staff. Nevertheless, strict hygienic precautions are recommended as spread is possible, especially in association with faecal incontinence. Although outbreaks of HAV are common in the community, they are rare in health-care settings, and hospital staff have a similar seroprevalence to other groups.

Protection against HAV is by passive immunization, with intramuscular normal immunoglobulin, or with hepatitis A vaccine. This is inactivated and highly immunogenic. Both methods of protection demonstrate efficacy when used as timely prophylaxis or post-exposure prophylaxis in outbreak situations (Centers for Disease Control, 1996).

HEPATITIS E VIRUS (HEV) INFECTION

Like HAV, HEV is enterically spread and has a similar clinical presentation, apart from its manifestation in the last trimester of pregnancy, when it is associated with up to 15% mortality. The reasons are currently unknown. Peak faecal shedding of virus occurs prior to the onset of symptoms. This infection is endemic in parts of India and Pakistan, Africa and South America, and all cases documented in the UK to date have recently returned from endemic areas. Diagnosis is by detection of HEV-specific IgM in serum. The risk of'nosocomial infection is rare, although hospital cases should be dealt with as for hepatitis A. No vaccine for HEV currently exists.

REFERENCES

Anon. (1996) Lessons from two linked clusters of acute hepatitis B in cardiothoracic surgery patients. *Communicable Disease Review* 6, R119.

Anon. (1997) Transmission of hepatitis B to patients from four infected surgeons without hepatitis e antigen. *New England Journal of Medicine* 336, 178.

Beckmann, S.E., Vlahor, D., Koziol, D.E. *et al.* (1994) Temporal association between implementation of universal precautions and a sustained progressive decrease in percutaneous exposures to blood. *Clinical Infectious Diseases* 18, 562.

Centers for Disease Control (1995) Case–control study of HIV seroconversion in health-care workers after percutaneous exposure to HIV-infected blood – France, United Kingdom and United States, January 1988–August 1994. *Morbidity and Mortality Weekly Report* 44, 929.

Centers for Disease Control (1996) Prevention of hepatitis A through active or passive immunisation. *Morbidity and Mortality Weekly Report* 45, RR15.

Centers for Disease Control (1998) Public Health Service guidelines for the management of health-care worker exposures to HIV and recommendations for post-exposure prophylaxis. *Morbidity and Mortality Weekly Report* 47, RR-7.

Crawshaw, S.C., Gill, O.N., Heptonstall, J. *et al.* (1994) Outcome of an exercise to notify patients treated by an obstetrician/gynaecologist infected with HIV-1. *Communicable Disease Report CDR Review* 4, R125.

Expert Avisory Panel on AIDS (1994) *AIDS/HIV-infected health-care workers: guidance on the management of infected health-care workers.* London: HMSO.

Gerberding, J.L. (1995) Management of occupational exposures to bloodborne viruses. *New England Journal of Medicine* 332, 444.

Hoofnagle, J.H. and Di Bisceglia, A.M. (1997) The treatment of chronic viral hepatitis. *New England Journal of Medicine* 336, 347.

Liang, J.T. (1998) Combination therapy for hepatitis C infection. *New England Journal of Medicine* 339, 1549.

National Health Service Executive (1996) *Addendum to HSG (93) 40. Protecting health care workers and patients from Hepatitis B.* London: HMSO.

UK Department of Health (1998) *Guidance for clinical health-care workers: protection against infection with blood-borne viruses.* London: Department of Health.

chapter 11

ASEPSIS IN OPERATING THEATRES

POST-OPERATIVE INFECTION

Surgical wound infection is mainly acquired during the operation, and may be endogenous from the patient's own flora, or exogenous from the operating-room staff or infrequently from the environment. Most post-operative infections are endogenous and are acquired from the skin, mucous membranes or gastrointestinal tract of the patient. Exogenous infections are mainly acquired from the nose or skin flora of the operating team and transmitted on the hands of the surgeon or through the air directly, or indirectly on instruments.

Other organisms may be transferred infrequently by staff during the operation (e.g. β-haemolytic streptococci from throat carriers or from other sites).

The clean wound infection rate is usually low (e.g. 1–3%) and infections are mainly caused by *Staphylococcus aureus,* coagulase-negative staphylococci or occasionally other organisms (e.g. Gram-negative bacilli), often in association with the normal skin flora (Cruse and Foord, 1980; Leigh, 1981; Ayliffe, 1994; Mangram *et al.*, 1999). Infections are more frequent in clean–contaminated or contaminated wounds (5–10%) and these are mainly endogenous, caused by *Bacteroides* species, *E. coli*, other Gram-negative bacilli and enterococci. The infection rates in these latter categories may be reduced to less than 5% by effective antibiotic prophylaxis. Coagulase-negative staphylococci, *Staphylococcus aureus, Proprionibacterium* species and other skin organisms are the main causes of infection following implants of artificial joints (Lidwell *et al.*, 1982). Patients who are colonized with hospital strains of antibiotic-resistant *Staphylococcus aureus* (e.g. MRSA) and antibiotic-resistant Gram-negative bacilli in the ward before operation may infect the wound with these organisms during operation. Although the organisms are hospital-acquired, the infections are likely to be classified as endogenous.

Infection from the theatre environment is rare (Ayliffe, 1991) and is usually due to failure of disinfection or sterilization (e.g. contaminated eyedrops or saline). *Clostridium perfringens* infections can often be isolated from the theatre environment, but clostridial infections following operation are usually acquired from the patient's own intestinal flora (Ayliffe and Lowbury, 1969; Parker, 1969). Some wounds are infected in the ward post-operatively. These are usually drained or moist wounds.

In recent years, much conventional open surgery has been replaced by endoscopic minimal-access surgery (e.g. for cholecystectomy, hernia repair, many gynaecological operations and surgery of the knee joint). Minimal-access surgery is not necessarily associated with a shorter operating time than conventional open surgery, but infection rates are usually lower (e.g. in cholecystectomies) (Dunn *et al.*, 1994; Watkins *et al.*, 1995). The reduced size of incisions should reduce the infection rate, but infection still occurs, particularly following bowel perforation (Goodwin, 1998).

PREVENTION OF INFECTION

In general the protection of the patient against the hazards of infection in the operating-theatre involves the application of a number of methods to prevent the contamination of wounds (Hambraeus and Laurell, 1980; Emmerson, 1992) and to enhance the patient's resistance. Some of the methods are described in more detail in the chapters on disinfection and sterilization in this handbook.

The risk factors associated with surgical wound infection have been considered in Chapter 3 (see Cruse and Foord, 1980; Bibby *et al.*, 1986, Culver *et al.*, 1991, Garibaldi *et al.*, 1991), but some important factors cannot be modified (e.g. the age and sex of the patient). The basic methods of prevention of infection consist of sterilization of instruments, disinfection of hands, wearing of sterile gloves and gowns by the operating team and disinfection of the skin of the operation site. Although not necessarily proven in prospective clinical trials, these methods are supported by microbiological studies and are accepted by surgeons (Leaper, 1995). Other methods of reducing infection that are supported by stronger clinical evidence include the following:

- surveillance and feedback of results to surgeons, presumably influencing surgical technique, which is an important risk factor (Cruse and Foord, 1980; Haley, 1995);
- reducing the pre-operative stay to a minimum;
- minimizing the length of operation;
- avoiding pre-operative shaving of the operation site. If removal of hair is considered necessary, use clippers, an electric razor or a depilatory cream. Shave immediately before the operation if shaving is required;
- avoiding wound drains. If this is not possible, use a closed drainage system and always remove drains as soon as possible;
- treating infection present at other sites on the patient;
- ensuring that the patient is as fit as possible;
- reducing excessive obesity or malnutrition if possible before surgery;
- using a good surgical technique (Mishriki *et al.*, 1990);
- giving peri-operative prophylaxis where applicable (Centers for Disease Control, 1985).

Methods of preventing infection in the operating suite can be considered under the following subheadings (Medical Research Council, 1968):

1 the operating suite and equipment;
2 preparation of the surgical team;
3 preparation and protection of the patient.

THE OPERATING SUITE AND EQUIPMENT

DESIGN

Although there is little evidence that the design of the operating suite has a major influence on the wound infection rate in general surgery (Maki *et al.*, 1982; Van Griethuysen *et al.*, 1996), it is rational to follow established principles, i.e. to:
- establish a protective zone around the sterile area;
- provide an airflow from the 'sterile' to less clean areas.

The zonal arrangement was described by the Medical Research Council (1962) and consists of separation of the suite into four zones:

- sterile or aseptic (operating-room and instrument lay-up room or sterile storage area);
- clean (anaesthetic room and scrub-up room or area);
- protective (entrance lobby and corridor, changing rooms and recovery room);
- disposal (sink, sluices and disposal corridor).

The zoning system is still commonly used (NHS Estates, 1991), but may be modified so long as rigorous microbiological principles are followed. The advice of the infection control team should be obtained at an early stage.

The disposal zone may not be required if dirty items or clinical waste are removed in sealed impervious bags. A single corridor should be adequate for transporting patients to and from the operating-rooms, and for removal of used instruments and waste, provided that appropriate traffic flows can be maintained. A trolley transfer area is not required (Ayliffe *et al.*, 1969).

A scrub-up area may be incorporated in a bay of the operating-room, but should be well away from the operating area, so that water splashes do not reach the operating team, instruments or operating site.

The number of operating-rooms should be based on the number of surgical beds (e.g. one theatre to 25–30 beds) and the throughput of patients. Allowance must also be made for cleaning, maintenance, and emergency and day surgery. A recovery ward should be in the operating suite, and the proximity of intensive care, sterile services, X-ray facilities and the Accident and Emergency department should be considered when upgrading a hospital or building a new one (Humphreys, 1993).

VENTILATION

Ventilation should remove airborne bacteria released in the theatre suite and prevent the entry of bacteria, especially from the corridors and other indoor areas, but also from outside the hospital. It should provide comfortable conditions for patients and staff, control the humidity to reduce the risk of electrostatic sparks, and remove anaesthetic gases. Although conventional ventilation systems for general surgery are unlikely to have a major influence on infection rates (Maki *et al.*, 1982; Ayliffe, 1994; Van Griethuysen *et al.*, 1996), a ventilation system will provide comfortable conditions, and it is rational to dilute the organisms released during an operation.

The air intake to the ventilation system should be in an area which is as free from dust and dirt as possible, and primary filters should be included to reduce the entry of dirt and larger particles into the ducts. Secondary filters need not be of the high-efficiency particulate air (HEPA) type unless there is an ultra-clean-air (see below) or other recirculating air system.

Recommended systems for most operating-theatres are plenum (positive pressure). The air is distributedly evenly within the space, usually via ceiling diffusers. Anaesthetic gases are commonly removed through a separate scavenging system.

The air flow in the operating-theatre should be 0.1–0.3 m/s (providing approximately 20 air changes per hour and the required pressure). The direction of the air flow is from the sterile area to the clean area and then to the protective and disposal zones (NHS Estates, 1994). A higher flow rate (e.g. providing 10–15 air changes per hour in a balanced system) than the protective zone as a whole is recommended for the recovery ward, to remove anaesthetic gases to the outside. Any flow from less clean to cleaner areas (e.g. on opening doors) should be minimized by ensuring a pressure gradient (e.g. a nominal pressure of 25 Pa in the sterile area, 14 Pa in the clean areas, 3 Pa in the protective zone and 0 to -5 Pa in any disposal areas). The relative humidity should be kept between 40 and 60%, using a steam injection system if possible.

The efficiency of the ventilation system should, when possible, be monitored daily by use of an airflow switch or a continuous monitoring system, which indicates on the theatre panel whether the correct volume of air is being supplied by the plant. When this equipment is not present, measurement of air flow at grilles (by an anemometer) and of room pressure at test points is desirable, and should be recorded in a log-book. Measurements of ventilation rates and pressures should be made periodically by an engineer. A reduced pressure and air turnover indicate probable blockage of filters, which require immediate replacement if they become blocked. Routine bacteriological testing is not required, but may be indicated when commissioning a new theatre or following maintenance, particularly if air is recirculated (Holton and Ridgway, 1993; Gosden *et al.*, 1998; see also Chapter 3). A hygrometer in the theatre should be read daily to ensure that the relative humidity does not fall below the required level.

If an operating suite is not used overnight or during a weekend, the ventilation system can be switched off, provided that it is switched on again for 1 hour before subsequent use (Clark *et al.*, 1985). A time clock is useful for this procedure.

Infections in clean undrained wounds should be reduced to 1–2% with good surgical technique in an operating-theatre with a conventional ventilation system, but in some instances a further reduction in infection rate is desirable because of the disastrous consequences of failure. In total hip or knee replacement operations (and possibly some other types of clean surgery), there is a strong case for the use of theatres or enclosures where the wound is protected against airborne infection by the provision of an ultra-clean air system. In a typical system, unidirectional (laminar) air-flow at about 300 changes per hour is recirculated through HEPA filters. The air flow is commonly vertical, but it could be horizontal. Charnley (1979) developed an ultra-clean air system for total hip replacement in which the operation was performed in an enclosure ventilated by a large turnover of filtered recirculated air, the operating team inside the enclosure wearing exhaust-ventilated bacteria-proof operating suits. Over a period of years, in which the system was progressively improved, there was a reduction in post-operative sepsis from about 10% to under 1%. This reduction was due, in Charnley's opinion, to the use of ultra-clean air.

Charnley's claim was disputed because, during the same period, he had introduced a number of other improvements which might have affected the infection rates, and because some other surgeons who did not use ultra-clean air reported infection rates no higher than his (Fitzgerald et al., 1977). These uncertainties were resolved by the results of a multicentre prospective controlled trial conducted by a Medical Research Council team, which showed that the incidence of deep joint sepsis was significantly lower in patients whose operations had been performed in ultra-clean air than it was in those who had their operations performed by the same teams but in conventional plenum-ventilated operating-rooms. The operations which showed the greatest reduction in joint sepsis (about 4 to 5-fold) were those performed in theatres showing the greatest reduction in the numbers of airborne bacteria and in the numbers present in washings from the operation wounds. These most marked reductions were obtained with unidirectional flow plus the use of bacteria-proof body-exhaust-ventilated clothing, and also by the use of surgical isolators (Lidwell et al., 1982, 1987; see also Salvati et al., 1982). A cost-benefit analysis has supported the use of ultra-clean air on economic as well as clinical grounds (Lidwell, 1984).

Similar reductions in joint sepsis rates have been obtained by the use of peri-operative antibiotic prophylaxis (Hill et al., 1981; Lidwell et al., 1982; An and Freeman, 1996). When antibiotic prophylaxis and ultra-clean air were used in combination in the Lidwell study, their effects were additive, leading (with the best ultra-clean air systems) to a reduction in wound sepsis from 3.4% to 0.19%. Charnley did not use prophylactic antibiotics as did the surgeons, whose results were as good as Charnley's without the use of ultra-clean air.

However, orthopaedic surgeons usually use both prophylactic antibiotics and an ultra-clean air system (Gosden et al., 1998). The studies of Lidwell et al. (1982) showed that, in conventional theatres, about 95% of the bacteria that contaminate the joint replacement operations are acquired from the air, but in other types of clean surgery a higher proportion may originate from the patient's skin. Although the role of ultra-clean air in other types of surgery remains uncertain, airborne infections are responsible for some infections in other types of implant surgery (e.g. cardiac valve replacement), and probably to a lesser extent in other types of clean surgery. It might therefore be reasonable to consider fitting a vertical flow system in all new operating-theatres, if this is not too expensive. Side walls would be unnecessary provided that the outer layer of air was directed outwards to ensure that organisms were not entrained in the downflow on to the operation site or instrument trolley (e.g. Exflow system; Howarth, 1985). Recirculation of most of the air would reduce running costs, and ventilation of other areas of the theatre – apart from the actual operating areas – would be unnecessary. The system could be extended to a large operating-theatre containing four or more operating-tables or enclosures in simultaneous use (Babb *et al.*, 1995). This would increase the opportunities for common use of facilities.

As much surgery is now minimally invasive, the risk of infection via the airborne route is decreased. The necessity for expensive ventilation systems in endoscopic surgery is doubtful. However, ultra-clean air systems are still likely to be required for implant surgery, and some other types of surgery will continue to be of the conventional type. Contamination of instruments from the air is also possible, and studies of new and less expensive ventilation systems for minimally invasive surgery are required.

STORAGE OF EQUIPMENT

The amount of equipment should be kept to a minimum, including the operating-table, lights, conduits for anaesthetic gases, diathermy and suction. An instrument table and trolley are also included if there is no lay-up room. Articles needed for servicing a list of operations are kept in the anaesthetic room, the scrub-up annexe or the lay-up room. Store items are arranged to require minimum movement by staff.

Maintenance of sterility in sterile supplies depends on adequate wrapping of packs and on the minimum exposure. Double-wrapping prevents contamination during opening of packs, which must also be protected against moisture. If not used promptly, packs should be kept in a cabinet or box with a well-fitting lid. Instruments and packs are now often kept in metal containers with a filter to prevent contamination. Items of equipment (X-ray, diathermy, etc.) must be stored under clean conditions and be cleaned or disinfected regularly.

Laying up of trolleys in advance of the operation involves some risk of contamination. When instruments are arranged for individual operations on pre-set trays, the wrapping can be removed in the operating-room immediately before use.

STERILIZATION OF INSTRUMENTS

The methods for sterilizing instruments are described in Chapter 4. These are mainly supplied by the SSD (see Chapter 17). Certain single-use items are obtained pre-sterilized from commercial sources (e.g. suture materials, syringes, needles, catheters and drip sets).

CLEANING OF THE OPERATING SUITE

The principles of cleaning and disinfection are described in Chapter 6. Surfaces should be kept free of visible dirt, and special attention should be given to areas which are likely to become heavily contaminated (i.e. upward-facing surfaces). It is advisable to clean the floor of the theatre after each operating session. A disinfectant should be used after known contamination of floors with material from infected patients, but for routine cleaning, mopping with water and a detergent is satisfactory. Floors should occasionally be rinsed with clean water after washing or disinfection, otherwise a deposit may build up and reduce antistatic properties. A suitable floor-scrubbing machine may be used at the end of the day (see Chapter 6). For other surfaces, normal housekeeping methods are adequate (e.g. daily damp cleaning of ledges and shelves). Walls with intact surfaces acquire very few bacteria even if left unwashed for long periods. However, they must not be allowed to become visibly dirty, and washing at least every 3–6 months should be adequate for this purpose (Ayliffe et al., 1967). If areas of paint peel off, the wall must be repainted or covered with a new wall finish. The operating lamp should be cleaned daily; oiling is unnecessary.

DISINFECTION OF ANAESTHETIC APPARATUS AND MECHANICAL VENTILATORS

Items which enter or come near to the patient's respiratory tract (e.g. endotracheal tubes, airways and face-pieces) should be disinfected after every use. Anaesthetic circuits (e.g. re-breathing bags and tubing) can be changed after each session. These items should be disinfected in the SSD, or in a special department with technical staff appointed for this work under the supervision of the manager of the SSD. Care must be taken to avoid contaminating the anaesthetic trolley, which should have a discard receptacle.

For details of disinfection of anaesthetic and respiratory ventilating equipment and of methods for preventing contamination of respirators and ventilators, see Chapter 6.

OPERATING-ROOMS FOR 'CLEAN' AND 'SEPTIC' CASES – ORDER OF OPERATION

The risk of transfer of infection from one patient to the next in a general surgical operating list is small. In conventional theatre suites with plenum ventilation, an interval of 10 minutes, during which the operating area is thoroughly cleaned, should make it safe for the next patient. No special 'septic' theatre is required. No special cleaning precautions are required after operations on patients with gas gangrene, as these do not contaminate the theatre any more than operations in which the intestine is opened. Septic patients should, when possible, and particularly if infected with MRSA, be placed at the end of an operating list. However, this should not be necessary if the operating area is thoroughly cleaned after removal of the infected patient from the theatre.

SUCTION APPARATUS (see also Chapter 6)

Contaminated aerosols from suction apparatus have frequently been described (Creamer and Smyth, 1996). A filter should be fitted between the collection bottle and the pump. This will prevent froth and spray contaminated by infective aspirates from being dispersed into the theatre. The filter should not be in the outlet to the atmosphere, because the pump may become clogged with coagulated protein if it is not protected by a filter.

If piped suction is installed, a filter at each peripheral suction point is required to prevent contamination of the pipeline and the exhaust discharge.

CONTAMINATION OF FLUIDS

To prevent contamination of fluids with *Pseudomonas aeruginosa, Serratia* species or other Gram-negative bacilli, aqueous solutions of cetrimide and chlorhexidine should be stocked in the pharmacy in concentrated solutions and diluted for issue with fresh distilled or sterilized water. If the solutions will withstand heat, the provision of sterilized antiseptic solutions is desirable. Stock and issue bottles should be covered with a screw cap without cork liners; cork must never be used. Once opened, a bottle should be in use for no longer than 1 day. All bottles should be sterilized or adequately disinfected before being refilled (unless disposable containers are used). Aqueous antiseptics are commonly supplied ready for use in sterile plastic packs. Fluids used in ophthalmic surgery should be supplied, whenever possible, autoclaved in their final containers and in small volumes, so that none of them are stored in bottles that have been opened for use. Heat-labile solutions should be sterilized by filtration.

Water 'sterilizers' and associated piped systems are liable to contamination and should be avoided.

Water-baths used in cardiothoracic operating-theatres for thawing of blood products have been found to be responsible for post-operative pseudomonas endocarditis. To prevent this lethal hazard, it has been recommended that water-baths should be effectively disinfected after use, changed 4-hourly and monitored for counts of bacteria, and also that blood products to be thawed should be double-bagged (Casewell *et al.*, 1981).

INFECTION TRANSMITTED IN BLOOD

See notes on hepatitis B and C and HIV infections in Chapter 10.

PREPARATION OF THE SURGICAL TEAM

Under this heading it is usual to consider only those measures which are taken to prevent the transfer of organisms from members of the surgical team to the wounds of patients in the operating-room. However, it is important to consider also those measures by which the surgeon and his or her assistants can be protected against pathogens carried by the patient, including HIV, HBV, HCV and other severe or dangerous infections (Joint Working Party of the Hospital Infection Society and the Surgical Infection Study Group, 1992). This subject is also considered in Chapter 10.

DEFINITIONS OF THE TEAM – MOVEMENTS

All individuals – surgeons, anaesthetists, operating-theatre nurses, and others – who enter the sterile zone of the theatre during an operation are described as members of the team. They are divided into 'scrubbed' and 'unscrubbed' members.

To reduce the hazard of contamination from dispersers of virulent staphylococci, the team should be kept as small as possible. No one whose presence is not essential should be admitted to the operating room.

Movements in the theatre should be reduced to a minimum. In particular, it should be unnecessary to fetch materials from outside the theatre or to remove instruments for resterilization before the end of an operation. Doors should be kept closed during the operation.

FITNESS OF THE MEMBERS OF THE TEAM FOR DUTY

No one with a boil or septic lesion of the skin or eczema colonized with *Staphylococcus aureus* should remain at work in an operating-theatre. Protection cannot necessarily be achieved by covering the lesion with an adhesive dressing. When the lesion is cured, it is desirable to use an antiseptic detergent preparation or soap for all ablutions, so that the staphylococci which caused the lesion can be removed from the skin.

When there has been an outbreak of infection with a particular type of *Staphylococcus aureus*, and there is evidence to suggest that the infection was probably acquired in the theatre, nasal or lesion carriers should be sought and treated. Nasal carriers should be treated with nasal antibacterial creams (e.g. mupirocin; see Chapter 9).

Respiratory infections in the team may cause respiratory infection in the patient at a time when he or she is particularly susceptible, and it is preferable for individuals with such infections to be excluded from the team. The hazard from respiratory infection applies especially to anaesthetists. A surgeon infected with *Streptococcus pyogenes* (e.g. streptococcal tonsillitis) must not operate.

Transmission of hepatitis B from a surgeon to a patient has been described. This is particularly associated with a carrier of the 'e' antigen (see Chapter 10).

BATHING AND SHOWERS

It has been shown that showers tend to increase rather than reduce the number of bacteria-carrying particles dispersed from the skin. Staff should therefore not take showers immediately before operations.

REMOVAL OF EVERYDAY CLOTHES

It is rational to remove the outer clothes before putting on operating-room clothes. However, there is no evidence that the removal of underclothes reduces the amount of contamination from the body, and this may be left to the discretion of the individual.

OPERATING-ROOM CLOTHES

With regard to operating suits and gowns (Whyte, 1988; Emmerson, 1992), the ideal requirements for operating-theatre clothing are as follows:
- an effective barrier to bacteria and other particles;
- 'breathability' of material to ensure comfort of wearers;
- ability to withstand repeated washing and autoclaving;
- ability to resist fluid penetration;

- antistatic;
- low linting;
- cost-effectiveness.

Clothing that meets all of these requirements is not necessarily available at reasonable cost, and may not be required for all types of operation.

Manufacturers will supply information on the results of tests for measuring pore sizes and penetration of bacteria and fluids through fabrics, although their interpretation in terms of prevention of infection is uncertain. A European Standard is currently being produced (Patel *et al.*, 1998).

Conventional cotton clothing gives some protection against contact contamination (if dry) and is comfortable to wear, but does not reduce airborne contamination with bacteria from the wearer's skin. Skin scales (average diameter about 20 μ) carrying bacteria escape through the large pores in the cotton fabric and, if trousers are worn, at the ankles. When cotton gowns are used, they must be changed if they become soaked with blood or other liquids.

Use of an operating suit made of tightly woven fabric (e.g. ventile) and the securing of trousers around the ankles reduces the dispersal of bacteria. This type of material can be made to reduce wetting, but it is uncomfortable to wear. With the Charnley–Howarth ultra-clean air enclosure, a body-exhaust ventilated operating suit made of small-pore woven fabric has been used by the operating team, but some surgeons find it uncomfortable. If the exhaust system is not used, a hood and mask should be worn in addition to closely woven or non-woven clothing for all implant surgery.

More comfortable disposable types of unwoven operating clothes have been developed, but they can be expensive. Clothing made from microfilament polyester is increasingly being used. These fabrics are effective in preventing transfer of organisms, and although they are not usually as comfortable as cotton, they are generally acceptable to theatre staff (Whyte *et al.*, 1990; Schiebel *et al.*, 1991). They are washable and can be autoclaved. Washable laminated fabrics which allow the passage of moisture but not fluids (e.g. Goretex) can also be considered, but are often expensive. Cheaper and more comfortable laminated clothing is now available. Preliminary trials should be conducted on any proposed new type of clothing to ensure that it is comfortable for the staff.

The necessity for such special operating clothing for routine general surgery in a conventionally ventilated theatre is doubtful, and it should only be introduced if it is comfortable and cost-effective. Routine wearing of headgear in a theatre is also of doubtful value, but it probably should be worn by the operating team (see below).

FOOTWEAR

Footwear with impervious soles (e.g. rubber or plastic boots, or overshoes made of waterproof material) should be worn in the sterile zone, and the shoes should fit properly, so that a bellows action is avoided. Overshoes are unnecessary for visiting staff who do not enter the aseptic area (Marshall *et al.*, 1991).

'TACKY' MATS

Mats with tacky or disinfectant surfaces at the entrance to theatres are not recommended, as they have been found to offer little protection against bacterial contamination of operating-room floors (Ayliffe *et al.*, 1967; Traore *et al.*, 1997). If they are not changed regularly, they may increase the numbers of organisms transferred into the theatre.

HEADGEAR

Hair is unlikely to be an important source of infection unless the member of staff is a heavy staphylococcal disperser (e.g. with colonized eczema). There is little evidence that the wearing of headgear reduces bacterial contamination in the theatre (Humphreys, 1991), unless it is part of an exhaust-ventilated suit. Routine wearing of headgear within the operating suite would seem to be unnecessary. However, it is rational for the operating team to wear headgear. If an exhaust-ventilated suit is not used for orthopaedic implant surgery, a hood covering the head, the side of the face and the chin would be desirable (for materials, see p. 228). It is also important for staff to keep their hair clean and tidy.

MASKS

To prevent the impaction of droplets from the mouth into the operation field, it is the usual practice to wear a mask. Formerly it was recommended that an impervious mask should be worn, but current practice is to use a disposable mask that acts as a filter and also to some extent as a deflector. Some disposable paper masks give poor protection. The mask should cover the nose and mouth, and should be changed after each operation or if it becomes damp (Belkin, 1997).

A mask does not reduce airborne contamination in the operating-theatre, and there is little evidence that a mask reduces the infection rate in general surgery. Few organisms are dispersed from the nose and mouth during normal breathing, and none were detected close to an operating table in a mock-up theatre with forced ventilation over the table (Mitchell and Hunt, 1991). Some surgeons do not wear masks for general surgery (Orr and Bailey, 1992), and a large controlled trial showed no difference in infection rates between operations during which masks were worn and operations in which they were not worn (Tunevall, 1991). Masks (or possibly visors) are required to protect the surgeon if splashing with blood is likely, and they should also be worn for implant surgery. However, it should be unnecessary for unscrubbed staff to wear masks.

HANDS AND GLOVES (see Chapter 7)

The clinical effectiveness of surgical handwashing/disinfection in preventing wound infection has not been proven, but it is accepted as a rational procedure and is supported by laboratory experiments. The optimal length of the handwashing/disinfection process is also unknown, but the following procedures have been found to be satisfactory in practice (Lowbury, 1992).

For the first handwash of the day, 3–5 mL (repeated if required) of an antiseptic detergent preparation (e.g. 4% chlorhexidine, 7.5% povidone iodine or 2% triclosan) is applied to moistened hands and forearms for approx 2 min and then rinsed off in running water and dried. The nails are scrubbed and a manicure stick can be used to remove dirt from beneath the fingernails if necessary. The disinfection process must be thorough and systematic, covering all areas of the hands and forearms. This process may be repeated before each operation, but for physically clean hands, a more effective alternative is to rub in two applications of 5 mL of 0.5% chlorhexidine, or another appropriate agent (e.g. povidone iodine), in 70% ethyl or isopropyl alcohol on to the hands and forearms until evaporated to dryness. Ethyl or isopropyl alcohol with an emollient but without an additional antibacterial agent is also effective, but does not have the possible advantage of residual action of deposited chlorhexidine.

A single application of an alcoholic preparation (5 mL) can be used on clean hands for subsequent operations on the operating list. A nailbrush should only be used for the first handwash of the day, to avoid damage to the skin.

On the basis of laboratory tests, many European countries recommend only the use of alcoholic preparations, especially n-propanol, applied for 3–5 min for surgical hand disinfection (Rotter, 1996), but good clinical evidence of an improved effect on the infection rate is not available.

Care must be taken to avoid contaminating the contents of soap or detergent containers (e.g. by the use of a foot-operated pump).

The use of gloves by the surgical team in addition to hand disinfection has not been shown to reduce wound infection, but provides protection to the operator. Glove punctures are frequent (e.g. 11.5%) (Church and Sanderson, 1980), but in the study of Cruse and Foord (1980) punctures could not be associated with wound infection. Nevertheless, on the appearance of a visible tear, gloves must be removed and replaced with new ones after disinfection of the hands with an antiseptic detergent or alcoholic preparation. A fresh gown must also be put on, because the sleeves may have become contaminated on changing the gloves. Waterproof sleeves are desirable to reduce the risk of blood soaking through the sleeves. It is desirable to remove rings before putting on surgical gloves. Double gloving is often recommended for operations on patients with HIV infection.

PREPARATION OF THE PATIENT AND PERFORMANCE OF THE OPERATION

FITNESS OF THE PATIENT FOR OPERATION – SUSCEPTIBILITY TO INFECTION

Risks of infection vary with the operation and with certain general factors. For example, there is a greater risk in the obese, cachectic or elderly, in those who spend a long time in hospital before operation, in patients with uncontrolled diabetes (especially in operating on limbs, because of impaired circulation), and in those treated with corticosteroids or immunosuppressive drugs. The likelihood of contamination is also greater in patients with existing infection. For such 'high-risk' patients, additional aseptic precautions are advisable, such as segregation and treatment for staphylococcal carriage before operation and, in some circumstances, specific chemoprophylaxis. Other factors such as the type and site of operation, length of operation and presence of drains influence the risk and have been incorporated into risk formulae (see Chapter 3). Indices measuring the state of the patient are also available and should be incorporated into any formula used for risk assessment (Bibby *et al.*, 1986, Culver *et al.*, 1991).

PROTECTION AGAINST 'SELF-INFECTION'

An operation wound may become infected with bacteria carried by the patient in the nose, gut or skin. For example, gas gangrene in patients having amputation of a leg with poor arterial blood supply is usually caused by faecal organisms present on the skin. Urinary infections and wound infections in bowel surgery are often due to coliform bacilli from the gut (see section on chemoprophylaxis on p. 234).

There is a particular hazard if the patient has an active staphylococcal infection, especially if it is near the operation site. In these circumstances, the patient's operation should, if possible, be delayed until the infection is over, or if this cannot be done, an appropriate antibiotic should be used for prophylaxis (see Chapter 13). Other measures, such as covering the lesions with a bacteria-impermeable dressing and disinfecting the surrounding skin, may also be helpful.

Early studies showed that staphylococcal nasal carriers developed post-operative sepsis more frequently than non-carriers. Pre-operative treatment (e.g. with mupurocin) may reduce post-operative infection, but further controlled studies are required (Mangram *et al.*, 1999). Pre-operative treatment of carriers of an epidemic strain during an outbreak should be considered, probably for a few days before the operation.

PROTECTION OF THE OPERATION SITE – DISINFECTION AND SHOWERING

Methods of cleansing and disinfection of the skin are described in Chapter 7. The agents recommended for routine use on skin are 0.5% chlorhexidine or 1% iodine in 70% alcohol or alcoholic povidone-iodine applied with friction for at least 2 min (Davies *et al.*, 1978). Alcoholic solutions are more effective and rapidly acting than aqueous ones, and are always preferable. Care is necessary to ensure that the skin is dry, particularly if diathermy is used.

If there is a special risk from clostridia, the application of a compress of 7.5% aqueous povidone-iodine for 30 min may be useful (as it kills many bacterial spores), but antibiotic prophylaxis is a more important measure. The skin should be washed with soap and water and dried before disinfection. Soap for shaving should be applied with a sterile gauze swab, not with a shaving brush. If it is considered necessary to shave the site of operation, this should be deferred until the day of operation because of the risk of causing small abrasions which may become heavily colonized with bacteria. Shaving should be avoided if possible;

clipping or the use of depilatory cream is preferable if removal of excess hair is considered to be essential (Seropian and Reynolds, 1971; Cruse and Foord, 1980).

For disinfection of mucous membranes, an aqueous solution of iodine (e.g. Lugol's or povidone-iodine) or aqueous chlorhexidine is generally recommended. Alcoholic solutions appear to be less effective on the oral mucous membranes, probably because of dilution by saliva.

For disinfection of the urethra, 1 mL of 1% chlorhexidine obstetric cream can be instilled immediately before the patient is taken to the theatre for cystoscopy or before catheterization. The instillation of a diluted solution (1/5000) of chlorhex-idine for disinfection of the bladder after gynaecological operations is also useful. A pad of plastic foam kept moist with chlorhexidine jelly may be attached to indwelling catheters at the urethral meatus in female patients, to prevent movement of the catheter (see Chapter 7).

PRE-OPERATIVE BATHS AND SHOWERS

It is customary for patients to have a bath or shower before elective operations. This cannot be expected to reduce the likelihood of post-operative infection unless an antiseptic detergent used at the time causes a significant reduction in the skin flora. Davies *et al.* (1977) found that a chlorhexidine detergent prepa-ration used in the bath or shower caused some reduction in the density of the skin flora. This effect, as would be expected, was much smaller than that of using the same preparation for disinfection of limited areas, namely the hands or the operation site. Assessments of the effect of the whole-body antiseptic ablutions on the incidence of post-operative sepsis have been varied. Cruse and Foord (1980) and Hayek *et al.* (1987) have reported a reduction in post-operative sepsis associated with pre-operative antiseptic baths and showers, but other studies, including some large-scale controlled trials, showed no such effect of one to three whole-body antiseptic baths or showers (Ayliffe *et al.*, 1983; Leigh *et al.*, 1983; Rotter *et al.*, 1988; Lynch *et al.*, 1992). The effect, if any, is marginal and sporadic.

TRANSPORT OF THE PATIENT TO THE OPERATING SUITE

The patient should be provided with freshly laundered theatre clothes and blankets immediately before he or she is taken to the operating suite. The porters should hand over the patient on his or her trolley to theatre staff in the inter-change area. There is no evidence that transfer of the patient to a clean trolley reduces the likelihood of contamination of the theatre, so this procedure (and the availability of a trolley transfer area in the theatre suite) can be omitted (Ayliffe *et al.*, 1969; Lewis *et al.*, 1990). The patient can be transferred in a bed from the ward to the anaesthetic room or to the operating-room without addi-tional risk of infection provided that ward bedding and clothing is removed before admission to the operating-room. Parents of small children may accompany the patient to the anaesthetic room without increasing the risk of infection.

DRAPES

Sterile drapes provide sterile cover for areas away from the immediate site of the operation and for instrument trays and other equipment. To prevent the loss of protectiveness on wetting, a layer of sterilized waterproof material under the drape or the use of waterproof towels is advantageous. Reusable drapes of microfilament polyester are available and may replace other materials. If necessary, new skin adhesion strips can be attached to the drape after each processing. Trilaminates with an absorbed layer next to the wound can also be used. There is evidence that adhesive plastic drapes do not protect the wound against contamination from the adjacent skin or reduce the incidence of sepsis. Their use for the prevention of infection of the operation wound is therefore of doubtful value (Whyte, 1988), although they are still widely used.

OPERATIONS ON CONTAMINATED ORGANS

The incidence and mortality from sepsis is higher after operations on the bowel than after operations on other sites. It is therefore rational to remove colonic bacteria when this can be done without risk. Colonic washouts have been widely used, but are unlikely to reduce the density of colonic bacteria or the incidence of sepsis. Non-absorbed aminoglycoside antibiotics (e.g. neomycin, framycetin) given by mouth can greatly reduce the aerobic flora, but they are ineffective against anaerobes. Metronidazole has been shown to reduce the incidence of anaerobic post-operative sepsis.

In operations involving sections of the alimentary tract or other heavily colonized viscera, gross soiling of tissue should be avoided by careful technique and by the use of packs (perhaps containing a layer of impervious material) and swabs. Instruments used on the opened viscus must be regarded as contaminated and should be kept separate from the rest of the instruments in the tray. They should be discarded after completion of anastomosis or excision.

TISSUE HANDLING TECHNIQUES

Good surgical technique is a major factor in reducing infection risk. Tissues must be handled gently, and no more foreign material must be left in a wound than is essential for the success of the operation. Careful haemostasis is important. Dead tissue and haematoma must be removed, and their formation must be prevented.

The practice of picking up with artery forceps only the bleeding vessel with little or no surrounding tissues, and the use of diathermy to coagulate the smaller bleeding points, reduces the amount of dead or foreign material in the wound. The thinnest ligature with the required strength should be chosen.

Whenever primary suture is intended, care must be taken to avoid contamination from the skin. Techniques to avoid sharps injuries have been developed to reduce the risk of acquisition of HIV infection (Sim and Jeffries, 1990; Joint Working Party of the Hospital Infection Society and the Surgical Infection Study Group, 1992).

WOUND DRAINAGE

A wound that is drained is more likely to become infected than a closed wound. Drainage should therefore only be used when there is a definite indication for it (e.g. to prevent accumulation of fluid, as for example when a serous cavity has been opened, when infection is present, when there is a fistula, or when there is much oozing of blood, lymph or serum into the wound).

The risk of infection may be reduced by the use of a closed system of drainage. The drain should be removed as soon as possible. For example, oozing of blood will stop after a few hours, and a drain inserted to meet this hazard can normally be removed after 24 hours or less. For deeper wounds, the drain should be long, extending to a bottle below the level of the bed. An underwater seal should be used for chest drains. Suction drainage provides a closed system which should help to prevent ascending infection.

DISPOSAL OF USED MATERIAL

Contaminated swabs and other articles should be placed in impermeable bags, which are sealed to prevent liberation of bacteria during handling and removal for cleaning and sterilization or removal to final disposal sites.

CHEMOPROPHYLAXIS (see also Chapter 13)

When the antibiotics were first introduced they were often used uncritically and needlessly for prophylaxis in surgery. This indiscriminate use encouraged the emergence of a predominantly resistant hospital flora. There was evidence, too, that patients were obtaining no clinical benefit from such prophylaxis, and when sepsis appeared it was likely to be caused by organisms that were resistant to the available antibiotics. The outcome was a general and somewhat uncritical condemnation of chemoprophylaxis in surgery.

A number of controlled trials and microbiological studies in recent years have led to a reappraisal of the situation. While routine systemic chemoprophylaxis is still seen as likely to do more harm than good, the use of selected patients, and of antibiotics which are likely to cover the range of probable invaders, can undoubtedly give valuable protection (Mangram *et al.*, 1999). Selective prophylaxis against known organisms of usually predictable sensitivity, used as an adjunct to careful asepsis, is appropriate when the consequence of infection would probably be serious.

The drug should be given in standard or large doses, covering the peri-operative period. A single dose should be adequate for most operations. Such a short period of treatment is unlikely to encourage the emergence of resistant variants, but it protects the patient during his or her most vulnerable period of exposure. There have been many publications which show the great importance of non-sporing anaerobic bacilli as a cause of post-operative sepsis after operations on the gastrointestinal tract. Such organisms greatly outnumber the aerobic organisms, including *E.coli*, in the faeces, and they are resistant to the aminoglycoside antibiotics (e.g. neomycin) which have been in common use for pre-operative disinfection of the gut. Prophylactic metronidazole may be expected to reduce anaerobic sepsis considerably after operations in which the anaerobic sepsis rates are usually high. Similar prophylactic results have been obtained in patients having appendicectomies and hysterectomies. The role of chemoprophylaxis for clean surgery remains uncertain and may not be cost-effective (Sanderson, 1999). Most surgeons would give prophylactic treatment for prosthetic surgery. Prophylactic regimes are discussed in Chapter 13.

REFERENCES

An, Y.H. and Freeman, R.J. (1996) Prevention of sepsis in total joint arthroplasty. *Journal of Hospital Infection* 33, 93.

Ayliffe G.A.J. (1991) Role of the environment of the operating suite in surgical wound infection. *Review of Infectious Diseases* 13 (**Supplement 10**), 800.

Ayliffe G.A.J. (1994) The role of ventilation systems in the prevention of infection. *Journal of the Institute of Medical Engineering* 48, 219.

Ayliffe G.A.J. and Lowbury E.J.L. (1969) Sources of gas gangrene in hospital. *British Medical Journal* 2, 333.

Ayliffe, G.A.J., Babb, J.R., Collins, B.J. and Lowbury, E.J.L. (1969) Transfer areas and clean zones in operating suites. *Journal of Hygiene* 79, 299.

Ayliffe, G.A.J., Collins, B.J., Lowbury, E.J.L. *et al.* (1967) Ward floors and other surfaces as reservoirs of hospital infection. *Journal of Hygiene* 65, 515.

Ayliffe, G.A.J., Noy, M.T., Babb, J.R. *et al.* (1983) A comparison of pre-operative bathing with chlorhexidine detergent and non-medicated soap in the prevention of wound infection. *Journal of Hospital Infection* 4, 237.

Babb, J.R., Lynam, P. and Ayliffe, G.A.J. (1995) Risk of airborne infection in an operating theatre containing four ultra-clean air units. *Journal of Hospital Infection* 31, 159.

Belkin, N.L. (1997) The evolution of the surgical mask: filtering efficiency versus effectiveness. *Infection Control and Hospital Epidemiology* 18, 49.

Bibby, B.A., Collins, B.J. and Ayliffe, G.A.J. (1986) A mathematical model for assessing post-operative wound infection. *Journal of Hospital Infection* 8, 31.

Casewell, M.W., Slater, N.P.G. and Cooper, J.E. (1981) Operating theatre water baths as a cause of pseudomonas septicaemia. *Journal of Hospital Infection* 2, 237.

Centers for Disease Control (1985) *Guidelines for prevention of surgical wound infections*. Atlanta, GA: Centers for Disease Control.

Charnley, J. (1979) *Low friction arthroplasty of the hip*. Berlin: Springer Verlag.

Church, J. and Sanderson, P. (1980) Surgical glove punctures. *Journal of Hospital Infection* 1, 84.

Clark, P.R., Reed, P.J., Seal, D.V. and Stephenson, M.L. (1985) Ventilation conditions and airborne bacteria and particles in operating theatres: proposed safe economics. *Journal of Hygiene* 95, 325.

Creamer, E. and Smyth, E.G. (1996) Suction apparatus and the suctioning procedure. *Journal of Hospital Infection* 34, 1.

Cruse, P.J.E. and Foord, R. (1980) The epidemiology of wound infection. A ten-year prospective study of 62 939 wounds. *Surgical Clinics of North America* **60**, 27.

Culver, D.H., Horan, D.C., Gaynes, R.P. *et al.* (1991) Surgical wound infection rates by wound class, operative procedure, and patient risk index. Nosocomial infections surveillance system. *American Journal of Medicine* **91 (Supplement 3B)**, 157S.

Davies, J., Babb, J.R., Ayliffe, G.A.J. and Ellis, S.H. (1977) Effects on the skin flora of bathing with antiseptic solutions. *Journal of Antimicrobial Chemotherapy* **3**, 473.

Davies, J., Babb, J.R., Ayliffe, G.A.J. and Wilkins, M.D. (1978) Disinfection of the skin of the abdomen. *British Journal of Surgery* **65**, 855.

Dunn, D., Fowler, S., Nair, R. and McCloy, R. (1994) Laparoscopic chlolecystectomy in England and Wales; result of an audit by the Royal College of Surgeons of England. *Annals of the Royal College of Surgeons* **76**, 269.

Emmerson, A.M. (1992) Environmental factors influencing infection. In Taylor, E.W (ed.). *Infection in surgical practice.* Oxford: Oxford University Press, 8.

Fitzgerald, R.H., Nolan, D.R., Ilstrup, D.M. and Van Scoy, R.E. (1977) Deep wound sepsis following total hip arthroplasty. *Journal of Bone and Joint Surgery* **59a**, 847.

Garibaldi, R.A., Cushing, D. and Lerer, T. (1991) Risk factors for post-operative infection. *American Journal of Medicine* **91 (Supplement 3B)**, 158S.

Goodwin, H. (1998) Minimal access surgery. *Journal of the Medical Defence Union* **14**, 12.

Gosden, P.E., MacGowan, A.P. and Banister, G.C. (1998) Importance of air quality and related factors in the prevention of infection in orthopaedic implant surgery. *Journal of Hospital Infection* **39**, 173.

Haley, R.W. (1995) The scientific basis for using surveillance and risk factor data to reduce nosocomial infection rates. *Journal of Hospital Infection* **30 (Supplement)**, 3.

Hambraeus, A. and Laurell, G. (1980) Protection of the patient in the operating suite. *Journal of Hospital Infection* **1**, 15.

Hayek, L.J., Emerson, J.M. and Gardner, A.M.N. (1987) A placebo-controlled trial of the effect of two preoperative baths or showers with chlorhexidine detergent on post-operative wound infection rates. *Journal of Hospital Infection* **10**, 165.

Hill, C., Flamant, R., Mazas, F. and Evrard, J. (1981) Prophylactic cephalozin versus placebo in total hip replacement. *Lancet* **1**, 795.

Holton, J. and Ridgway, G.L. (1993) Commissioning operating theatres. *Journal of Hospital Infection* **23**, 153.

Howarth, F.H. (1985) Prevention of airborne infection during surgery. *Lancet* **1**, 306.

Humphreys, H. (1991) The effect of surgical theatre headgear on bacterial counts. *Journal of Hospital Infection* **19**, 175.

Humphreys, H. (1993) Infection control and the design of a new operating theatre suite. *Journal of Hospital Infection* **23**, 61.

Joint Working Party of the Hospital Infection Society and the Surgical Infection Study Group (1992) Risks of surgeons and patients from HIV and hepatitis:

guidelines on precautions and management of exposure to blood and body fluids. Working Party Report. *British Medical Journal* 305, 1337.

Leaper, D.J. (1995) Risk factors for surgical infection. *Journal of Hospital Infection* 30 (Supplement), 127.

Leigh, D.A. (1981) An eight-year study of post-operative wound infection in two general hospitals. *Journal of Hospital Infection* 2, 207 .

Leigh, D.A., Stronge, J.L., Marriner, J. and Sedgwick, J. (1983) Total body bathing with 'Hibiscrub' (chlorhexidine) in surgical patients: a controlled trial. *Journal of Hospital Infection* 4, 229.

Lewis, D.A., Weymont, G., Nokes, C.M. *et al.* (1990) A bacteriological study of the effect on the environment of using a one or two trolley system in theatre. *Journal of Hospital Infection* 15, 35.

Lidwell, O.M. (1984) The cost implication of clean air systems and antibiotic prophylaxis in operations for total joint replacement. *Infection Control* 5, 36.

Lidwell, O.M., Lowbury, E.J.L., Whyte, W. *et al.* (1982) Effect of ultraclean air in operating-rooms on deep sepsis in the joint after operation for total hip or knee replacement: a randomised study. *British Medical Journal* 285, 10.

Lidwell, O.M., Elson, R.A., Lowbury, E.J.L. *et al.* (1987) Ultra-clean air and antibiotics for prevention of post-operative infection. *Acta Orthopaedica Scandinavica* 58, 4.

Lowbury, E.J.L. (1992) Special problems in antisepsis. In Russell, A.D., Hugo, W.B., Ayliffe, G.A.J. (eds), *Principles and practice of disinfection, preservation and sterilization,* 2nd edn. Oxford: Blackwell Scientific Publications, 310.

Lynch, W., Davey, P.G., Malek, M. *et al.* (1992) Cost-effectiveness analysis of the use of chlorhexidine detergent in preoperative whole-body disinfection in wound infection prophylaxis. *Journal of Hospital Infection* 21, 179.

Maki, D.G., Alvarado, C.J., Hassemer, C.A. *et al.* (1982) Relation of the inanimate environment to endemic nosocomial infection. *New England Journal of Medicine* 307, 1562.

Mangram, A.J., Horan, T.C., Pearson, M.L. *et al.* (1999) The Hospital Infection Practices Advisory Committee guidelines for the prevention of surgical site infection. *Infection Control and Hospital Epidemiology* 20, 247.

Marshall, R.J., Ricketts, V.E., Russell, A.J., and Reeves, D.S. (1991) Theatre overshoes do not reduce theatre floor bacterial counts. *Journal of Hospital Infection* 17, 125.

Medical Research Council (1962) Design and ventilation of operating suites. *Lancet* 2, 943.

Medical Research Council (1968) Aseptic methods in the operating suite. *Lancet,* 1, 705, 763, 931.

Mishriki, S.F., Law, D.J.W. and Jeffrey, P.J. (1990) Factors affecting the incidence of post-operative wound infection. *Journal of Hospital Infection* 16, 223.

Mitchell, N.J. and Hunt, S. (1991) Surgical masks in modern operating-rooms – a costly and unnecessary ritual. *Journal of Hospital Infection* 18, 238.

NHS Estates (1991) *Health Building Note. Operating departments.* London: HMSO.

NHS Estates (1994) Health Technical Memorandum 2025. *Ventilation in healthcare premises*. London: HMSO.

Orr, N.W. and Bailey, S. (1992) Masks in surgery (letter). *Journal of Hospital Infection* 20, 57.

Parker, M.T. (1969) Postoperative clostridial infections in Britain. *British Medical Journal* 3, 671.

Patel, S.R., Urech, D. and Werner H.P. (1998) Surgical gowns and drapes into the 21st century. *Institute of Sterile Services Management Journal* 3, 19.

Rotter, M.L. (1996) Handwashing and hand disinfection. In Mayhall, G.C. (ed.), *Hospital epidemiology and infection control*. Baltimore, MD: Williams and Wilkins, 1052.

Rotter, M.L., Larsen, S.O., Cooke, E.M. *et al.* (1988) The European Working Party on Control of Infection. A comparison of the effects of preoperative whole body bathing with detergent alone and with detergent containing chlorhexidine gluconate on the frequency of wound infections after clean surgery. *Journal of Hospital Infection* 11, 310.

Salvati, E.A., Robinson, R.P. and Zeno, S.M. (1982) Infection rates after 3175 total hip and total knee replacements performed with and without a horizontal filtered air-flow system. *Journal of Bone and Joint Surgery* 64-A, 525.

Sanderson, P.J. (1999) Assessing the role of prophylactic antibiotics in clean surgery. *Journal of Hospital Infection* 42, 7.

Schiebel, J.H., Jensen, I. and Pedersen, S. (1991) Bacterial contamination of air and surgical wounds during joint replacement operations. Comparison of different types of staff clothing. *Journal of Hospital Infection* 19, 167.

Seropian, R. and Reynolds, B.M. (1971) Wound infections after pre-operative depilatory versus razor preparation. *American Journal of Surgery* 121, 251.

Sim, J.W. and Jeffries, D.J. (1990) *Aids and surgery*. Oxford: Blackwell Scientific Publications.

Traore, O., Eschapasse, D. and Laveran, H. (1997) A bacteriological study of a contamination control tacky mat. *Journal of Hospital Infection* 36, 158.

Tunevall, T.G. (1991) Post-operative wound infections and surgical masks: a controlled study. *World Journal of Surgery* 15, 383.

Van Griethuysen, A.J.A., Spies-van Rooijen, N.H. and Hoogenboom-Verdegaal, A.M.M. (1996) Surveillance of wound infections and a new theatre: unexpected lack of improvement. *Journal of Hospital Infection* 34, 99.

Watkins, D.S., Wainwright, A.M., Thompson, M.H. and Leaper, D.J. (1995) Infection after laparoscopic cholecystectomy: are antibiotics really necessary? *European Journal of Surgery* 161, 509.

Whyte, W. (1988) The role of clothing and drapes in the operating-room. *Journal of Hospital Infection* 11 (Supplement C), 2.

Whyte, W., Hamblen, D.L., Kelly, I.G. *et al.* (1990) An investigation of occlusive polyester surgical clothing. *Journal of Hospital Infection* 15, 363.

chapter 12

LAUNDRY, KITCHEN HYGIENE AND CLINICAL WASTE DISPOSAL

LAUNDRY HYGIENE AND HANDLING OF CONTAMINATED LINEN (Barrie 1994)

Clothing or bed linen used by hospital patients is a possible infection risk to staff handling it on the ward and during transport to or processing in the laundry. Inadequately disinfected or recontaminated clean laundry may also be a risk to subsequent users.

Used linen may be heavily contaminated with bacteria, but these are mainly Gram-negative bacilli from the intestinal tract or coagulase-negative staphylococci from the skin. These organisms are common environmental contaminants and are unlikely to cause infection in staff handling linen. *Staphylococcus aureus* may be present, usually in small numbers (less than 1% of the total), and presents little hazard if normal precautions are taken. Large numbers of *Bacillus cereus*, not killed by the routine heating process, have been isolated from clean laundry and have been responsible for rare outbreaks of infection (meningitis following neuro-surgery and umbilical infections in neonatal units) (Birch *et al.*, 1981; Barrie *et al.*, 1992).

Used linen that has been in contact with patients infected with specific pathogens (e.g. *Salmonella* species and *Shigella* species) is a potential infection hazard if excretions or secretions are present (Standeert *et al.*, 1994). Linen from patients who are infected with or carriers of HBV or HIV is unlikely to be hazardous unless it is bloodstained. The risk of acquiring infection from linen, even if it is contaminated with blood, body fluids or excreta from infected patients, is low if it is handled with gloves and sealed in an impermeable bag or container.

CURRENT UK RECOMMENDATIONS

The present UK recommendations categorize laundry as follows: 1, used; 2, 'infected'; 3, heat-labile (Department of Health NHS Executive, 1995).

Used linen (soiled or foul)
This includes all used linen, irrespective of state, but on occasion contaminated by body fluids or blood and often with excreta. It excludes linen from patients in linen category 2 ('infected').

Visibly fouled linen is usually contaminated with the same range of organisms as other used linen, although the numbers are usually much higher. The linen from some geriatric establishments may contain many items of fouled linen (Taylor, 1982). Fouled linen, if handled with reasonable care, is unlikely to infect laundry workers. However, sorting is unpleasant and undesirable. Fouled linen may be included with infected linen and not sorted if agreed by the laundry manager and approved by the Infection Control Team (ICT). The main problems with avoiding sorting fouled linen are the possible presence of extraneous items (e.g. scissors) which could damage the washing-machine, and of heat-labile linen which might be ruined by the heating process.

'Infected linen'

This is linen from patients with specified infections with a potential to infect healthy staff as well as other patients (see Chapter 9). 'Infected' is a convenient if incorrect term for linen potentially contaminated with organisms from patients with or suspected of suffering from enteric fever, other salmonella infections, dysentery, open pulmonary tuberculosis, hepatitis A, B or C, HIV infection, other notifiable diseases, including infections in hazard groups 3 and 4 (Advisory Committee for Dangerous Pathogens, 1990), or other infections specified by the ICT. Although the risk from handling linen in most of these categories is small, especially if it is not visibly contaminated, it was felt that handling by laundry workers should be avoided. Linen from patients with most notifiable diseases (e.g. measles, chicken-pox) is not hazardous and could be treated as used linen. Linen from patients contaminated with hazard group 4 pathogens should be treated as 'infected' (Advisory Committee on Dangerous Pathogens, 1996), but if there is any doubt about the safety of routine processing, treatment should be discussed with the ICT.

Linen from 'infected' patients should be sealed in an alginate stitched or hot-water-soluble bag, or a bag with a water-soluble membrane, as soon as it is removed from the patient. This bag should then be placed in a clearly identifiable impermeable outer bag for storage or transport. On arrival in the laundry, the alginate or water-soluble bag should be removed from its outer bag, or bags and placed unopened in a washing-machine with a suitable heat-disinfection cycle. Alginate or water-soluble bags, or bags with a water-soluble membrane, are designed to dissolve or partly dissolve, releasing their contents into the washing-machine at an early stage in the cycle. Infested linen (e.g. with lice or fleas) should be dealt with in the same way. The outer bag should be washed at the same time as the contents. The potential problem with insoluble plastic bags is that they may stick to the inner surface of the washing-machine, particularly during drying.

There is evidence that levels of contamination are similar in linen from isolation rooms to those in linen from other areas of the hospital, and that double bagging is unnecessary (Maki *et al.*, 1986). In the USA, linen is not segregated as described above, and water-soluble or similar bags are not usually recommended (McDonald and Pugliese, 1996). As it is often unknown whether or not linen is from an infected patient, sorting of all used linen is carried out using universal precautions, and there is no evidence of acquired infection in laundry workers provided that precautions are taken. However, in the UK the existing guidelines should be followed unless evidence-based alternatives are available.

It is recommended that all hospital linen should be heat-disinfected during the wash process by raising the temperature to either 65°C for 10 min or 71°C for 3 min. This has been found to be effective, but in practice higher temperatures or longer times are usually used (e.g. 80°C for 1 min or more). Mixing times of 4–8 min should be included in the cycle, depending on the machine.

Experimental evidence suggests that temperature differences as great as 20°C can occur throughout the load. These recommended times and temperatures were calculated from the killing of over 10^6 enterococci, which are more resistant to heat than most other vegetative organisms and viruses. More resistant strains of enterococci than the test strain have been isolated, but as yet are unlikely to be a major problem (Bradley and Fraise, 1996). A temperature of 71°C for 3 min associated with thorough washing should be adequate (Wilcox and Jones, 1995). Dilution and rinsing, followed by drying, will remove or kill most organisms. However, if there is a problem with heat-resistant strains in the hospital, temperatures and times of disinfection should be reviewed by the ICT.

Measurement of temperatures at the interface between water and linen is difficult. All washing-machines should be fitted with accurate heat sensors to indicate the temperature reached during the disinfection cycle. The relationship between the indicated temperature and the coolest part of the load should be established.

The efficiency of the disinfection cycle should be checked when commissioning new machines, at regular intervals (e.g. every 6 weeks), during major outbreaks, and in disputes with private laundries. Because of the difficulties in measuring load temperatures accurately, microbiological methods may be required in some of these situations (e.g. in disputes with private laundries) (Collins et al., 1987).

Tests for survival of relatively heat-resistant vegetative organisms, (e.g. cultures of enterococci applied to patches of material or sealed in narrow-bore plastic tubing and attached to an item of linen in the load) are commonly used (Collins et al., 1987). The latter test measures the effect of heating only, and does not take into consideration removal and dilution. Although microbiological testing of linen after processing is rarely required, it may also occasionally be useful if there is evidence or suspicion that infection has been transmitted by this route. Contact plates taken from processed linen awaiting distribution should not normally show more than one colony-forming unit (cfu)/cm^2 and should not average more than 2 cfu/cm^2. The organisms isolated should be predominantly Gram-positive cocci and aerobic spore-bearing bacilli. Gram-negative bacilli should not be present. As some of the bacteria on linen are destroyed during the heat-drying and finishing process, counts taken from the load after washing, but before drying, are likely to be higher. The presence of substantial numbers of Gram-negative bacilli or spore-bearing bacilli in these samples taken after washing may be evidence of recontamination from the surrounding environment or from contaminated water used to rinse after heat disinfection. Tests on a number of machines, including batch, tunnel and continuous batch washers, if properly adjusted, have shown that all would adequately disinfect the load (Collins *et al.*, 1987).

Continuous batch washing machines or tunnel washers are now commonly used. These should disinfect the load, but organisms can grow in wet linen kept in the machine overnight. Machines should preferably be emptied at the end of the day and rinse sections should be heat-disinfected before production starts each day. If linen remains in the machine it should be disinfected. It is recommended by the NHS Executive that continuous batch washers are not used for infected linen. Blockages may occur in the pre-wash section before disinfection has taken place, and may require entrance into the machine by maintenance staff. It is recommended that infected linen should be washed and disinfected in a washer extractor connected by a closed pipe to the drainage system to avoid the release of aerosols. However, separate machines for 'infected' linen should be unnecessary, and continuous batch washers could be used for 'infected' linen provided that these difficulties are overcome.

HEAT-LABILE LINEN

The requirement to heat-disinfect all linen is becoming more difficult to achieve because of the increasing use of fabrics that are likely to be damaged at disinfecting temperatures (e.g. knitted polyester). Thorough washing and rinsing at low temperatures (e.g. 40–50°C) will remove most organisms and should be sufficient in most circumstances, particularly in domestic washers. Disinfection can be achieved by chemical disinfectants. A chlorine-producing agent to give a final concentration or 150 ppm available chlorine can be introduced into the penultimate rinse. These chlorine compounds should not be used on fabrics treated for fire retardance. Other agents may be used (e.g. hydrogen peroxide), but further research is necessary. Heat-labile linen should be enclosed in a white bag with an orange stripe. This bag could be labelled with a prominent label marked 'infected' if sorting is to be avoided.

Since all used linen is likely to be contaminated, and may contain sufficient moisture to allow microbes present to continue to multiply, it should be enclosed as soon as possible in bags which are impermeable to microbes. All used linen should be handled with minimum disturbance to avoid dispersal of organisms. Once enclosed in a suitable bag, it can be safely transported through wards and corridors. The bag, if not disposable, should be processed through a suitable heat-disinfection cycle before reuse. Used linen is usually enclosed in white bags, and the water-soluble bags containing infected linen are placed in red bags, or in white bags with a red line, and marked 'infected' on a yellow label. If temporary storage of used linen is necessary, it should be stored in a properly designated area where it is secure from pilfering and protected from pests. Facilities for keeping the area clean must be available (e.g. by installing hose points for water/steam). There is probably no reason for providing separate storage facilities for infected linen where it is enclosed in water-soluble bags contained in a secure identifiable outer bag.

When handling used linen, laundry staff should wear aprons, gloves and overalls, and should be provided with adequate facilities for washing and changing when starting and finishing each shift of work. Staff handling used linen should be given training to ensure that they understand the measures required to protect themselves and others. Staff should be offered immunization against poliomyelitis, tetanus, hepatitis B and BCG vaccination if they are tuberculin-negative. Staff with unhealed lesions, rashes or any exfoliative skin condition should not handle clean laundry unless the lesions can be covered with an impermeable dressing.

Linen returned after processing should not normally be carried in the same vehicle as used linen of any category. Exceptions could be made if the vehicle is divided into two compartments with separate loading doors and the partition is impervious and complete. In small units where the use of two vehicles is uneconomical, a single vehicle may be used if it is adequately cleaned between loads.

Domestic-type washers used in some small units for personal clothing may be acceptable if the patients are physically healthy, but arrangements must be made for the adequate disinfection of items that would normally be classified as infected if the machines fail to reach disinfection temperatures.

Education of ward staff should make it less common for laundry bags of used linen to contain objects that should not have been placed in them. The presence of sharp objects, particularly needles, represents a major hazard to laundry sorting staff. Labelling bags with their ward of origin may help to reduce these hazardous practices.

If an outside contractor is responsible for hospital laundering, a similar policy to that used in hospital should be employed, including immunization and training of staff in hygienic methods. The laundry should be periodically visited by infection control staff to ensure that standards are acceptable.

A written quality control system should be introduced and regularly monitored. Although the infection risks are much lower than those in catering, a hazard analysis critical control points (HACCP) method should be introduced. Temperatures and times of disinfection and other processes and chlorine concentrations could be included.

KITCHEN HYGIENE (Hobbs and Roberts, 1993; Department of Health NHS Executive, 1996)

All patients commonly receive food from a single kitchen, and poor hygiene in food preparation may be followed by an outbreak of infection involving the whole hospital. The cook–chill method of preparation may include staff meals possibly in more than one hospital, and could further increase the risk, although if controls are adequate the risks may be less than with conventional catering. Infection from contaminated food is particularly hazardous in debilitated or elderly people, and can cause severe illness or even death. It is also important to prevent foodborne infection among the staff, as subsequent transfer to patients would have similar unfortunate results.

Outbreaks of bacterial food poisoning are usually caused by *Salmonella* species, or the toxins of certain strains of *Staphylococcus aureus, Clostridium perfringens* and *Bacillus cereus. Campylobacter* species are now the most common cause of foodborne infection, although outbreaks in hospitals are infrequent. Outbreaks caused by *E. coli* 0157:H7 have been increasingly reported, but mainly occur in the community. The small numbers of organisms required to initiate an infection increase the problem of controlling an outbreak of this organism. These organisms, especially *Salmonella* species, may be transferred to the patient directly from contaminated raw foods (e.g. meat and poultry if inadequately cooked), or indirectly from initially contaminated food via the hands of staff, or from inadequately cleaned surfaces or equipment. Staphylococcal and salmonella carriers on the staff may also contaminate food if their personal hygiene is poor, but are infrequently responsible for outbreaks. Inadequately cooked food which is left without refrigeration for several hours, particularly if it is subsequently warmed, is an important source of infection. Any food that is capable of supporting bacterial growth should be stored either below 8°C or above 63°C, and should not normally be allowed to remain between these temperatures for more than 2 hours, and sufficient time must be allowed for complete thawing before cooking. Food hygiene regulations in the UK Food Safety (Temperature Control) Regulations 1995 (Department of Health NHS Executive, 1996) state that 8°C is satisfactory for cold storage, but 5°C is preferable if possible. Some bacterial species (e.g. *Listeria*) can grow slowly at low temperatures, and chilled food should be kept at a temperature of 0–3°C

Good personal hygiene of kitchen staff and effective methods of cleaning food preparation areas and equipment are of major importance in preventing the spread of infection. The general kitchen structure, (e.g. walls, floors and ceilings), although of little direct relevance in the spread of infection, should be kept clean and in good condition.

MEDICAL EXAMINATION OF STAFF

The prospective employee should be questioned about any past history of typhoid or paratyphoid fever, dysentery, persistent diarrhoea, or attacks of diarrhoea and vomiting lasting for more than 2 days within the past 2 years, tuberculosis, boils, skin rashes, discharges from the eye, ear, nose or other site, and also the place and date of all visits abroad. A questionnaire on the above illnesses and other relevant information is filled in by the catering manager or a member of the occupational health department and signed by the proposed employee (see Appendix 12.1). The catering manager may provisionally accept the applicant pending a satisfactory assessment by a medical officer, who may require a more detailed medical examination. A tuberculin skin test is advisable and, if negative, BCG should be offered. Examination of blood, faeces, other laboratory tests or a chest X-ray need not be performed unless indicated by past history. The Microbiologist or Infection Control Doctor should be consulted if laboratory tests are considered necessary. If an examination of faeces is required, at least three samples taken on successive days should be examined.

SICKNESS

A system for recording all incidents of diarrhoea and vomiting in both patients and staff is required, and is of particular importance for catering staff. An example of a reporting scheme for staff is shown in Appendix 12.2. General practitioners may regard hospital staff as fit to return to work when they are still excreting salmonella or shigella. An assessment of fitness to return to food-handling duties may therefore have to be made in the hospital. In addition, all catering staff who have been exposed to enteric infection require counselling on handwashing technique and on other measures required to prevent possible spread.

Food-handlers suffering from diarrhoea and/or vomiting while at work should immediately be referred to an appropriate authority for assessment. This could be the occupational health or infection control department, or the Consultant in Communicable Disease Control, depending on the system used. They should, where possible, be referred before leaving for home to ensure that specimens are obtained where appropriate, and that the incident is properly documented. If it is then decided that they are unfit for further duty, they should be reminded that they must report back before returning to normal duties. Skin rashes, boils and other lesions or rashes should be reported in a similar manner.

All food handlers should report to the Occupational Health Department, staff medical officer, or Infection Control Nurse:

1 if they have been off sick with one of the above conditions;
2 if they have suffered from diarrhoea or vomiting lasting more than 2 days while on leave;
3 if other members of the household are suffering from diarrhoea or vomiting.

If, on reporting, they are considered to be fit for return to work, they should be counselled on the importance of a good handwashing technique and general hygiene, and given a note for their manager specifying whether they can or cannot return to food preparation duties. To encourage prompt reporting of such conditions, staff should be made aware that being sent off duty will not lead to loss of salary.

TRAINING

All food handlers should be given training in personal and kitchen hygiene both on employment and at intervals thereafter. A booklet containing rules of hygiene should be provided for each member. Posters demonstrating different aspects of hygiene should be prominently displayed in catering food storage areas and changed at frequent intervals (see Appendix 12.3).

PERSONAL HYGIENE

The main route of transfer of infection to food is via the hands of staff. Hands should be washed frequently, especially after using the toilet and before handling food. In addition to the hands and fingernails, the face and other parts of the body should be kept clean, including the hair and scalp, and the forearms when short sleeves are worn. The nose, lips and hair should not be touched while handling food, and nails should be kept short. Hands cannot be assumed to be free from pathogenic organisms after washing, and food should be handled as little as possible. Non-sterile disposable gloves should be worn when handling food which is to be eaten without further processing (e.g. sandwiches). Hands should be washed in hot water using the recommended soap or detergent, and must then be well rinsed and thoroughly dried on a fresh paper towel. As they may damage the skin, nail-brushes should only be used if they are essential to remove heavy soiling. Nailbrushes lying in soap-dishes are likely to be heavily contaminated with Gram-negative bacilli. Their use may then both damage the skin and inoculate it with bacteria. A small number of sterile or adequately decontaminated nail brushes should be available on request, and arrangements should be made for these to be reprocessed after use. Wash-basins must be provided in each food preparation area, together with plain bar or liquid soap or detergent. Bar soap should be kept in a dry state between uses. If liquid soap dispensers are used, they must be thoroughly cleaned at regular intervals and must not be refilled without prior cleaning and disinfection. The liquid soap should contain a preservative. Antibacterial soaps and detergents (e.g. chlorhexidine-detergent preparations, iodophors, triclosan) may be required during an outbreak of infection, but should only be used on advice from the infection control staff. The catering staff should be provided with good changing and sanitary accommodation. Food handlers should keep their personal clothing and overalls clean, and should change their protective clothing daily or more frequently if necessary. Protective clothing should only be worn for catering duties, and should not be worn in other departments. Laundering should be arranged by the hospital authorities. Uniforms and other protective clothing should not be taken home for laundering or for any other purpose unless this is unavoidable. Staff should not smoke while handling food or while in a room where food is exposed. All cuts and grazes must be completely covered with a waterproof dressing.

CLEANING AND MAINTENANCE

Detailed schedules should be produced defining methods and responsibility. Floors should be constructed to facilitate cleaning, and they should be well maintained. Walls and ceilings should have smooth impermeable surfaces, and cooking equipment should be sited so that areas below and around it can be easily cleaned. All cleaning should be carried out with a freshly prepared and accurately diluted detergent solution. Cleaning equipment (e.g. scrubbing machines and mops) should remain in the kitchen but not in the food preparation area (for methods of disinfection, see Chapter 6), and should be examined at defined intervals. If it becomes worn or damaged, equipment should be repaired or replaced. Special attention should be paid to the cleaning of food preparation surfaces and meat slicers. Preparation surfaces should be impervious to water and should be maintained in a good condition. Stainless-steel surfaces are advised, although composition chopping boards and blocks are suitable. Wherever possible, preparation surfaces should be used for one purpose only and colour coded. In small units with limited working areas, it may be necessary to use surfaces for more than one purpose. Thorough cleaning and drying between different uses is required in such cases. In any case, food that requires no further cooking (e.g. sandwiches, cooked meat, etc.) must not be prepared on surfaces which have previously been used for preparation of raw meat, fish, poultry or vegetables. Preparation surfaces should always be cleaned with a recently prepared hot cleaning solution and a fresh disposable or freshly laundered cloth. There is little point in providing separate surfaces for different types of food if all surfaces are cleaned with the same cleaning solution and cloths, as contamination will be transferred from one surface to another. Each individual surface should be dried with a disposable or freshly laundered dry cloth, as most Gram-negative bacilli die on drying if the surface is initially clean.

Disinfectants are usually unnecessary, but may be recommended by the Infection Control Doctor or Microbiologist during outbreaks of infection (chlorine releasing solutions containing at least 250 ppm available chlorine are often used).

Transfer of contamination from one product to another is particularly likely with meat mincers and slicers. Cooked and uncooked meats must never be processed with the same machine without thorough cleaning between operations.

CROCKERY AND CUTLERY: POTS AND PANS

Crockery and cutlery should be machine-washed at a minimum temperature of 60°C and a final rinse of at least 80°C for 1 min or another appropriate temperature and time (see Chapter 5). A central washing-up machine is preferred, and washing up by hand on the ward should be avoided whenever possible. However, a washing-up machine on the ward is a satisfactory alternative provided that a machine with a disinfection cycle is available. If machine-washing facilities are not available and crockery and cutlery have to be washed by hand, twin sinks should preferably be used to ensure efficient rinsing. Detergent solutions and rinsing water should be changed frequently and should be as hot as possible. Reusable washing-up cloths should not be used unless they are thoroughly washed and dried after each use. They should preferably be replaced by disposable cloths. Nylon brushes, washed and thoroughly dried after each use, are preferable to non-disposable cloths, but should not be used in preference to disposable materials.

It is important that all crockery, cutlery, pots and pans and kitchen equipment should be thoroughly dried after cleaning. The use of linen drying cloths (tea towels) should be discontinued whenever possible and replaced by a system of heat-drying or air-drying in racks. When drying by hand is necessary, a disposable or recently laundered towel is preferable.

Crockery, cutlery, pots and pans should be examined regularly. Worn, chipped, stained or broken items should be replaced. When not in use, they should be stored clean and under conditions in which recontamination is reduced to a minimum. If heat disinfection is not possible, disposable cutlery and crockery may be recommended by the infection control team for certain infections (e.g enteric fever and gastrointestinal infections).

STORAGE AND TRANSPORTATION OF FOOD

Certain food (e.g. raw meat, fish and poultry) may carry harmful bacterial contaminants, and should be prepared and cooked in such a way that these organisms are destroyed before serving. Periodic checking of temperatures with a probe thermometer in the coldest part of the food is recommended. A temperature of at least 70°C for 2 min should be achieved. Poultry may be contaminated with *Salmonella* species, and inadequate thawing of frozen poultry before cooking may enable these organisms to survive the cooking process. The multiplication of bacteria should be prevented by careful storage of food at the correct temperature before and after cooking. For example, *Clostridium perfringens* is a common cause of food poisoning, and its spores may survive the cooking process. These bacteria may multiply if cooked food is left unrefrigerated for longer than 2 hours. Subsequent reheating may further increase the numbers of bacteria, and when large numbers are eaten, toxins may be released into the intestine and cause food poisoning. Food must be stored so that raw meat, fish and uncooked vegetables (whether prepared or unprepared) do not come into contact with food which is to be served without further heat treatment. These foods must be separated by storing them in separate refrigerators or in closed compartments within the same refrigerator or cold room. Food must not be stored on the floor of cold rooms or below foods which may leak or be spilt. The temperatures of cold rooms and refrigerators (including ward refrigerators) should be routinely monitored.

Food that requires cooling must not be left in the kitchen area but should be transferred to a cooling area and cooled rapidly to at least 8°C (see also section on cook–chill foods). Stored food should be protected from recontamination. Food which is transported within the hospital (e.g. from stores to kitchen), or from kitchen to ward, should be transported under clean conditions and properly covered to prevent contamination. It should be carried in a clean closed container, especially if the vehicle is used for other purposes. Vehicles used for this purpose should be appropriately designed and kept clean and in good repair. Contaminated materials (e.g. refuse or soiled linen) must not be carried in these vehicles.

Refuse and food waste (swill) must not be allowed to accumulate in the kitchen, and should be removed at frequent intervals.

The length of time for which food is allowed to stand on hot plates and trolleys must be kept to a minimum. Trolleys, hot cupboards and containers must be maintained at the correct temperature (over 63°C) and checked at regular intervals (e.g. monthly).

Food should be served by staff trained in food hygiene. Clean overalls or plastic aprons should be worn and adequate serving equipment provided in order to prevent unnecessary handling. Patients should not take part in food preparation or washing-up procedures unless this is agreed by the ward sister. Leftover food in ward refrigerators should be discarded daily; swill must not be retained or stored on the ward.

GOOD CATERING PRACTICE

A policy for safe handling and processing of food should be available in all catering departments. This should be prepared by the catering staff with advice from the infection control team or environmental health officer. Where possible, standardized recipes should be used so that internal temperatures can be measured and reproduced to ensure adequate cooking. Policy decisions should be made for each type of food with regard to the minimum internal temperature required, the maximum time allowed at room temperature after cooking, and how long it can be kept refrigerated before use or disposal. Whenever possible, meat should be cooked on the day that it is to be served. There should also be a strict policy on the maximum time for which sandwiches, salads, etc., are kept at room temperature or in chilled storage before they are discarded.

RETAINING FOOD FOR TESTING

Food poisoning organisms, when present, are not uniformly distributed throughout contaminated food and, whatever the conditions of storage, the numbers of bacteria/g of food will vary from sample to sample examined over the storage period. The absence of food-poisoning organisms in a sample does not indicate that the item contained no such organisms, and the numbers present at the time of testing does not necessarily reflect the numbers present when the food was eaten. The results obtained from stored samples can be misleading. Sampling requires careful planning, proper supervision and extensive documentation. The amount and type of food stored and the particulars of the storage container should be defined. The full co-operation of the microbiologist is necessary. Even if only representative samples of those items that are likely to be associated with food poisoning are saved, the value of sampling for intestinal pathogens is unlikely to justify the substantial resources required, and cannot be recommended as a routine procedure. Although outbreaks of food poisoning in an individual hospital are very rare, some monitoring may be required, particularly during the setting up of a cook–chill service. Control of processes by good techniques is much more important than microbiological sampling.

COOK–CHILL MEAL SERVICES (Department of Health, 1989)

Good catering practices should be followed as with conventional catering. A flow-chart should be prepared at each stage and examined for potential infection risk. Monitoring systems should be set up to ensure that agreed standards are met, and all stages should be documented. A system of monitoring based on hazard analysis critical control points (HACCP) is now commonly used. This involves defining and controlling microbiological or other hazards at certain critical points during the processing of food (Wilkinson et al., 1991). The responsibility for maintaining standards should be clearly defined. The present Department of Health guidelines should generally be followed, and should not be modified unless the microbiologist or environmental health officer agree that a modification is acceptable. The following precautions should be observed.

1 Raw foods of good microbiological quality should be chosen and correctly stored.
2 Areas for handling raw and cooked foods should be separate.

3 During cooking, food should reach a temperature of 70°C (and preferably be retained at this temperature for 2 min to destroy listeria).

4 The food should be chilled to a temperature of 0–3°C within 90 min. Special arrangements may be required for joints and poultry. They should either be sliced hot and transferred to a rapid chiller within 30 min, or else the temperature of joints should be reduced to 10°C or less in 2.5 hours. When the temperature has reached this level the joints should be sliced in a temperature-controlled room and transferred to the rapid chiller without delay.

5 Food should be stored at 0–3°C for no longer than 5 days. If the temperature exceeds 5°C but remains less than 10°C, the food should be eaten within 12 hours. If the temperature exceeds 10°C, destruction of the stored food should be considered. Advice should be obtained from the microbiologist before destroying the food.

6 Food should be transported in a refrigerated or insulated trolley and the temperature should not exceed 10°C before reheating to 70°C. If refrigeration is not available, maximum transport times should be agreed.

7 Food containers should either be disposable or cleaned, disinfected by heat and dried after use. Times and temperatures should be regularly checked and recorded to ensure that no bacterial growth can occur during the process. A probe thermometer should be used to confirm that the necessary temperatures are reached in each of the processes. Most pathogenic organisms fail to grow at temperatures below 5°C, and significant growth is unlikely to occur within less than 2 hours at room temperature.

Although routine microbiological testing should be unnecessary if process control is reliable, tests are usually performed with a recently set up service, or if changes are made a suggested standard is as follows.

A sample of 100 g of each item of food from each batch to be tested should be taken immediately before reheating.

The following criteria are suggested (Sandys and Wilkinson, 1988):

1 total aerobic count – less than 100 000/g (agar plates incubated at 37°C for 48 hours);

2 *Salmonella* species and *Listeria monocytogenes* should not be detected in 25 g;

3 *E. coli* – less than 10/g; *E.coli* 0157:H7 should not be detected;

4 *Staphylococcus aureus* and *Clostridium perfringens* – less than 100/g.

Listeria monocytogenes has recently emerged as a potential hazard, as it will grow at lower temperatures than most other pathogens. It is commonly found in the environment and as a contaminant of raw foods, but the number of foodborne infections remains low. Although the number of clinical infections reported has increased in recent years, the overall number is still relatively small. Nevertheless, susceptible groups (e.g. pregnant women or immunocompromised patients) should not eat food that is likely to contain listeria.

HAZARD ANALYSIS CONTROL POINTS (HACCP)

Hospitals are advised to set up this system for conventional food services as well as cook–chill meal services. HACCP is a structured system set up to analyse potential hazards and identify the points where hazards may occur, implementing changes as required and periodically reviewing the system (Richards *et al.*1993; Barrie, 1996; Department of Health NHS Executive, 1996). The system should identify and assess microbiological and other hazards in production, processing, preparation, storage and distribution of food. A critical point is a point in the operation at which control can be exercised to eliminate or minimize a hazard (e.g. the temperature of food during cooking, time spent at room temperature and refrigerator temperatures). The system should rapidly detect any failures in procedures.

RESPONSIBILITY

Managers should ensure that written operational policies are in place and functioning satisfactorily. These should cover training of staff, pest control, critical control systems, cleaning and waste disposal. Ward staff who handle or serve food should comply with regulations and be adequately trained and supervised. The catering manager is responsible for hygiene and cleaning in his or her department. The responsibility for maintenance of structure and equipment should be clearly defined. At least one annual inspection should be made by the catering manager, Infection Control Doctor or a member of the infection control team, and a member of the engineering or building staff to examine aspects of hygiene in the catering area. A check-list for kitchen inspections is shown in Appendix 12.4. Occasional inspections should also be made by an environmental health officer. The Infection Control Doctor and committee are responsible for advising the district manager or administrator on all hygienic matters, including catering, and reports should be referred to them before action is taken.

LEGISLATION IN THE UK

All food provided by the National Health Service must comply with food safety requirements, i.e. the Food Safety Act 1990, Food Safety (General Food Hygiene) Regulations 1995 and Food Safety (Temperature Control) Regulations 1955 (Department of Health NHS Executive, 1966). Recent changes in food regulations are based on European Community Council Directives. The Food Safety Act 1990 empowers an authorized officer (e.g. an environmental health officer) to serve an improvement notice requiring measures to remedy defects and to serve emergency prohibition notices if it is considered that an imminent risk to health exists. If premises and equipment belonging to the NHS are used by a contractor providing food services, the contractor will have legal responsibilities, but the health service will also retain some responsibility.

Liaison between health services and the environmental health departments is important, as closure of health-care establishments can have severe repercussions, and the costs can absorb funds required for patient care. A risk assessment should be made before closures are enforced. The Food Safety Act 1990 provides a defence if defendants are able to prove that they took 'all reasonable precautions and exercised all due diligence' to avoid committing an offence.

Hospital managers should hold meetings with the infection control team and the local authority environmental health officer to review issues such as training, works programmes, pest control and any problems following routine inspections. Food premises should be registered with local authorities.

PESTS: ERADICATION AND CONTROL

The infestation of hospital premises (e.g. kitchens, staff restaurants, laundries, nurses' homes, etc.) with pests, particularly cockroaches, Pharaoh's ants and mice, is a common but undesirable occurrence. Although it may be difficult to keep some old premises free of pests, every effort should be made to achieve a reasonable level of control or eradication, whichever is practicable. This will depend on the type of pest, the extent of infestation, the complexity of the buildings and other local factors (Baker, 1981).

The role of pests in the transmission of hospital-acquired infection is uncertain, but reports indicate that carriage of specific pathogens, including *Salmonella* species, may occur. Apart from the possibility of disease transmission, food may be tainted and spoiled, and fabrics and building structure damaged. Pharaoh's ants have been responsible for the penetration of sterile packs and the invasion of patient's dressings, including those in use on a wound. Treatment with insecticides and rodenticides alone is seldom sufficient, and attention must also be paid to good hygiene and structural maintenance. Pests require food, warmth, moisture, harbourage and a means of entry. Therefore hospital staff should be encouraged to keep food covered, to remove spillage and waste, and to avoid accumulations of static water. Buildings should be of sound structure and well maintained, drains should be covered, leaking pipework must be repaired, and damaged surfaces should be made good. Cracks in plaster and woodwork, unsealed areas around pipework, damaged tiles, and badly fitting equipment and kitchen units are all likely to provide excellent harbourage. Close-fitting windows and doors and the provision of fly screens and bird netting all help to exclude pests from hospital buildings.

Many pests are nocturnal (e.g. cockroaches and mice), and infestation surveys are best conducted at night and when the rooms are unoccupied. In addition to seeing the pests themselves, droppings, nests, runs, rodent smears, insect fragments, structural and fabric damage are all signs of infestation. Sticky detectors or traps are also now available for monitoring the control of cockroaches and other crawling pests. Pyrethrum aerosols are useful for flushing cockroaches and other insects from their harbourage, and liver baiting is useful for assessing infestation with Pharaoh's ants.

In most hospitals, the task of pest control is given to a commercial company that specializes in this work. Nevertheless, the hospital should appoint an officer to co-ordinate local pest control activities, initiate a reporting system, conduct preliminary and routine assessments of control measures, and negotiate with and follow up the recommendations of the servicing company (Department of Health NHS Executive, 1992).

Standard NHS Pest Control Contracts require that premises be 'rid' of certain pests within a finite period of time. Thereafter there is a contractual obligation upon the servicing company to ensure that the premises remain free of those pests. Integrated into this type of strategy are inspection and reporting procedures.

The pesticides used will have been approved under the Pesticides Regulations, and furthermore will have been considered by the health authority to be suitable for use within its premises.

Advice on all aspects of pest control is available from the Environmental Health and Food Safety Division (EHF4A) of the Department of Health.

DISPOSAL AND MANAGEMENT OF CLINICAL WASTE

Every effort should be made to reduce the total waste by employing more reusable items and recycling, and by minimizing clinical waste by better segregation.

Hospital waste is classified into two categories, namely household and clinical. Clinical waste in some countries may be referred to as *medical waste*, or may include a separate category of *infectious waste*. Definitions are correspondingly viable, and in the UK, legislation is increasingly influenced by European Union Directives (Collins and Kennedy, 1993). Clinical waste is defined in the UK Controlled Waste Regulations 1992. Other relevant Acts include the Environmental Protection Act (Duty of Care) Regulations 1991, the Health and Safety at Work Act 1974 and the Control of Substances Hazardous to Health Act (COSHH) 1988 (Moritz, 1995).

There is no evidence that waste as a whole from hospitals poses a greater infection risk than waste from domestic and commercial premises, or that clinical waste, apart possibly from sharp instrument injuries, has been the cause of infections in hospital staff or in the community (Ayliffe, 1994). Nevertheless, some waste is potentially more hazardous (e.g. used needles, untreated microbiological waste and clinical waste from certain highly contagious or hazardous infections) and these items require special treatment (Rutala and Mayhall, 1992).

Categorization of waste should preferably be based on scientific evidence. Infection risk is related to the number and type of organisms present in the waste, their likelihood of survival in the environment, and the probability that those organisms will reach a susceptible site in sufficient numbers or with sufficient virulence to set up an infection. All of these conditions are required for infection to occur, and they will rarely be met in the handling of clinical waste, apart possibly from a needlestick or other sharp instrument injury. Waste handled by staff who are wearing suitable protective clothing and taking adequate hygienic precautions should pose only a minimal risk and, if sealed in an impermeable plastic bag, presents no risk to the handler. However, aesthetic aspects and public perception of risk may differ from the actual infection risk. Human tissues, although not usually infectious, would be unacceptable if exposed on a landfill site, and should be adequately contained and incinerated. Some items in bulk (e.g. incontinence pads) are unpleasant and should if possible be incinerated, although deep burial would be adequate in terms of infection risk.

Guidance based on existing legislation has been given in the UK by the Health Services Advisory Committee (Health and Safety Commission, 1992) and the London Waste Regulation Authority (1994). Other countries have produced somewhat similar guidelines (Rutala and Mayhall, 1992; Collins and Kennedy, 1993).

CATEGORIZATION OF CLINICAL WASTE (Health and Safety Commission, 1992)

Group A

This includes all human tissues, including blood (whether infected of not), animal carcasses and tissues from veterinary centres, hospitals and laboratories, and all related swabs and dressings. It also includes waste materials, where the assessment indicates a risk arising from, for example, infectious diseases cases, and soiled surgical dressings, swabs and other soiled waste from treatment areas.

Group B

This includes discarded syringe needles, cartridges, broken glass and any other contaminated disposable sharp instruments or items.

Group C

This includes microbiological cultures and potentially infected waste from pathology departments (laboratory and post-mortem rooms) and other clinical or research laboratories.

Group D

This includes certain pharmaceutical products and chemical wastes.

Group E

This includes items used to dispose of urine, faeces and other bodily secretions or excretions assessed as not falling within group A, including used disposable bedpan liners, incontinence pads, stoma bags and urine containers.

Groups A and B must be incinerated or otherwise rendered safe, and this is the preferred option for the other groups as well.

- Recognizable animal or human tissue (e.g. amputated limbs) should be transported under supervision to an incinerator for immediate disposal. If transport outside the hospital is necessary, the bag should be placed in a rigidly locked container labelled with instructions as to who should be contacted in the event of a breakdown or accident to the vehicle.
- Used sharp instruments must be disposed of in containers to an approved standard (e.g. see Department of Health NHS Executive, 1982). Containers should be stored under secure conditions to prevent any unauthorized access (syringes and needles are an attraction to children).
- Laboratory waste is usually autoclaved in the laboratory before disposal. This will render it safe for transport, but secure storage to prevent spread of infection by pests prior to autoclaving requires consideration. Incineration without prior autoclaving could be acceptable provided that adequate safety

precautions are taken during transport and subsequent storage before incineration.

Special arrangements are also required for radioactive, cytotoxic materials and pharmaceuticals. Those who are involved with the use of these materials should be aware of the legislation.

Potentially offensive materials (e.g. incontinence pads, babies' diapers, stoma bags and most soiled dressings) in category E are unlikely to be an infection risk to handlers, as the organisms present, even in large numbers, are likely to be present in any moist waste in the hospital or the community. Although incineration is preferable, other arrangements (e.g. deep landfill) could be acceptable. The subdivision of clinical waste into groups A to E is generally reasonable but causes some problems, particularly in the community, and is not always scientifically valid. It is illogical to include group E as clinical waste, as urine and faeces (and other bodily fluids) are discharged untreated into the sewage system without evidence of harm to sewage workers of the environment. The subdivision of clinical waste into infectious and non-infectious categories, as used with laundry, would be more cost-effective (see p. 239). The main difficulties with the present classification are in the domestic situation. Sharps should obviously be contained and incinerated as in hospital, but other items (e.g. incontinence pads, babies' diapers and tampons) can be enclosed in a plastic bag and discarded safely in household waste. Whether other items (e.g. wound dressings) should be treated as clinical waste and collected by the local authority is debatable, and this would certainly not be cost effective or necessary with regard to the infection risk. However, although national guidelines are not legally enforceable, any major deviations should be discussed with the legal enforcement agencies before implementation.

Legally acceptable, environmentally safe incinerators are expensive and are now not available in most hospitals, so incineration of clinical waste by commercial contractors or local authorities is usually required. This is also expensive, and other methods of rendering waste safe are being investigated (e.g. chemical, macerating and steaming methods, and microwaving) (London Waste Regulation Authority, 1994: Blenkharn, 1995). Disinfection of clinical (infectious) waste, and not sterilization, is required to render it microbiologically safe.

MANAGEMENT OF WASTE IN HOSPITALS

A clinical waste control officer should be appointed, and he or she should be accountable to the Chief Executive or Senior Manager in the hospital. The hospital is responsible for reviewing and proposing improvements in waste handling and disposal, for carrying out COSSH assessments on waste disposal, for investigating and reviewing incidents involving waste handling, and for identifying the training requirements of staff who handle waste (Health and Safety Commission, 1992). The officer should liaise with clinical services, the training officer, the occupational health department, the supplies and service managers and the pharmacist, and he or she should be a member of the infection control committee. A waste management committee, consisting of representatives from these departments and the risk manager, would be useful. The officer should be advised by the infection control team, particularly on the assessment of infection risks, and in some cases the duties of officer will be carried out by the Infection Control Nurse or Doctor.

The following are important requirements.

- A written policy should be produced and regularly updated and audited.
- Staff handling waste should be trained (particularly in the handling of spillage), provided with appropriate protective clothing and immunized against poliomyelitis, hepatitis B and A, and tuberculosis if they are not already tuberculin positive or have previously received BCG.
- Clinical waste should be sealed in a strong impermeable bag or container (e.g. yellow bag in the UK) and labelled with the place and date of origin. Clinical waste suitable for deep landfill should be contained in a yellow bag with black stripes, waste to be autoclaved in a light blue bag or clear bag with blue lettering. A black bag is used for domestic waste.
- Disposal of clinical waste is more expensive than disposal of domestic waste, and good segregation at source is cost-effective. Mistakes in segregation and in bag colours will occur, but these should be kept to a minimum. Legal enforcement officers should where possible make scientific assessments of risks (e.g. on spillage and errors in segregation, when called to investigate incidents and before taking legal action).

WASTE STORAGE AND TRANSPORT

Clinical waste should be regularly removed from clinical areas (e.g. twice daily) to secure storage areas. These should be easy to clean, roofed, properly drained and bird and rat proof. A water supply for hosing down is essential.

Producers of clinical waste will either use an on-site incinerator or arrange for transport to an off-site incinerator. They are responsible for ensuring that these arrangements are adequate and that a contractor is authorized to transport and dispose of waste. A transfer note which includes a description of the waste should be completed and signed (Health and Safety Commission, 1992).

APPENDIX 12.1 QUESTIONNAIRE FOR CATERING STAFF

	Yes	No	When (year)?	How long off work?	If yes, name of doctor or hospital
1 Have you ever had any of the following? Typhoid fever Paratyphoid fever Dysentery Persistent diarrhoea Tuberculosis					
2 Have you suffered from any of the following within the past 2 years? Diarrhoea and/or vomiting for more than 2 days Skin rash Boils Discharge from eye Discharge from ear Discharge from nose Other infections					
3 Have you ever been abroad? If yes:	Yes Where?	No When?			

I declare that all the foregoing statements are true and complete to the best of my knowledge and belief.

. . . .

4 *Investigations:*
  Chest X-ray
  Faeces
  Blood
  Other

Comments

APPENDIX 12.2 CATERING STAFF AGREEMENT TO REPORT INFECTION

I agree to report to the Catering Officer or his or her deputy

1 If suffering from an illness involving:
   vomiting
   diarrhoea
   skin rash
   septic skin lesions (boils, infected cuts, etc., however small)
   discharge from ear, eye or nose.
2 After returning and before commencing work following an illness involving vomiting and/or diarrhoea, or any of the above conditions.
3 After returning from a holiday during which an attack of vomiting and/or diarrhoea lasted for more than 2 days.
4 If another member of my household is suffering from diarrhoea and/or vomiting.

I have read (or had explained to me) and understood the accompanying rules on personal hygiene.

Signed   Date

APPENDIX 12.3 KITCHEN AND FOOD-HANDLING STAFF – RULES OF PERSONAL HYGIENE

Patients in hospital may develop severe infection with germs which are not harmful to healthy people.
   The following rules must be observed to prevent germs from entering food.
1 **WASH THE HANDS FREQUENTLY**, ESPECIALLY AFTER USING THE TOILET AND BEFORE HANDLING FOOD. THIS IS THE MOST IMPORTANT METHOD OF PREVENTING THE SPREAD OF INFECTION. In addition to hands and particularly nails, the face and other parts of the body likely to come into contact with food should be kept clean (e.g. the hair and scalp, and the forearms when short sleeves are worn). Avoid touching the nose, lips and hair while handling food.
2 Personal clothing and overalls must be kept clean. Protective clothing provided by the hospital must be worn.
3 All open cuts and grazes must be completely covered with a waterproof dressing.
4 You must not smoke while handling 'open' food or while in a room where there is such food.
5 Observe other hygienic rules as indicated by the Catering Manager.

APPENDIX 12.4 INSPECTION OF KITCHENS

A check-list should be produced from the following guidelines.

DELIVERY

Food should be properly transported, delivered in good condition and at the right temperature.

Check that:

1 transport is clean, not used for any other purpose, and refrigerated if specified;
2 food is properly contained and at the right temperature (deep-frozen food should be at –18°C or below; chilled food should be between 0°C and +3°C);
3 a probe thermometer should be used to check the temperature, which should be recorded. Is the food properly wrapped and handled? Does packaging give any information on origin? Is it dated? Is the person unloading the van wearing clean clothing, etc.?

HANDLING ON ARRIVAL

Food should be transferred to the correctly designated storage area at the appropriate temperature as soon as possible. It should be transferred with minimal handling and without coming into contact with other foods.

Check wet stains on the bottom of boxes of frozen food, which suggest that it has been defrosted and refrozen. If boxes are stacked, check their contents to ensure that thawing meat is not dripping into butter, cheese, etc.

STORAGE TEMPERATURE

Any food capable of supporting microbial growth should be stored either below 8°C or above 63°C (cook-chilled food should be stored below 3°C).

Check the temperature at which food items should be stored. Question staff if food is at room temperature – ask two different people, not present at the same time, how long it has been there. Use a probe thermometer to check the temperature of food being served or plated.

FOOD STORES

Food stores should be generally clean, uncluttered and with good access for cleaning. Food in boxes or sacks should not be stored directly on the floor. Shelving should be easy to clean and, if not moveable, easy to clean under, around and behind.

Check for evidence of infestation, lids left off bins, packets left open, etc. Ensure that there is a proper stock rotation system and that products are clearly identified. There should be no staff clothing, handbags, etc., in the storage area. Any opening skylights or windows should be bird-proofed, door bottoms should be rat-proofed, and all pipes, etc., should be sealed into the wall.

FOOD SEPARATION

Any food that is likely to be naturally contaminated with organisms capable of causing food poisoning (e.g. raw poultry, meat and fish) should be prevented from coming into direct or indirect contact with any food that will be eaten without further cooking.

Question staff closely on requirements for food separation.

Look out for the use of the same surface for preparation of different foods, the use of common cloths or knives, and staff not washing their hands.

Note that good practice includes the use of separate bays for each task, colour-coded cloths, and satisfactory cleaning of knives, preparation surfaces and chopping blocks.

ADEQUATE COOKING

The use of approved detailed recipes should include minimum internal temperatures both before starting cooking and at the end. The type of container used should also be specified. For each type of food there should be clear guidelines on whether unserved portions can be used as a basis for other dishes and whether all processes for the particular meal are completed on the same day. Clear guidelines must also exist as to how long the food can be retained after it has been cooked and before it is served, and at what temperature it should be stored. Is reheating allowed? If so, under what circumstances and to what temperature.

Check the details of at least one commonly prepared dish, and question staff in detail to ensure that guidelines are known, understood and followed.

STAFF HYGIENE

All staff who are handling food should be trained in personal and catering hygienic methods.

Check the numbers of hand wash-basins and whether they are correctly sited, the presence of soap and paper towels, and evidence of recent use. Is it the clearly defined responsibility of a named individual to ensure that soap and towels are always available? Are staff aware under what conditions they should report sick, and to whom? Is counselling on the need for care in handwashing given after each absence for illness if diarrhoea or vomiting is involved? What is the availability of clean uniforms, and are they sufficient?

Question staff on training courses and their content, and on their existing knowledge.

WARD KITCHENS, ETC.

Ensure that all the food preparation and service areas (including ward kitchens) are included in inspections, and that they are covered by an agreed policy.

CLEANING

Every area and item in the kitchen should have an agreed cleaning procedure. Methods, materials and frequency should be defined, including an order of priority during periods of staff shortage. These should be displayed and known by all staff concerned. It should be clearly understood where the cleaning equipment is stored and who is responsible for cleaning and notifying any need for repair or replacement.

REFERENCES

Advisory Committee for Dangerous Pathogens (1990) *Categorisation of pathogens according to hazard and categories of containment.* London: HMSO.

Advisory Committee for Dangerous Pathogens (1996) *Management and control of viral haemorrhagic fevers.* London: HMSO.

Ayliffe, G.A.J. (1994) Clinical waste: how dangerous is it? *Current Opinion in Infectious Diseases* 7, 499.

Baker, L.F. (1981) Pests in hospitals. *Journal of Hospital Infection* 2, 5.

Barrie, D. (1994) Infection control in practice: how hospital linen and laundry services are provided. *Journal of Hospital Infection* 27, 219.

Barrie, D. (1996) The provision of food and catering services in hospital. *Journal of Hospital Infection* 33, 13.

Barrie, D., Wilson, J.A., Hoffman, P.N. and Kramer, J.M. (1992) *Bacillus cereus* meningitis in two neurosurgical units: an investigation into the source of the organism. *Journal of Infection* 25, 291.

Birch, B.R., Perera, B.S., Hyde, W.A. *et al.* (1981) *Bacillus cereus* cross-infection in a maternity unit. *Journal of Hospital Infection* 2, 349.

Blenkharn, J.I. (1995) The diposal of clinical wastes. *Journal of Hospital Infection* **30 (Supplement)**, 514.

Bradley, C.R. and Fraise, A.P. (1996) Heat and chemical resistance of enterococci. *Journal of Hospital Infection* 34, 91.

Collins, B.J., Cripps, N. and Spooner, A. (1987) Controlling microbiological decontamination levels. *Laundry and Cleaning News* 30, 31.

Collins, C.H. and Kennedy, D.A. (1993) *The treatment and disposal of clinical waste.* Handbook No. 13. Leeds: H and H Consultants Ltd.

Department of Health (1989) *Chilled and Frozen. Guidelines on cook-chill and cook-freeze catering systems.* London: HMSO.

Department of Health NHS Executive (1982) *Specifications for containers for disposal of needles.* London: HMSO.

Department of Health NHS Executive (1992) *Pest control management for the health service.* London: HMSO.

Department of Health NHS Executive (1995) *Hospital laundry arrangements for used and infected linen.* Heywood: Health Publications Unit.

Department of Health NHS Exectuve (1996) *Management of food hygiene and food services in the National Health Service.* London: Department of Health.

Health and Safety Commission (1992) *The safe disposal of clinical waste.* London: HMSO.

Hobbs, B.C. and Roberts, D. (1993) *Food poisoning and food hygiene,* 6th edn. London: Edward Arnold.

London Waste Regulation Authority (1994) *Guidelines for the segregation, handling and disposal of clinical waste,* 2nd edn. London: London Waste Regulation Authority.

McDonald, L.L. and Pugliese, G. (1996) Laundry service. In Mayhall, C.G. (ed.) *Hospital epidemiology and infection.* Baltimore, MD: Williams and Wilkins, 805.

Maki, D.G., Alvado, C. and Hassemer, C. (1986) Double-bagging of items from isolation rooms is unnecessary as an infection control measure: a comparative study of surface contamination with single- and double-bagging. *Infection Control* 11, 535.

Moritz, J.M. (1995) Current legislation covering clinical waste. *Journal of Hospital Infection* 30 (Supplement), 521.

Richards, J., Parr, E. and Risborough, P. (1993) Hospital food hygiene: the application of hazard analysis critical points to conventional hospital catering. *Journal of Hospital Infection* 24, 273.

Rutala, W.A. and Mayhall, C.G. (1992) SHEA position paper: medical waste. *Infection Control and Hospital Epidemiology* 13, 38.

Sandys, G.H. and Wilkinson, P. (1988) Microbiological evaluation of a hospital-delivered meals service using precooked chilled foods. *Journal of Hospital Infection* 11, 209.

Standeert, S.M., Hutcheson, R.H. and Schaffner, W. (1994) Nosocomial transmission of salmonella to laundry workers in a nursing home. *Infection Control and Hospital Epidemiology* 15, 22.

Taylor, L.J. (1982) Is it necessary to treat foul linen from geriatric patients as infected? *Journal of Hospital Infection* 3, 209.

Wilcox, M.H. and Jones, B.L. (1995) Enterococci and hospital laundry. *Lancet* 344, 594.

Wilkinson, P.J., Dart, S.P. and Haddington, C.J. (1991) Cook–chill, cook–freeze, cook–hold, *sous vide*: risks for hospital patients? *Journal of Hospital Infection* 18 (Supplement A), 222.

chapter 13

USE OF ANTIBIOTICS AND CHEMOTHERAPEUTIC AGENTS

In this chapter the word *antibiotic* refers to both synthetic compounds (antimicrobial chemotherapeutic agents) and naturally produced agents (antibiotics). Some of these substances (e.g. the penicillins) are almost without toxicity to humans (except for those individuals who are hypersensitive to them) but will kill many pathogenic bacteria. Certain antibiotics (e.g. bacitracin) are so toxic to humans that they cannot safely be given parenterally, and are reserved for topical treatment of superficial infections, or are given orally to disinfect the gut, if non-absorbed.

If a patient is known or suspected to be suffering from an infection, the clinician must decide which organism is known or likely to be responsible, and to which antibiotic it will or will probably be sensitive. Other factors which need to be considered include the expected value of treatment and the possible side-effects of the antibiotic.

The aim of chemotherapy is principally to aid the natural defences of the body to eliminate the microbes from tissues by preventing their multiplication. In order to have this effect, the blood and infected tissues must contain a concentration of the antibiotic which is ideally 2–5 times higher than the *minimal inhibitory* (i.e. bacteriostatic) *concentration* (MIC) of the antibiotic for the infecting organism. There are a limited number of circumstances where chemotherapy must aim to kill the infecting organisms (i.e. tissue fluids must contain more than the *minimal bactericidal* (i.e. killing) *concentration* (MBC) of the antibiotic). Such situations include endocarditis and infections in patients who are immunosuppressed.

Antibiotic-resistant strains of certain organisms are common in hospital. *Staphylococcus aureus* and certain Gram-negative bacilli that cause hospital infection have become increasingly resistant to the commonly used antibiotics. These resistant organisms may have appeared either as a result of the selection of intrinsically resistant strains by extensive and often indiscriminate use of antibiotics, or by mutation of previously sensitive bacteria, and selection following exposure to the antibiotics. Some resistant organisms, especially Gram-negative bacilli, can transfer antibiotic resistance to other bacteria. These antibiotic resistance genes can reside on plasmids or on segments of DNA which are capable of moving between organisms (transposons).

Whereas the majority of hospital staphylococci and also most strains in the community are now resistant to penicillin, all haemolytic streptococci of group A (*Streptococcus pyogenes*), clostridia and the treponema of syphilis remain sensitive to this antibiotic – an example of the extreme variability of bacterial resistance.

In view of the large number of available antibiotics, there is need for guidance on their use. This chapter provides concise information about antibiotics and recommendations for their safe and effective administration in treatment and (where indicated) in prophylaxis. Methods of delaying the emergence of resistance (especially by avoidance of unnecessary or inefficient use) are emphasized. (For detailed information on antibiotics, see Kucers *et al.*, 1997; O'Grady *et al.*, 1997.)

CLASSIFICATION OF ANTIBIOTICS

Antibiotics have been classified in many different ways. The most useful approach for clinical use is to classify them according to which micro-organism they are likely to affect. In practice, the acquisition of resistance may render antibiotics less useful, and knowledge of the local epidemiology of resistant bacteria is necessary in selection of the most appropriate agent. Table 13.1 is a summary of the classification used in Parker and Collier (1990), and indicates which groups of bacteria are sensitive to the different classes of antibiotics.

Although much has been written about the importance of bactericidal activity (i.e. the ability to kill bacteria) compared to bacteriostatic activity (prevention of growth), the clinical significance of this distinction is questionable. Many agents which are bacteriostatic become bactericidal if used in higher doses, and the clinical situations in which bactericidal activity is required are limited. Similarly, *in vitro* tests can demonstrate antagonism between cell-wall-active antibiotics such as penicillins and bacteriostatic agents, but the clinical significance of this is probably not great.

Although it is tempting to use broad-spectrum antibiotics for the treatment of many infections and thus cover a large range of less common pathogens, this has the disadvantage of selecting out resistant organisms. In particular, the use of broad-spectrum antibiotics can increase the risk of antibiotic-associated diarrhoea and other infections caused by *Clostridium difficile*. Broad-spectrum antibiotics should therefore not be used to treat specific pathogens that are sensitive to narrow-range agents (e.g. *Streptococcus pyogenes*).

USE OF INDIVIDUAL ANTIBIOTICS

For guidance on complex treatment and its control, the clinician should consult a clinical microbiologist or a physician experienced in chemotherapy. The *British National Formulary,* which should be available in all wards and departments, contains up-to-date information on all available antibiotics.

Table 13.1 Classification of antimicrobial agents according to activity

Activity against Gram-positive bacteria and Gram-negative cocci	Main activity against Gram-negative bacteria	Broad-spectrum antibiotics	Specific antibacterial agents	Antifungal and antiviral agents
Benzylpenicillin	Ampicillin[a]	Sulphonamides	*Anaerobes*	*Antifungals*
Phenoxymethyl-penicillin	Mezlocillin[a]	Co-trimoxazole	Clindamycin	Nystatin
	Piperacillin	Cephalosporins	Metronidazole	Amphotericin B
Flucloxacillin	Ciprofloxacin	Imipenem	*Tuberculosis*	5-Fluorocytosine
Erythromycin	Ofloxacin	Tetracyclines	Isoniazid	Imidazoles
Clindamycin	Temocillin	Chloramphenicol	Rifampicin	Griseofulvin
Rifampicin	Aztreonam	*Meropenem*	Ethionamide	*Antivirals*
Vancomycin	Gentamicin	*Imipenem*	Pyrazinamide, etc.	Acyclovir
Teicoplanin	Amikacin		*Chlamydia*[c]	Ganciclovir
	Nitrofurantoin[b]			Zidovudine
	Nalidixic acid[b]		Erythromycin	
			Tetracycline	
			Chloramphenicol	
			Campylobacter species	
			Erythromycin	
			Ciprofloxacin	
			Legionella species	
			Erythromycin	
			Rifampicin	

[a] Some activity vs. Gram-positive cocci.
[b] Urinary tract infection only.
[c] Also *Mycoplasma*, *Rickettsia*.

APPLICATION OF ANTIBIOTICS TO TISSUES

Most infections with sensitive organisms respond to systemic antibiotic therapy. However, there are times when local application of chemotherapeutic agents may be indicated. Chloramphenicol is used for the treatment of purulent conjunctivitis. Suppurative external ear conditions are treated with antibiotic eardrops. Silver nitrate solution (0.5%) is an effective chemoprophylactic agent for severe burns. Silver sulphadiazine cream is a more convenient and very effective application for this purpose, although sulphonamide-resistant bacteria may be selected through its use in a burns unit. Gentamicin should not be used topically for routine prophylaxis because of the risk of promoting resistance. Streptococcal infections of burns should be treated with a systemic antibiotic (flucloxacillin or erythromycin; see Chapter 16, p. 302) and not topical therapy. In general, it is best to avoid applications of penicillins or neomycin to the skin, as sensitization may result. Furthermore, neomycin should not be applied to severe burns, as it may lead to absorption and subsequent deafness through damage to the auditory nerve. Intrathecal administration of antibiotics is potentially hazardous and should be avoided. Antibiotics may be instilled into the pleural and peritoneal cavity in addition to parenteral therapy in the treatment of purulent effusions or peritonitis. This route of administration of antibiotics is particularly useful in the treatment of peritonitis associated with continuous ambulatory peritoneal dialysis (CAPD).

ANTIBIOTIC COMBINATIONS

Most infections respond satisfactorily to treatment with a single antibiotic. In the following circumstances, however, combined therapy may be valuable.

PREVENTION OF DEVELOPMENT OF BACTERIAL RESISTANCE

Tuberculosis is the outstanding indication for obligatory combined chemotherapy for this purpose.

INFECTIONS CAUSED BY MORE THAN ONE ORGANISM (POLYMICROBIAL SEPSIS)

Intra-abdominal sepsis is usually caused by both aerobic and anaerobic bacteria, and for this reason a combination of gentamicin or a cephalosporin with metronidazole is commonly used.

SEPTICAEMIA AND ENDOCARDITIS

Combinations of antibiotics are sometimes required for treatment of septicaemia and certain forms of endocarditis. A combination of penicillin and gentamicin should be used to treat endocarditis caused by viridans streptococci. Fully sensitive strains of streptococci can be treated with 2 weeks of penicillin plus gentamicin, followed by 2 weeks of oral amoxycillin. If the organism shows reduced susceptibility to benzyl penicillin, the British Society for Antimicrobial Chemotherapy Working Party (1990) recommend a combination of penicillin and gentamicin for a total of 4 weeks.

Penicillin or ampicillin plus gentamicin is suitable for *Enterococcus faecalis* endocarditis. Ceftazidime, piperacillin or ticarcillin may be used in combination with gentamicin (they must be injected separately) for the treatment of pseudomonas septicaemia, and combined therapy (e.g. flucloxacillin and fusidic acid) has been suggested for staphylococcal septicaemia. However, most infections mentioned under this heading can be treated successfully with a single antibiotic.

WHEN A COMBINATION IS SUPERIOR TO A SINGLE AGENT (SYNERGY)

Combination therapy is often useful in serious sepsis such as endocarditis or septicaemia because the mixture of two agents has greater activity than the sum of the individual activities of the agents. This phenomenon is called synergy, and laboratory methods are available for testing of chemotherapeutic agents for this interaction.

SELECTION OF AN ANTIBIOTIC

The selection of an antibiotic should never be a haphazard choice, but must be based on careful consideration of the following factors.

THE SENSITIVITY (OR PROBABLE SENSITIVITY) OF THE INFECTING ORGANISM

Before the infecting organism and its sensitivity are known, it is useful to make a presumptive diagnosis of its possible identity and the antibiotic sensitivity of the organism by consideration of the clinical picture, so that treatment with a potentially appropriate antibiotic can be started; (e.g. in infective endocarditis, where the commonest infecting organism is a viridans streptococcus, or in purulent meningitis, in which the organisms are usually meningococci or pneumococci). *Haemophilus influenzae* is now a rare cause of meningitis since the introduction of the childhood vaccine against type b strains (Hib). Severe infections such as endocarditis require detailed sensitivity testing, including the determination of the MIC and MBC of the organism.

THE CLINICAL PHARMACOLOGY OF THE VARIOUS ANTIBIOTICS

Particularly important factors are absorption, excretion and distribution. Certain antibiotics (e.g. ampicillin) are excreted in the bile and urine, while some (e.g. chloramphenicol and the penicillins) penetrate the inflamed 'blood–brain barrier' and pass in to the cerebrospinal fluid (CSF). For drugs which are predominantly excreted by the renal route, it is important to be aware that renal failure will delay excretion. It is also important to know how different antibiotics are cleared by haemodialysis and haemofiltration so that dosages can be adjusted appropriately.

ROUTE OF ADMINISTRATION

Oral therapy is satisfactory for the treatment of many infections. However, severe infections may require intravenous injections. To achieve adequate blood levels, antibiotics given intravenously should normally be administered by 'bolus'. IV infusion is the recommended method of administration for some antibiotics (e.g. vancomycin). Topical application of antibiotics may be sufficient for certain eye, superficial skin and external ear infections.

TOXICITY OF ANTIBIOTICS

All antibiotics have side-effects, and toxic drugs should not be used when safer agents are available. For example, chloramphenicol can cause fatal aplastic anaemia and is thus rarely indicated systemically.

Aminoglycoside antibiotics cause eighth-nerve damage if blood concentrations are allowed to exceed accepted safe levels. In the presence of renal failure, longer intervals between doses are required to prevent toxic blood levels. Recent data on the efficacy and toxicity of different dosage regimes for aminoglycosides have demonstrated that giving large doses (4–6 mg/kg) once daily results in equal efficacy with lower toxicity compared to standard 3 times daily regimes.

PROPHYLAXIS

There are several well-defined indications for prophylactic antibiotics (see p. 272).

COST OF ANTIBIOTICS

When other factors are equal, the least expensive drug should be selected.

TREATMENT OF SPECIFIC INFECTIONS

URINARY TRACT INFECTIONS

In domiciliary practice most urinary tract infections are caused by *E. coli,* 60% of which will be resistant to ampicillin. Trimethoprim is usually effective against ampicillin-resistant strains, although the incidence of resistance in the community is approximately 20%. Patients with chronic or recurrent infections and those with hospital-acquired infections often have organisms in their urine that are resistant to many antibacterial agents, and the choice of antibiotic must then be made when the results of sensitivity testing are available. Acute pyelonephritis must be treated as soon as the diagnosis is suspected with a parenteral drug active against a wide range of Gram-negative bacilli (e.g. a cephalosporin or Augmentin). Treatment for pyelonephritis should continue for 14 days in order to avoid an unacceptable relapse rate.

ALIMENTARY TRACT INFECTIONS

Antibiotics are not indicated for the treatment of most gastrointestinal infections. Exceptions to this rule include the following:
1 Invasive salmonella infections and those which are clinically severe. Typhoid fever is treated with ciprofloxacin or chloramphenicol. Trimethoprim and ciprofloxacin are effective in invasive and non-invasive severe infections caused by salmonella organisms other than *Salmonella typhi* and *Salmonella paratyphi B.*
2 Trimethoprim or ciprofloxacin are indicated for severe bacillary dysentery.
3 Perforation of the bowel (including the appendix) leads to peritonitis, often with a mixed flora, the principal organisms being Gram-negative bacilli and anaerobic bacteria, especially *Bacteroides* species. The treatment of choice is cefuroxime plus metronidazole (or clindamycin), or cefoxitin. Augmentin is an alternative.

4 Acute cholecystitis and cholangitis should be treated with gentamicin or a cephalosporin.

5 Campylobacter enteritis, if severe, should be treated with erythromycin or ciprofloxacin, although antibiotics probably have no effect on the course of the disease unless they are started early.

TUBERCULOSIS

Material such as pus, sputum or CSF, from which tubercle bacilli may be cultured, should be sent to the laboratory before chemotherapy is commenced. Tubercle bacilli readily acquire resistance when exposed individually to one of the four principal drugs (isoniazid, rifampicin, ethambutol and pyrazinamide), and also to the drugs of second choice (e.g. streptomycin) which are used when the infecting strain is resistant to the standard drugs. For this reason, at least three drugs must always be used in combination. Treatment should be supervised by a physician with experience in the management of tuberculosis.

RESPIRATORY TRACT INFECTIONS (OTHER THAN TUBERCULOSIS)

Upper respiratory tract infections are frequently viral, and antibiotic therapy is only indicated when a bacterial aetiology is known or suspected. The commonest bacterial cause of acute sore throat is the haemolytic streptococcus of group A, for which benzylpenicillin or phenoxymethylpenicillin are the drugs of choice (except in mixed infections with β-lactamase-producing *Staphylococcus aureus* (e.g. in burns), when flucloxacillin or erythromycin are indicated). Acute sinusitis and otitis media usually respond satisfactorily to erythromycin or ampicillin. For oral candidiasis (thrush), local applications of nystatin are effective. However, fluconazole is available orally and is more acceptable to the patient.

Acute infections of the lower respiratory tract acquired outside hospital are usually due to *Streptococcus pneumoniae* or *Haemophilus influenzae*. Both organisms are usually sensitive to ampicillin and co-trimoxazole. Benzylpenicillin is the drug of choice for pneumococcal infections, although pneumococci with decreased sensitivity to penicillin are increasing in prevalence. In debilitated patients or those suffering from viral infections such as influenza, *Staphylococcus aureus* may cause a fulminating pneumonia which should be treated with high doses of flucloxacillin and fusidic acid. Acute epiglottitis is a very serious and sometimes fatal condition which is usually caused by *Haemophilus influenzae* and should be treated with parenteral cefotaxime, although this infection is fortunately rare since the introduction of Hib vaccine. Acute bronchitis and exacerbations of chronic bronchitis are treated with amoxycillin or trimethoprim. Specific pneumonias are initially treated as follows:
- staphylococcal – flucloxacillin, fusidic acid or Augmentin;
- pseudomonas – gentamicin, ticarcillin, azlocillin or ciprofloxacin;
- mycoplasma – erythromycin or new quinolone;
- chlamydia – tetracycline or new quinolone;
- legionella – erythromycin (plus rifampicin if severe).

WOUND INFECTIONS

Wounds are frequently colonized by bacteria without being grossly infected, and respond satisfactorily to local measures such as removal of sutures, drainage, application of antiseptics and frequent saline bathing.

Severe wound infections with spreading cellulitis and/or systemic illness are usually due to *Staphylococcus aureus* or group A streptococcus infections, and are treated with an antibiotic, depending on sensitivity testing. Infected abdominal wounds in patients who have had operations of the gastrointestinal tract (including appendix and gall-bladder) are likely to be due to the patient's bowel flora, including aerobic and anaerobic organisms, and should be treated with combinations of metronidazole and cefuroxime. Infections of clean stitched wounds when the intestine has not been opened are usually staphylococcal and should be treated with flucloxacillin. A combination of gentamicin or cefuroxime plus metronidazole may be necessary for 'mixed' wound infections or those where the severity is such that treatment must be commenced before the results of sensitivity testing are available. Augmentin is an alternative.

Burns must be cultured regularly and treated according to the results obtained. The isolation of *Staphylococcus aureus, Pseudomonas aeruginosa* or other Gram-negative bacilli is not an indication for chemotherapy except when there is evidence of clinical sepsis (e.g. severe illness, septicaemia, cellulitis). Flucloxacillin, erythromycin or clindamycin should be used rather than penicillin G for *Streptococcus pyogenes* (haemolytic streptococci of Group A) burns infections because of the co-existence of *Staphylococus aureus*. Chemotherapy is obligatory on all full-thickness lesions infected with a group A streptococcus because of destruction of skin grafts by this organism.

MENINGITIS

Bacterial meningitis caused by identified organisms should be treated as follows:
- meningococcal – benzylpenicillin, 2.4 grams IU every 4–6 hours by 'bolus' injection;
- pneumococcal – cefotaxime;
- *Haemophilus influenzae* – because of the increasing prevalence of penicillinase (β-lactamase)-producing strains of *Haemophilus influenzae*, cefotaxime has become the initial therapy for presumptive *Haemophilus infuenzae* meningitis.

Other forms of meningitis are treated according to the predicted or known sensitivity of the organism. If the organism is unknown, give cefotaxime and ampicillin to neonates and cefotaxime to adults.

INFECTIONS IN NEONATES

Most superficial infections, such as septic spots, 'sticky' eyes and umbilical sepsis, respond to local treatment. Systemic infections are frequently caused by Gram-negative bacilli, including *Pseudomonas* species and also by penicillin-resistant staphylococci. A combination of penicillin with gentamicin, or a cephalosporin such as cefotaxime, should be used to treat seriously ill neonates with an undiagnosed infection.

PUERPERAL SEPSIS (AND SEPTIC ABORTION)

Infection is usually due to streptococci or anaerobic organisms, but is also sometimes caused by Gram-negative bacilli. It should be treated initially with a combination of metronidazole and cefuroxime until the results of cultures are available.

EYE INFECTION

Gonococcal ophthalmia is treated with a combination of topical and parenteral penicillin. Most other forms of purulent conjunctivitis respond to topical chloramphenicol.

EAR INFECTION

Acute bacterial otitis media is usually caused by *Streptococcus pyogenes,* pneumococci and *Haemophilus influenzae.* The majority of cases respond to amoxycillin, Augmentin or erythromycin; children under the age of 5 years should be given amoxycillin, as *Haemophilus influenzae* is a common pathogen of that age group. It should be noted that erythromycin does not penetrate well into the middle ear, and levels at this site are insufficient to treat most strains of *Haemophilus influenzae.*

SEPTICAEMIA

This is a serious and potentially fatal condition which should be treated with a parenteral bactericidal antibiotic as soon as the diagnosis is suspected on clinical grounds. It is often possible to infer from the clinical features of the illness what organism is probably causing the infection. For example, acute pyelonephritis or cholangitis may be complicated by Gram-negative septicaemia, and segmental pneumonia may be associated with pneumococcal septicaemia. Acute osteomyelitis is frequently secondary to staphylococcal septicaemia which can also accompany wound infection and skin sepsis. *Enterococcus faecalis* may enter the patient's bloodstream during operations on the genito-urinary tract or catheterization. It may cause endocarditis in elderly males after cystoscopy of prostatectomy, and in young women following gynaecological procedures.

When an organism is cultured from the blood, it is important to carry out detailed sensitivity testing. If endocarditis is suspected, this should include MIC and MBC determinations for appropriate antibiotics. When there is a lack of response to treatment, serum levels of the selected antibiotic should be determined during treatment of endocarditis or septicaemia to ensure that adequate concentrations are obtained in the blood. Many laboratories examine the activity of the patient's blood (taken immediately before and 1 hour after the dose of antibiotic) against the patient's own isolate. This test is called the serum bactericidal titre (SBT), and high levels are predictive of cure in endocarditis.

The blind initial therapy of septicaemia requires the selection of a broad-spectrum agent such as cefuroxime. If the patient has had previous treatment with the cephalosporins, it is appropriate to use a quinolone (e.g. ciprofloxacin) or a carbapenem. Metronidazole should be added if abdominal sepsis is present.

ENDOCARDITIS (British Society of Antimicrobial Chemotherapy, 1985, 1990)

Infective endocarditis can be caused by many different organisms. However, the commonest are the viridans group of streptococci and *Staphylococcus aureus*.

VIRIDANS STREPTOCOCCAL ENDOCARDITIS

If the organism is fully sensitive to penicillin, treatment is with 14 days of intravenous penicillin plus low-dose (60 or 80 mg a day) gentamicin followed by 14 days of amoxycillin. For streptococci of reduced sensitivity to penicillin, continue treatment with penicillin and gentamicin for 4 weeks.

STAPHYLOCOCCUS AUREUS ENDOCARDITIS

Treatment is with two antibiotics, usually flucloxacillin plus gentamicin or fusidic acid for 4 weeks.

FUNGAL INFECTIONS AND ACTINOMYCOSIS

Most fungal infections seen in the UK involve skin, nails or mucous membranes. Systemic fungal infections (or mycoses) are relatively rare, although they occasionally occur in debilitated patients, in immunodeficient patients or following gastrointestinal surgery.

The commonest superficial fungal infection is candidiasis or thrush caused by *Candida albicans,* which responds satisfactorily to topical applications of nystatin or miconazole. Systemic candida infection is treated with intravenous injections of amphotericin B, a relatively toxic antibiotic which may cause drug fever, nausea, vomiting and an increase in blood urea levels. Fluconazole is also effective against serious candida infections, and has the advantage that it is available in an oral formulation. Flucytosine may be used in combination with amphotericin B. Actinomycosis is treated with benzylpenicillin. Griseofulvin has a specific action against dermatophytes, and is used for the treatment of fungal infections of hair and nails. Terbinafine is an oral medication which is active against dermatophytes and results in a quicker cure than griseofulvin.

INDICATIONS FOR PROPHYLAXIS WITH ANTIBIOTICS

SYSTEMIC CHEMOPROPHYLAXIS

There is a limited range of clinical conditions – both medical and surgical – in which the prophylactic use of antibiotics is indicated both because there are special hazards of infection in such cases, and because of the probable or known benefits of chemoprophylaxis. When chemoprophylaxis is not indicated (e.g. in most clean surgical operations) it should, for obvious reasons, be avoided. Routine prophylactic use of antibiotics leads to an increase in the proportion of resistant organisms, and may cause the replacement of sensitive strains by resistant ones and species in the patient's flora, increasing the hazards of infection. When prophylaxis is indicated, it is important that the most appropriate antibiotic or antibiotics are given, and that the dosage, duration of course and route of administration should be optimal. In prophylaxis against post-operative infection this involves very short peri-operative administration, which is most unlikely to cause the selection of resistant strains. In the early years of antimicrobial chemotherapy, antibiotics were often used for prophylaxis without such precautions. Such courses proved ineffective, and the concept of antibiotic prophylaxis fell under a cloud, from which it was eventually rescued by studies that demonstrated the value of antibiotic prophylaxis used with rational care.

When chemoprophylaxis is used, attention must be given to a number of factors, including the clinical state of the patient at operation, the procedure to be carried out and the presence or absence of existing infection. In the choice of antibiotics, alternatives must be available for patients who are hypersensitive to the agents of first choice, and the choice between oral and parenteral administration should take into account any side-effects that may appear. It may be necessary to change the regimen in order to meet changes in the pathogens carried by patients (e.g. the emergence of MRSA and highly resistant enterococci).

In open heart surgery there is a very low incidence of infection, but the risk of mortality is high if infection (e.g. with coagulase-negative staphylococci) occurs. On theoretical grounds it should be possible to prevent lodgement at key sites in the heart or sternum at the time of the operation, and antibiotic prophylaxis is almost always given for this purpose. Some clinical trials suggest that this is beneficial.

Medical indications for systemic prophylaxis
These include the following:
1 prevention of endocarditis in patients with heart valve lesions, septal defect, patent ductus or prosthetic valve; (see *British National Formulary*)
2 for non-immune diphtheria contacts, give erythromycin 500 mg four times a day for 1 week;
3 for contacts of meningococcal infection, give rifampicin 600 mg twice a day for 2 days or ciprofloxacin 500 mg as a single dose;
4 following acute rheumatic fever for at least 5 years or until the child leaves school, give phenoxymethyl penicillin (penicillin V) at a dose of 125 or 250 mg twice a day by mouth;
5 following splenectomy, especially in children, give long-term oral penicillin (and/or immunization against pneumococcal infection).

Indications for systemic prophylaxis in clean surgery
These include the following:
- arterial grafts;
- cardiac surgery;

- neurosurgical operations involving foreign materials;
- joint prostheses;
- severe injuries and burns (e.g. *Clostridium tetani* and *Clostridium perfringens*);
- high amputation of ischaemic legs (*Clostridium perfringens*).

PROPHYLAXIS AGAINST SURGICAL SEPSIS (see Chapter 11)

Indications

Prophylaxis against surgical sepsis is advisable whenever an internal organ, the contents of which contain high concentrations of bacteria, is opened. The type and extent of bacterial colonization within the gastrointestinal tract are related to the site and nature of any underlying disease. Prophylaxis should be used for the following groups of operations:

1 operations on the stomach or oesophagus in patients with carcinoma or bile reflux gastritis;
2 cholecystectomy in selected patients who may have infected bile. Patients at risk for sepsis can be selected on the basis of a history of jaundice, rigors, recent acute cholecystitis, age over 70 years, or a previous biliary operation;
3 all intestinal operations in patients with inflammatory bowel disease;
4 all colorectal operations involving resection and/or anastomosis;
5 patients with a perforated gangrenous appendix should be given a therapeutic course of antibiotic. The need for prophylaxis in non-perforated, non-gangrenous appendicitis is not yet established;
6 pelvic operations: there are also other indications for prophylaxis for which there is often no general agreement:
   - recurrent cystitis in women of child-bearing age with a normal upper urinary tract;
   - infants of mothers with sputum-positive tuberculosis (if the child cannot be separated from the mother);
   - siblings of patients with whooping cough;
   - all instrumentations in the presence of bacteriuria;
   - transrectal prostatic biopsy;
   - urethral dilatation.

Timing and route of prophylaxis in surgery

Prophylaxis is only effective if high blood and tissue levels of an appropriate antibiotic are present at the time of bacterial contamination of the surgical wound. Prophylaxis should not continue after completion of the operation. Intramuscular drugs should be given 1 hour before the start of the surgery, and IV drugs should be given during the induction of anaesthesia.

Choice of chemotherapeutic agent

This should be based on the nature of the organisms that are likely to contaminate the operative field. For patients in groups 1 and 2, the organisms most likely to cause sepsis are streptococci, *E.coli* and other aerobic Gram-negative bacilli.

Operations in groups 3, 4 and 5 require antibiotics active against anaerobic bacteria, *E.coli* and other aerobic Gram-negative bacilli. Anaerobic and micro-aerophilic bacteria are mainly responsible for pelvic sepsis in group 6 patients. Suitable prophylactic regimens for the above groups are as follows:

- group 1 – a single pre-operative dose of gentamicin or a cephalosporin by IM or IV injection;
- group 2 – a single pre-operative injection of gentamicin or cephalosporin IM or IV;
- groups 3 and 4 – a single pre-operative injection of gentamicin IM or IV and metronidazole is recommended. Pre-operative oral bowel preparation with antibiotics is often effective, but is not recommended because of the risk of emergence of resistant Gram-negative bacilli;
- group 5 – metronidazole given as a suppository or IV is the most rational prophylactic for appendicectomy;
- group 6 – metronidazole combined with cefuroxime is effective prophylaxis against pelvic sepsis.

Chemoprophylaxis with antibiotics will almost inevitably lead to the selection of bacteria that are resistant to the prophylactic agent. For this reason indiscriminate prophylaxis should be avoided. Narrow-range rather than broad-spectrum antibiotics should be used whenever possible (e.g. in prophylaxis against a particular pathogen, such as *Streptococcus pyogenes or Clostridium perfringens*). Short-term or single-dose prophylaxis should be used to cover short periods of hazard, such as exposure to microbial contamination during an operation, and a careful watch must be kept for the appearance of resistant bacteria.

PERITONEAL DIALYSIS

The dialysis fluid is an excellent culture medium for bacteria, and may become infected from the outside (due to faulty technique) or the inside (due to pre-existing peritoneal infection or transperitoneal spread). Prophylactic addition of antibiotics to dialysis fluid is not recommended, but is a useful route of administration should peritonitis occur. Intraperitoneal therapy with vancomycin and a cephalosporin is often started on clinical evidence of infection, and treatment is then modified when cultures are available (see Chapter 17).

TOPICAL CHEMOPROPHYLAXIS

Local treatment of severe burns with 0.5% silver nitrate compresses, one of the most effective means of preventing infection with *Pseudomonas aeruginosa* and *Proteus* species, is now used infrequently. Patients who receive this treatment need supplements of electrolytes by mouth and laboratory control of serum electrolyte levels. Silver sulphadiazine cream is less effective against *Pseudomonas aeruginosa* and *Proteus* species, but more effective against many other Gram-negative bacilli (see Chapter 16). It is a valuable alternative to silver nitrate compresses, easier to use and more appropriate for the treatment of infants, and also for smaller burns. Mafenide acetate (11%) cream applied daily and left exposed is an alternative to 0.5% silver nitrate compresses which can be used if silver nitrate solution is not appropriate (e.g. if serum electrolytes cannot be maintained at normal levels). It is painful on burns in which the nerve endings are not destroyed, and may cause acidosis, and patients require daily baths to remove the dried cream. A cream containing 0.5% silver nitrate and 0.2% chlorhexidine gluconate is also effective and involves less risk of emergence of resistant bacteria (Lowbury, 1976).

FORMULATION OF ANTIBIOTIC POLICY

There are several reasons for having in each hospital an agreed policy for prescribing antibiotics.
1 It is a way of ensuring that patients receive appropriate therapy.
2 The restrained use of antibiotics means that the appearance of resistant organisms is delayed and their incidence in hospital is kept low. Resistant staphylococci remain a problem, and strains resistant to methicillin are found increasingly. Gentamicin-resistant Gram-negative bacilli, especially *Klebsiella aerogenes* and *Pseudomonas aeruginosa,* have caused cross-infection problems in urological, intensive-care and burns units. Resistance is commonly transferred from one organism to another, even when the organisms are unrelated. Transferable resistance to one antibiotic is often linked to resistance to other antibiotics, so that excessive use of one antibiotic may be the cause of a high incidence of resistance to several others.
3 Up-to-date information should be provided for the prescriber, and the incidence of adverse reactions should be reduced by restricting the use of certain potentially toxic agents.
4 Prescribing costs are reduced by controlling the use of expensive agents.

The type of policy must be adapted to the needs of the staff, the type of patients treated and the prevalent organisms in the hospital or unit. It must therefore be flexible and, where necessary, adapted to the needs of individual units (e.g. burns and intensive care). The policy could have the components described in the following paragraphs.

PERSONAL ADVICE AND EXAMPLE

This refers to the effect that daily discussion between senior and junior doctors has on prescribing habits. Effective use of antibiotics requires experience, and this is not readily obtained. Most hospitals have doctors (usually a medical microbiologist or infectious diseases consultant) with a special interest in and knowledge of antibiotics which should be available to other members of staff.

GENERAL ADVICE AND EDUCATION

The education of antibiotic prescribers can also be enhanced if some aide-mémoire is available on the wards. The *British National Formulary* is one source of information. Some hospitals or even regions have their own booklets. It is particularly important that advice is available on the use of topical agents, on prophylaxis and on expensive preparations. Postgraduate lectures on chemotherapy are also helpful, but are less important than personal advice and discussion.

PROVISION OF SURVEY DATA

The antibiotic policy depends to a considerable extent on the sensitivity pattern of currently isolated strains of bacteria. The percentages of *Staphylococcus aureus* and Gram-negative bacilli that are resistant to a number of antibiotics varies greatly both from one hospital to another, and between different units in the same hospital. Similar variations will occur from time to time in the same hospital. Regular reports can be prepared from information available in most laboratories where sensitivity tests are performed, and knowledge of the current resistance patterns gives the clinician a valuable guide to the therapy that is most likely to be of use. This type of information is complementary to that provided by the individual report on a particular patient.

The same type of information can be made available to general practitioners. Of particular use is the resistance pattern of urinary tract organisms isolated from domiciliary urinary tract infections. Such information need only be made available once a year in general practice because of the small changes in resistance of bacteria among the general community compared to those found in hospitals.

RESERVATION OF ANTIBIOTICS

Some hospitals may find it valuable to group antibiotics into different categories in order to hold some in reserve for particular organisms or specific types of patient. There is no doubt that such a policy of restricting the use of specific compounds can preserve the useful life of an antimicrobial agent. In large hospitals, where there is a resident population of organisms 'waiting to acquire resistance', and large amounts of antibiotics may be used, it is essential to keep some in reserve.

Examples of the ways in which antibiotics can be classified for this purpose are shown in Tables 13.2 and 13.3, which summarize the policy adopted in a general hospital (Table 13.2) and in a hospital with many specialized services and departments (Table 13.3).

PURCHASING POLICY

New agents should be carefully considered by a drug and therapeutics committee, and should only be purchased if they are superior in one or more respects to existing drugs. In particular, by this means the clinician can be guided in the use of the numerous antibiotic preparations now available.

Table 13.2 Example of antibiotic policy used in a general hospital

Unrestricted use
Penicillin
Ampicillin and derivatives
Flucloxacillin
Tetracyclines
Erythromycin
Metronidazole
Gentamicin
Cefuroxime
Co-trimoxazole (or trimethoprim)

Restricted use (on advice of infectious disease physician or microbiologist)
Azlocillin
Ceftazidime
Netilmicin
Clindamycin
Vancomycin
Chloramphenicol
Ciprofloxacin

Not recommended (and not in stock in the hospital)[a]
All other cephalosporins
Amikacin
Tobramycin
Ureidopenicillins

[a] Some of these agents (e.g. amikacin) may be on the restricted list in some hospitals.

CHANGES IN ANTIBIOTIC POLICIES

ACTION WHEN RESISTANCE TO AN IMPORTANT ANTIBIOTIC BECOMES COMMON

Sometimes stopping the use of the antibiotic in question will lead to a large reduction or even elimination of the resistant organisms. This happened more often in the early years of the antibiotic era, before multiple and genetically linked resistance became common in hospital bacteria. When multiple resistance is present, all of the antibiotics involved in the resistance pattern may need to be withdrawn and not be used again until these strains have been eliminated. In some outbreaks, withdrawal of antibiotics has not been effective. Transfer of all patients carrying or infected with strains which show the resistance pattern to one ward, which is kept closed to new admissions until all carriers of the resistant strain have been discharged, may be effective in such a situation.

The antibiotic resistance pattern in hospital is constantly changing, and it is necessary to change a policy in response to alterations in resistance. Often one unit

Table 13.3 Antibiotic policy employed by a complex teaching district with many specialist units[a]

Category A	Category B
Amoxycillin (O+P)[b]	Ampicillin/sulbactam (surgical prophylaxis)
Phenoxymethyl penicillin	Cefotaxime (STD; paediatrics)
Cephalexin	Ceftazidime (ITU)
Erythromycin stearate	Dapsone (dermatology)
Flucloxacillin (O+P)	Doxycycline (STD; dermatology)
Fusidic acid	Minocycline (dermatology)
Metronidazole (O+P)	Netilmicin (renal unit)
Nalidixic acid	Vancomycin (haematology, renal unit)
Nitrofurantoin	Piperacillin (haematology)
Ciprofloxacin	Anti-TB drugs (chest unit)
Trimethoprim	
Chloramphenicol	
Cefixime	
Co-amoxiclav	
Benzylpenicillin	
Cefuroxime	
Erythromycin lactobionate	
Gentamicin	
Piperacillin	
Teichoplanin	
Nystatin	

Category C	Category D
(a) Amikacin	Variable list
Aztreonam	
Ciprofloxacin (inj)	**Category E**
Clindamycin	Variable list
Imipenem	
Rifampicin (inj)	
(b) Category B compounds used for non-listed indications	
(c) Antivirals: Acyclovir, Ganciclovir, Ribavirin, Zidovudine	
(d) Antifungals: Fluconazole, Amphotericin	

[a] The antibiotics are divided into five categories with different degrees of accessibility. (A) Oral and parenteral compounds which are available for prescription by all doctors. (B) Compounds which are restricted to certain units or indications. (C) Compounds which can only be started by senior doctors, usually consultants. (D) Drugs which are undergoing trial in the hospital and only available to trialists. (E) All other antibiotics available in the UK. These are not in stock and can only be ordered via consultants.

[b] (O+P) Oral and parenteral prescriptions of these compounds are available to all doctors.

in the hospital may require a policy which is different to that used by other units. For example, methicillin-resistant *Staphylococcus aureus* or cephalosporin-resistant enterobacteria may appear in one unit but not in others. A change could then be made to a reserve antibiotic in the ward with the newly acquired resistant strains.

ANTIBIOTICS AND THE LABORATORY

The hospital clinician can only use antibiotics rationally if adequate laboratory services are available. There are several ways in which the laboratory can provide such assistance. Most important is the provision of accurate sensitivity tests on the relevant isolates from individual patients to the most appropriate antibiotics. The choice of agents and the susceptibility guidelines employed should be kept under regular review. In addition, the laboratory should provide regular summary data on the prevalence of resistant bacteria, and facilities for monitoring of certain antibiotic levels (particularly aminoglycosides) should be available. Laboratories should report a limited number of sensitivities to appropriate antimicrobial agents to the clinicians in order to restrict the range of antibiotics used (e.g. the sensitivity of *Staphylococcus aureus* could be reported to flucloxacillin and erythromycin only).

REFERENCES

British Medical Association and Royal Pharmaceutical Society of Great Britain (revised twice yearly) *British National Formulary*. London: British Medical Association and Royal Pharmaceutical Society of Great Britain.

British Society for Antimicrobial Chemotherapy (1985) Working Party Report. Antibiotic treatment of streptococcal and staphylococcal endocarditis. *Lancet* 2, 815.

British Society for Antimicrobial Chemotherapy (1990) Antibiotic prophylaxis of infective endocarditis. Recommendations from the Endocarditis Working Party. *Lancet* 1, 88.

Kucers, A., Crowe, S.M., Grayson, M.L. and Hoy, J.F. (1997) *The use of antibiotics. A clinical review of antibacterial, antifungal and antiviral drugs*, 5th edn. Oxford: Butterworth-Heinemann.

Lowbury, E.J.L. (1976) Prophylaxis and treatment for infection in burns. *British Journal of Hospital Medicine* 16, 566.

O'Grady, F., Lambert, H.P., Finch, R.G. and Greenwood, D. (1997) *Antibiotic and chemotherapy. Anti-infective agents and their use in therapy*. Edinburgh: Churchill Livingstone.

Parker, M.T. and Collier, L.H. (1990) *Topley and Wilson's principles of bacteriology, virology and immunity*, 8th edn. London: Edward Arnold.

chapter 14

IMMUNIZATION AND SPECIFIC PROPHYLAXIS

Immunization is important in the control of hospital infection:

1 for the protection of certain members of staff against tuberculosis, poliomyelitis, rubella, diphtheria, hepatitis B and certain other infectious diseases which could be contracted from patients;
2 for the protection of patients, when a patient suffering from a communicable disease is accidentally admitted to an open ward;
3 for the protection of patients who, because of their illness or treatment, are particularly susceptible to infection;
4 for the protection against tetanus of patients with open wounds.

For the protection of staff, active immunization with a vaccine or toxoid is the method of choice, and immunity should be established in so far as is practicable before the individual is employed in an area of potential risk (e.g. a paediatric ward). Non-immune patients exposed to certain infections can be given immediate protection against that infection by passive immunization with immunoglobulin, but not by active immunization, which takes time to develop. The importance of both active and passive immunization, prophylactic antibiotics and surgical techniques must be integrated for the prevention of tetanus in hospital.

IMMUNIZATION OF HOSPITAL STAFF (see also Chapter 15 and Department of Health [1996])

GENERAL POLICY

The risks of staff contracting infection vary according to the type of hospital, tuberculosis being a special risk in chest wards of hospitals, enteric fever and poliomyelitis in infectious disease units, hepatitis B in renal and liver units, and all of these infections in pathology departments. The person in charge of a unit or department must be responsible for ensuring that measures are taken to avoid infection in staff, and also for ensuring that their immunization status is appropriate for their work.

It is neither practicable nor desirable to immunize all members of staff against all diseases for which vaccines are available. This is because the risk may not be great (e.g. typhoid fever in the UK), or the vaccine may not be very effective or may have unpleasant side-effects. The risks of side-effects from immunization must be balanced against the potential hazard of spread of the infection from patient to staff in a unit at a particular time, account being taken of the fact that intestinal infections in particular are effectively contained by good hygiene and barrier nursing. Secondly, account must be taken of the effectiveness of specific treatment should infection arise (e.g. antibiotics are effective against typhoid fever, but not against poliomyelitis). Thirdly, the usual rapid turnover of nursing and domestic staff can make it impossible to ensure that well-immunized staff are always available. In the average infectious disease unit only the senior nursing staff tend to be permanent. In view of these difficulties, it is impossible to ensure immunity of all staff to meet the chance admission of a patient with unrecognized infectious disease. Good hygienic practice is usually a better safeguard for the staff than reliance on an immunity which may not exist. However, there are circumstances where immunization is useful and necessary. For example, in units that deal with open pulmonary tuberculosis it is important to ensure that all staff have evidence of previous BCG (usually identified by the presence of a scar) or are tuberculin positive.

ACTIVE IMMUNIZATION OF HOSPITAL STAFF

Active immunity results from naturally acquired disease or from immunization. It usually takes at least 10–14 days for active immunity to develop, and it may take longer, depending on the vaccine; immunity develops much more rapidly with some vaccines. Immunity may be good and highly protective (e.g. diphtheria) or rather poor in the face of a large infective dose of bacteria (e.g. cholera).

Hepatitis B immunization
All hospital staff involved with invasive procedures or who come into contact with blood or body fluids or contaminated materials should be immunized (see Chapter 10).

Smallpox vaccination
In 1980 the World Health Organization formally declared the world free from smallpox – the very successful conclusion to its smallpox eradication programme. There is thus no medical reason whatsoever to vaccinate anyone against smallpox.

The vaccinia virus may be used as a carrier for certain other vaccine antigens. Laboratory staff working with the virus should be vaccinated, but preferably only those requiring re-vaccination should be used in these studies. If primary vaccination is essential, the member of staff should be fully informed of the risks (e.g. a severe local reaction) and be prepared to accept them. Further advice is available from the Public Health Laboratory Service (PHLS) Virus Reference Division.

BCG and tuberculosis
All hospital staff employed either continuously or intermittently in high-risk areas (defined below) must have their resistance to infection tested by the presence of a BCG scar or a positive tuberculin reaction (ideally the Mantoux test) before being employed in such areas (Joint Tuberculosis Committee of the British Thoracic Society, 1994). However, as tuberculosis is likely to be present in many general hospitals, it may be advisable to include all staff in contact with patients, in

addition to those working in high-risk areas. Screening of health-care staff is most effectively performed using a health questionnaire rather than routine chest X-ray examination. If staff have no BCG scar and are tuberculin negative, they must be given BCG vaccine. If they have a grade 4 Mantoux test they should be referred to a chest physician for further investigation. If, after having had a successful BCG vaccination, the individual is tuberculin tested 1 year or more later and is found to be negative, he or she should be referred to a chest physician for an opinion. BCG should not be re-administered without such an opinion, for this can produce a severe reaction (chronic ulceration at the site, etc.).

High-risk areas include the following:
- wards, clinics and isolation units where patients with open (i.e. transmissible) tuberculosis are commonly seen;
- laboratories where processing of specimens for isolation and culture of the tubercle bacillus takes place;
- post-mortem rooms.

Staff of other departments (e.g. radiographers and physiotherapists) who visit patients in the tuberculosis wards should be similarly screened and immunized if indicated. Screening of staff should be the responsibility of the occupational health physician who will keep the necessary records.

Immunization does not exclude the need for methods of surveillance or for instruction of staff about potential hazards and how to avoid them, including details of when to seek medical advice, and chest X-ray if indicated.

Poliomyelitis
Although most young adults in the UK will have been immunized against poliomyelitis, it is desirable to maintain immunity by re-vaccination, as the disease in the adult is often of the paralytic type and also because no specific treatment exists. Immunization with the Sabin, living attenuated vaccine is easily administered, safe, has minimal side-effects and is effective. It should be offered to all hospital staff who are non-immune. It is also recommended that a booster be given to staff who may be in contact with cases during their day-to-day work. The vaccine is given by mouth, and three doses must be given at intervals of 4–8 weeks. Although the vaccine contains strains of the three serotypes of poliomyelitis virus, only one of these generally infects the recipient at a time to produce immunity to that serotype. Thus to confer immunity to all types, three doses are required. It is incorrect to assume that two doses will necessarily confer some degree of immunity to all strains. Booster doses can be offered every 10 years or more often if there is a continuing risk of infection. It is recommended that individuals over about 30 years of age who have never previously had poliomyelitis immunization should be given their primary immunity with the formalin-killed or Salk-type vaccine. This is because occasionally primary immunization with the Sabin vaccine (containing live attenuated virus) can give rise to mild paralytic disease in older people, although the risk of this is small.

Diphtheria
Most adults born in this country after 1941 will have residual immunity to diphtheria as a result of childhood immunization. Although the vaccine is effective in

preventing disease, its administration to adults is not without occasional unpleasant reactions such as painful brawny induration of the arm. Diphtheria vaccine is therefore not recommended routinely even for staff of infectious disease units. Staff who may be exposed to diphtheria as a result of their work (e.g. some laboratory workers) should have their immune status determined by serology. Vaccination of those who are susceptible with boosters at 10-year intervals should be advised. If vaccination is necessary, adults should always be given a low dose vaccine.

If diphtheria is diagnosed in a patient in hospital, he or she should be transferred immediately to an infectious diseases unit. Staff in close contact should be given a 5-day course of oral erythromycin and placed under surveillance for 7 days after contact. Following the course of antibiotic, nose and throat swabs should be taken to detect any possible carriers.

Typhoid and paratyphoid (enteric) fevers

It is not essential to immunize staff routinely against typhoid fever, even in infectious diseases units. These diseases are not very communicable, are adequately contained by efficient nursing and hygienic techniques, and are treatable with antibiotics.

Laboratory staff who handle specimens that may contain typhoid organisms are at slight risk. These staff should be offered immunization. Typhoid (monovalent) vaccine has replaced TAB, which also contained the killed bacteria of paratyphoid fevers and was of unproven efficacy. Two doses of monovalent vaccine give protection for 3 years or more. There is now an active oral vaccine containing the attenuated strain Ty21a which is of similar efficacy to typhoid vaccine.

Rubella (German measles)

The Joint Committee on Vaccination and Immunization of the Department of Health has recommended that routine rubella vaccination should be offered to children of both sexes along with a combined measles/mumps/rubella vaccine (MMR) at the age of 12–15 months. Women of childbearing age should be tested for immunity. Those who are found to be susceptible (seronegative) and who are not pregnant should be offered rubella vaccination (Department of Health, 1996). Those who are susceptible and pregnant should be employed in other units and immunized after delivery. Because of the theoretical possibility (not proven) that live rubella vaccine might damage the fetus, pregnancy must be excluded at the time of vaccination and should be avoided for 8 weeks thereafter.

Influenza

When epidemics of influenza are predicted, those responsible for the health of hospital staff often find themselves under pressure to have the staff vaccinated against this infection. However, such immunization is not recommended as a routine. When a new strain of virus appears and an epidemic is expected, the new strain is usually incorporated into the vaccine, although this takes some time. Flu vaccine is recommended for those at risk of serious illness or death, and offers 70–80% protection.

Measles

This is given as MMR and can be given to any non-immune adult, although in practice it is rarely given to hospital staff. Passive immunization with human normal immunoglobulin (HNIG) is available for children and adults with compromised immunity who come into contact with measles.

Varicella (chicken-pox)
An effective live vaccine is available, but not in the UK. When it is available, this should be given to high-risk staff who are antibody negative.

Other diseases
Active immunization against tetanus should be given to all staff, and should be maintained by booster doses. Hepatitis B vaccine should be offered to certain staff (see Chapter 10).

PASSIVE IMMUNIZATION OF STAFF

Passive immunization is conferred by the injection of human normal immunoglobulin (gamma-globulin), hyperimmune human specific immunoglobulin (e.g. hepatitis B immunoglobulin) or specific immunoglobulins from animal sources (usually horse) (e.g. diphtheria antitoxin). The purpose is to confer immediate but short-term immunity to certain diseases. In this situation antibodies are not made by the person immunized (hence the term passive), but are provided from other human or animal sources. Pooled human normal immunoglobulin therapy is effective against measles (adult dose 750 mg), and probably also against poliomyelitis (adult dose 1500 mg). It will also give some protection for about 4 months against hepatitis A but not against hepatitis B. However, a specific hyperimmune gamma-globulin has been developed for protection against hepatitis B (see Chapter 10). Varicella Zoster immune globulin (VZIG) is prepared from pooled plasma of blood donors with a history of recent chicken-pox or herpes zoster, and can be used for protection against chicken-pox. Human normal immunoglobulin is not generally indicated for adult contacts of measles, rubella, mumps or chicken-pox (see below).

DOCUMENTATION

When immunization of staff is mandatory, a record must be kept in the hospital. It is desirable that records of other immunizations should also be held in the occupational health department of the hospital (see Chapter 15).

IMMUNIZATION OF PATIENTS

There are few circumstances in which immunization of patients against infectious disease is indicated. When applicable, passive immunization which is immediately effective should be used. Passive immunity conferred by human immunoglobulin or antitoxin of animal origin is applicable to the following diseases in the circumstances mentioned. (For protection against tetanus, see the section below on protection against tetanus.).

Measles
When a case of measles is inadvertently admitted or develops in a paediatric ward, human normal immunoglobulin should be given to patients on immunosuppressive

drugs or to those with debilitating diseases, or in whom the clinician considers that it is clinically indicated (e.g. cystic fibrosis, primary tuberculosis, hypogammaglobulinaemia and after splenectomy). Children who have not had measles or been vaccinated against it, and who have been given passive immunization, should be given active immunization at a later date. Immunoglobulin, 250 mg given within 7–10 days of contact, will probably modify an attack of measles. The disease may often be prevented with doses of between 250 and 750 mg, depending on age. Active immunization is contraindicated for compromised patients such as those with malignant disease or on immunosuppressive therapy (including high-dose steroids).

Poliomyelitis
If a case of acute poliomyelitis is accidentally admitted to or develops on a ward, all individuals who have not been immunized with a vaccine (Sabin or Salk) should be given human normal immunoglobulin. With the exception of close contacts within a family, live polio vaccine is now a much more effective agent for preventing spread in the community.

Hepatitis A
When this disease is diagnosed in a ward, certain patients (e.g. those with chronic diseases requiring a long stay in hospital) can be treated with human normal immunoglobulin, which may be used to help in the control of an outbreak. Patients who are on immunosuppressive drugs or who have had extensive radiotherapy should also be protected. It may be desirable to protect staff who are especially at risk. The recommended doses are 250 mg for a child and 500 mg for an adult, which gives protection for about 4 months.

It is not generally possible or necessary to offer protection to all patients, apart from those in the categories mentioned above, as stocks of immunoglobulin have to be conserved. Hepatitis A can probably be controlled to some extent by good hygiene.

Hepatitis B, C and E
See Chapter 10.

Chicken-pox
Although chicken-pox is not a serious disease in the otherwise healthy person, it will occasionally be necessary to attempt to prevent (or attenuate) an attack in the newborn or in individuals on immunosuppressive therapy or on cytotoxic drugs. Human normal immunoglobulin is probably not very effective, but limited supplies of hyperimmune anti-varicella/zoster immunoglobulin (ZIG) are available for such patients.

ZIG may attenuate an attack of chicken-pox, but cannot be relied upon to prevent it. There is no evidence of the efficacy of ZIG in the treatment of chicken-pox. In herpes zoster, patients normally possess antibodies to the causative virus, so administration of ZIG is not indicated. As a routine measure, patients who are at long-term risk (e.g. leukemia and transplant patients) and who have no history of chicken-pox should be tested for varicella-zoster antibodies. If they are found to be immune, then if they are subsequently exposed to chicken-pox, ZIG will be unnecessary. However, if they are bone-marrow-transplant recipients, their previous immunity will be ablated and they should receive ZIG (dose of ZIG for prophylaxis is as follows: 0–5 years, 250 mg; adults, 1000 mg) (see also page 285).

Gas gangrene

An antitoxin prepared in the horse against the toxins of *Clostridium perfringens* (welchii), *Clostridium septicum* and *Clostridium oedematiens* is available. There is no evidence that this has any value in prophylaxis against gas gangrene when used in patients with open wounds, but the use of a polyvalent antitoxin containing 10 000 units of *Clostridium oedematiens* antitoxin (IV or IM) has been advocated by some authorities for extensive soiled wounds. In established gas gangrene it may have some value (dose $\geqslant 75\ 000$ units IV) when used together with the most important measures, namely wide excision of affected muscle and high dosage of penicillin. These are probably of greater value than the antiserum, which carries a risk of allergy, including anaphylaxis.

Rabies

If a patient is thought to be at risk from rabies (e.g. after being bitten by an animal while abroad), the nearest Public Health Laboratory will give advice on the current requirements for post-exposure prophylaxis (see also Chapter 9).

Mumps

Convalescent mumps immunoglobulin may occasionally be available, but is in short supply. Human normal immunoglobulin has sometimes been used to modify or prevent an attack of mumps, but the efficacy of this measure is doubtful.

Rubella

Human normal immunoglobulin is of no value in the prevention of rubella in pregnant women exposed to infection.

PROTECTION AGAINST TETANUS

The risk of tetanus varies with the type and severity of wound or injury, the place where the patient was when they were injured (e.g. there is a special risk to agricultural workers) and the presence or absence of immunity induced by a course of toxoid. Thorough surgical toilet of the wound is necessary irrespective of the tetanus immunization history.

ASSESSMENT OF THE STATE OF IMMUNITY TO TETANUS

If a patient does not know whether he or she has received tetanus toxoid in the past, consult the patient's general practitioner. If he or she does not know, the patient must in most situations be considered non-immune. Many district health authorities hold a record on immunizations, especially of children, so that it may be possible to discover an individual's immune status by telephoning the appropriate authority.

The procedure is outlined in the Table 14.1 and can be summarized as follows:

1 booster doses of adsorbed toxoid (vaccine) for all patients known to have been actively immunized, unless they are known to have completed a course or a booster dose of toxoid within the previous 10 years;

2 the use of human antitetanus globulin (HTIG) for all patients not known to be actively immune;
3 active immunization with adsorbed toxoid for all patients if there is evidence that they are not actively immune;
4 the first dose of adsorbed toxoid administered at the same time as HTIG, but injected separately at another site.

ACTIVE IMMUNIZATION – USE OF TETANUS TOXOID

The patient is considered to be actively immune (a) for 10 years after three injections (the full immunizing course) of toxoid or diphtheria/tetanus/pertussis (DTP) vaccine or (b) for 10 years after a boosting dose of toxoid given to an actively immune individual. Patients with open wounds who by the above criteria are actively immune do not require a boosting dose of toxoid, but they may be given a dose of HTIG if the risk of infection is considered to be high (e.g. contamination with stable manure).

Immunizing procedure

1 Active immunity is induced by three intramuscular or deep subcutaneous injections of 0.5 mL of toxoid (adsorbed), the doses being separated by intervals of 1 month.

Table 14.1 Prophylaxis against tetanus in patients with open wounds (Birmingham Accident Hospital) (Lowbury *et al.*, 1978)

Type of wound	Other relevant circumstances	Procedure
1 Superficial wound or abrasion		Cleanse and cover No HTIG Start active immunization if not actively immune Cleanse toilet and cover
2 Puncture wound	If *known* to be actively immune	Toxoid (adsorbed) booster[a]
3 Deep laceration Animal or human bites Wound with devitalized tissue Wound more than 4 hours old Infected traumatic wound	If *not known* to be actively immune Admit to hospital if (a) severe if (b) heavily contaminated	Cleanse toilet and cover HTIG 250 IU (or 500 IU if 24 hours delay) Antibiotic (except for wounds that have had prompt and effective treatment, including HTIG, and are not heavily contaminated or septic) Start active immunizaton

[a] Not necessary if last dose of toxoid in course of active immunization or last booster dose was given less than 1 year previously.
HTIG human, antitetanus globulin.

2 A patient so immunized should have a booster dose of 0.5 mL of toxoid (adsorbed) 3 years after the primary course, and at intervals of 10 years. A patient who has received a primary course and two boosters at 10-year intervals can be regarded as permanently fully immune. If a patient with a wound is known to have had a dose of toxoid (the last dose in a course or a booster) within the last 10 years, it is not necessary to give a booster dose at the time of injury.

3 Any patient who is given HTIG should be actively immunized, the first dose of tetanus toxoid (adsorbed) being injected into the other arm at the same time as HTIG is given.

4 Forms – a card is used to record injections of toxoid during the course of immunization.

5 Out-patients:
   - if active immunization has been started, the patient is given a card and told to take it to his or her doctor for the second toxoid injection in 4 weeks;
   - if a booster dose of toxoid is given, the date of this is entered on the card and duplicates will be sent to the general practitioner.

6 In-patients – active immunization will be carried out as far as the length of hospital stay allows. According to the stage reached at the time of discharge, patients will be given a card suitably inscribed, and the duplicate cards will be sent to the patient's general practitioner and health authority.

PASSIVE IMMUNIZATION AGAINST TETANUS

Use of human antitetanus globulin (HTIG)

HTIG ('Humotet', Wellcome) is available for prophylaxis of patients who are not known to be actively immune. A single dose of 1 mL (250 IU) IM can give a protective level of antitoxin for 4 weeks. A dose of 500 IU is given if 24 hours have elapsed since injury or there is a risk of heavy contamination.

Tests for hypersensitivity to ATG are not required, but ATG should be avoided if patients have had adverse reactions to human gammaglobulin. Such reactions are very rare.

USE OF ANTIBIOTICS IN PROPHYLAXIS AGAINST TETANUS

Patients who cannot be adequately protected with toxoid because they are not actively immune, or for whom HTIG is not available, will have to rely for protection on surgical cleansing, and supportive prophylaxis by systemic antibiotics. It is essential that the antibiotic treatment is started as soon as possible after injury. Patients with severely contaminated wounds and those in whom there has been delay in starting treatment should be given antibiotic prophylaxis together with HTIG.

The antibiotic used should be one which is highly active against *Clostridium Tetani*. Suggested schedules are a 7–10 day course of IV metronidazole, erythromycin or flucloxacillin.

STORAGE AND DISPOSAL OF VACCINES

POTENCY AND STORAGE OF VACCINES

Vaccines are biological products and have a limited effective life. Conditions of storage must be controlled to maintain the potency of the vaccine for as long as possible. Vaccines are normally given an expiry date by the manufacturer, and all staff involved in immunization programmes should take great care to ensure that the product is not out of date. Rotation of stocks to avoid expiry is essential.

The optimum storage temperature for most vaccines is between 4°C and 10°C (39°F and 50°F) and the manufacturer's instructions must be followed. Vaccines should not be left at room temperature for a long time, particularly in the summer, nor should they be allowed to freeze, as they may lose potency. Modern domestic refrigerators may be used to store immunizing preparations, and these are sometimes set at a temperature which is too low for the storage of vaccines, e.g. 2°C (35°F). The thermostat should be reset to approximately 6°C (43°F) to prevent loss of potency. The temperature of storage refrigerators should be monitored closely.

DISPOSAL OF UNWANTED VACCINES AND DOSES

Time-expired vaccines containing live organisms (e.g. BCG, measles, poliomyelitis [oral], rubella and yellow fever) should be incinerated or inactivated by autoclaving or boiling prior to disposal or pouring down a sink drain. Residues of vaccine remaining after an immunizing session must be discarded.

REFERENCES

Department of Health (1996) *Immunisation against infectious diseases.* London: HMSO.

Joint Tuberculosis Committee of the British Thoracic Society (1994) Control and prevention of tuberculosis in the United Kingdom. Code of Practice 1994. *Thorax* 49, 1193.

Lowbury, E.J.L., Kidson, A., Lilly, H.A. *et al.* (1978) Prophylaxis against tetanus in non-immune patients with wounds: the role of antibiotics and human antitetanus globulin. *Journal of Hygiene* 80, 267.

chapter 15

OCCUPATIONAL HEALTH SERVICES IN THE CONTROL OF INFECTION

Occupational health departments will vary according to the size of the hospital and the number of staff, but most will have at least one trained occupational nurse and a physician (NHS Health Service Guidelines, 1994). Occupational health staff will give advice on all forms of staff illness and injury where these have either been caused by the job or may be a risk to patients, but this chapter will deal mainly with infective aspects. Transmission of infection from staff to patients and from patients to staff is well recognized (Bolyard *et al.*, 1998). The modes of spread are described in Chapter 8.

The main responsibilities of the occupational health department with respect to infection control are as follows:

- screening of new staff (mainly by use of questionnaires);
- providing relevant vaccinations and immunizations;
- keeping records and immunization schedules;
- health education, counselling and training in control of infection issues;
- collaboration with infection control staff in monitoring infections and investigating outbreaks;
- management of staff infections in collaboration with general practitioners and the infection control team;
- issuing policies on the prevention and control of staff infection;
- identification of work-related infections and infection risks to staff in the hospital environment;
- co-ordinating of health care of staff in all departments of the hospital and the community.

RISKS TO THE STAFF FROM PATIENTS

Members of hospital staff are exposed to risks of acquiring many kinds of infection (see Chapter 8), but some infections, notably tuberculosis, meningococcal infection, poliomyelitis, HIV, HBV and HCV infection, enteric fever, other salmonella infections and viral gastroenteritis, present special hazards.

The risk of acquiring HIV infection is small, but the serious outcome of such an infection has had a major influence on preventative measures (see Chapter 10). These measures include the wearing of disposable gloves for handling blood and body fluids, and care in handling sharps (e.g. not recapping needles and the use of puncture-proof sharp containers). A high incidence of staphylococcal or strepto-coccal infection among the patients may sometimes lead to outbreaks among nurses and other members of hospital staff. However, most staphylococci that cause infections in hospital patients, as well as Gram-negative bacilli (e.g. *Pseudomonas aeruginosa* and *Klebsiella* species), are unlikely to infect staff or be transmitted to their relatives. Epidemics of respiratory virus diseases in the community necessitating admissions of patients to hospital may lead to outbreaks of the disease in hospital. Certain infections (e.g. herpetic whitlow) occur predom-inantly in members of hospital staff. Head lice and scabies may occasionally be a hazard to staff – the latter especially in units for those with learning impairment.

In addition to overt clinical infections, carrier states may arise. The acquisition of hospital staphylococci in the external nares and on the hands is not uncommon, particularly in burns units and dermatological wards.

RISKS TO PATIENTS FROM STAFF

The commonest infections transmitted to patients by hospital staff, apart from upper respiratory viral infection, are staphylococcal sepsis, streptococcal sore throat and infective diarrhoea. *Candida* species may be transmitted to neonates by staff with paronychia. The spread of pulmonary tuberculosis from a member of staff is a rare but important hazard. The transmission of HIV, HBV or HCV infection to a patient is rare, and usually only occurs where there has been an invasive procedure, and normally carriers are able to continue with their usual work. However, HIV has been transferred to patients by a dentist and a surgeon, and HCV and HBV have been transferred during an operation. A difficult decision as to whether to allow the member of staff to continue operating has to be made, and counselling and follow-up are always necessary (see Chapter 10; UK Departments of Health, 1998). Staff in the UK who are HBe Ag carriers should not carry out invasive procedures. However, recommendations in different countries are inconsistent, particularly with regard to Hb_sAg and HCV.

Symptomless carriers of virulent pathogenic bacteria among members of staff are also a potential hazard of infection to patients. Outbreaks of staphylococcal infection in neonatal departments, or of wound sepsis acquired in the operating-theatre, may originate from a nasal or a skin carrier of a virulent strain of *Staphylococcus aureus*. An important source of infection, especially in surgical wards, may be a member of staff with eczema colonized by an epidemic strain of *Staphylococcus aureus*. Nose, throat or rectal carriers of Group A β-haemolytic streptococci have been responsible for outbreaks of puerperal sepsis in maternity wards, particularly if carried by delivery-room staff, and surgical operations. Kitchen staff who carry dysentery bacilli or *Salmonella* species may also be a hazard, although outbreaks of infection arising initially from staff in hospital kitchens are uncommon.

Salmonella carriers are normally allowed to return to work after the acute symptoms have resolved. However, a common requirement is that they do not work with food or babies and are instructed in good hygiene. This also applies to catering staff if they are known to be conscientious in their personal hygiene, although microbiological clearance is usually required. Carriers of *Salmonella typhi* should be kept off duty. Treatment with a quinolone (e.g. ciprofloxacin) will often eliminate salmonella carriage.

During an outbreak of infection in hospital, epidemiological evidence may point to staff members being involved in the occurrence or spread of infection. In these circumstances, a search for carriers or cases among staff may be necessary. Apart from this situation, routine and regular monitoring of otherwise healthy staff members is not required. Food handlers should be required to report any episodes of vomiting and diarrhoea.

INITIAL SCREENING OF STAFF ON APPOINTMENT

All staff (e.g. medical, nursing, administrative, ancillary (laboratory, and other technicians, physiotherapy, X-ray, etc.), domestic, portering and mortuary staff, SSD staff, catering and laundry staff should be included in the initial screening and immunization programme. This usually involves the completion of a questionnaire (see p. 257). Enquiry should be made for diarrhoeal diseases, recurrent sepsis, tonsillitis, chronic skin diseases, bloodborne infections or symptoms of possible tuberculosis. It is advisable that applicants suffering from certain chronic conditions (e.g. severe eczema) should not be accepted for nursing or other duties that bring them into close contact with patients, because of the likelihood of colonization with antibiotic-resistant organisms. For those coming into contact with patients the BCG scar should be checked and, if absent, a tuberculin (e.g. Heaf) test for susceptibility to tuberculosis may need to be performed. BCG vaccination should be offered to tuberculin-negative individuals who have not previously received BCG vaccination and shown conversion of the tuberculin test. Conversion of the tuberculin test to a positive reaction should be demonstrated before close contact with tuberculous patients or laboratory specimens which might be considered to be tuberculous is allowed. A chest X-ray should only be taken if indicated in the questionnaire or if there are suggestive symptoms (Subcommittee of the Joint Tuberculosis Committee of the British Thoracic Society, 1994; Department of Health Welsh Office, 1996 (see below and Chapter 14).

Bacteriological examination of the nose, throat and faeces and chest X-ray are not recommended as routine, but may be indicated in special circumstances (see Chapters 2 and 12). Other past infections should be recorded, especially chicken-pox.

IMMUNIZATION OF STAFF

All staff who perform invasive procedures or are in contact with blood, body fluids or contaminated procedures are strongly recommended to be immunized against hepatitis B. The principles involved in selecting immunization procedures are discussed in Chapter 14 (see also Department of Health, 1996). For most general hospitals the following are suggested.

All staff should be offered protection against tuberculosis and poliomyelitis. Non-pregnant susceptible women of childbearing age should also be offered rubella vaccination. The Health Services Advisory Committee (1991) Report suggests that tetanus toxoid should be given to laboratory staff and to engineering staff who service laboratory equipment. It seems reasonable to offer tetanus immunization to all engineering and gardening staff, and to other staff who request it. This may be given by the individual's general practitioner.

In general hospitals there is no need for routine immunization against typhoid fever or hepatitis A unless there is an increased risk. Rubella vaccination is intended for staff in contact with children, but due to rotation of staff it is usually more practicable to offer vaccination to all female members of staff who are at risk. Rubella antibody-negative women should not work in a maternity unit until they have been immunized. Rubella vaccine should also be offered to non-immune male staff who are likely to come into contact with women in the early antenatal period. Antibody levels should be tested for varicella in staff in neonatal and paediatric wards and in units for immunosuppressed patients.

Measles vaccine should be offered to staff in paediatric, infectious diseases or leukaemia wards if they have not already had the disease or been previously immunized. Diphtheria immunization should be offered to laboratory staff who are at risk.

CONTINUING SURVEILLANCE AND ADVICE

In addition to initial screening, the occupational health service or practitioner and nurse responsible for staff health should be concerned with the following:
- training of staff of all grades in personal hygiene (e.g. handwashing, mode of transmission of infection, handling contaminated materials, prevention of inoculation incidents);
- immunization and vaccination of existing staff at the required time interval (Department of Health, 1996);
- making decisions on exclusion of staff from work and examination of staff returning to work after absence due to diarrhoea or sepsis, to ensure that the infection has cleared and to give advice to carriers;
- arranging tests and possibly treatment for staff with sepsis of hospital origin, or who are carriers of pathogens which may be harmful to patients;
- keeping accurate records of work-related infections in the staff;
- keeping records of inoculation incidents, arranging for prophylaxis and counselling of staff at risk of infection (e.g. HIV, HBV, HCV, cytomegalovirus, etc.);
- determining staff contacts of infectious disease, and checking immunity and follow-up if necessary;
- surveys of potential infective and toxic hazards to staff in hospital.

The responsibilities described above are mainly concerned with risks of infections, and are only a part of the work of the occupational health department. The implementation of the COSHH regulations (see Chapter 2) is an example (Health and

Safety at Work Act, 1974) (Boucher, 1979). Staff are exposed to potential toxic hazards of disinfectants, especially aldehydes, in addition to risks from micro-organisms. Another example is allergy to latex gloves.

Where an occupational health department exists, a close working relationship must be established between the infection control doctor and nurse and the staff of the occupational health department. A member of the occupational health department should be on the infection control committee.

The infection control and occupational health nurses should work together in tracing contacts of infectious diseases, providing advice and educating staff.

STAFF WITH OR IN CONTACT WITH INFECTIOUS DISEASES

The recommended periods of isolation for patients with infectious disease (see Chapter 8) are also appropriate periods of time for members of staff with such infections to be kept away from patients in the hospital. Staff who are in contact – either at home or in hospital – with infectious disease need not be excluded, but when they are or have been in contact with cases of typhoid fever, diphtheria, meningococcal meningitis and other potentially dangerous diseases, the infection control doctor should be consulted for advice. Diphtheria contacts should be given prophylactic erythromycin and kept under surveillance. Poliomyelitis and diphtheria contacts should be offered active immunization. Contacts of childhood infections, particularly chicken-pox, should not work where there are high-infection-risk patients unless they are immune or otherwise protected against the infection to which they have been exposed. Very close contacts with patients with meningococcal infection (e.g. following mouth-to-mouth respiration) should be given a course of rifampicin (600 mg bd) or ciprofloxacin (500 mg single dose).

Staff receiving an inoculation incident should report immediately to the occupational health department or inform the duty microbiologist if outside normal working hours (the required action is outlined in Chapter 10). Special precautions may be required for pregnant staff, and immunizations and prophylaxis should be discussed with infection control staff (see also Bolyard et al., 1998).

REFERENCES

Bolyard, E.A., Tablon, O.C., Williams, W.N. et al. (1998) Guidelines for infection control in healthcare personnel. Infection Control and Hospital Epidemiology 19: 407

Boucher, B.J. (1979) Guidance on preparing local rules to help implement the Health and Safety at Work Act, etc. British Medical Journal i, 599.

Department of Health (1996) Immunization against infectious diseases. London: HMSO.

Department of Health Welsh Office (1996) The prevention and control of tuberculosis in the United Kingdom. Recommendations for the prevention and control of tuberculosis at local level. London: Department of Health.

Health Services Advisory Committee (1991) *Safe working and the prevention of infection in clinical laboratories: model rules for staff and visitors.* London: HMSO.

Joint Tuberculosis Committee of the British Thoracic Society (1994) Control and prevention of tuberculosis in the United Kingdom: code of practice. *Thorax* 49, 1193.

NHS Management Executive (1994) *NHS Health Service Guidelines: Occupational health services for NHS staff.* London: Department of Health.

UK Departments of Health (1998) *Guidance for clinical health care workers. Protection against infection and bloodborne viruses.* London: Department of Health.

chapter 16

SPECIAL WARDS AND DEPARTMENTS. I.

INTENSIVE CARE UNITS AND HIGH-DEPENDENCY UNITS

Infection is one of the principal hazards to which patients in intensive care units (ICUs) are exposed. A patient who requires intensive care may be defined as one who requires support of a vital function until the disease process is arrested or ameliorated. Such a patient may need ventilation (in which case they will be nursed in an intensive care unit) or not (in which case they will usually be in a high-dependency unit). They are likely to have poor resistance to infection, sometimes due to immunosuppressive or steroid therapy, or due to depression of the immunological response (often seen in such patients with multiple organ failure). In addition to being more susceptible, they are exposed in the intensive care unit to greater hazards of contamination and cross-infection than most patients in ordinary wards. This is due to the fact that they receive much more nursing attention and handling, and various forms of instrumentation, particularly tracheostomy, mechanical ventilation, aspiration of bronchial secretions, catheterization of the urinary tract, treatment of open wounds and central venous catheterization. Special difficulties arise in emergencies (e.g. respiratory obstruction requiring immediate clearing of the patient's airway) and the sudden excessive pressure of work which occurs when several patients are admitted at the same time. In such circumstances it may be difficult or impossible to observe all of the recommendations of asepsis. Even so, cross-infection is in many cases probably due to thoughtlessness or staff shortages. Intensive therapy requires what is sometimes considered to be an inordinate number of trained nursing staff, but if such a complement is not available, nurses inevitably have to move rapidly between patients without having time even to wash their hands. The amount of technical assistance and the number of domestic staff in intensive therapy units (ITU) is much greater than it is in normal wards, but these are essential if nursing skills are to be used effectively and if meticulous cleanliness of equipment is to be maintained.

The micro-organisms which cause infection in intensive care units include any of those which are associated with hospital infection, but as the patients are often deficient in resistance to infection, many organisms which have little or no pathogenicity to healthy individuals and tissues are potentially important as causes of infection in intensive care patients. The commonest infecting organisms in an ITU

are *Staphylococcus aureus* (including MRSA), *Staphylococcus epidermidis,*
Escherichia coli, Pseudomonas aeruginosa, Klebsiella species, *Proteus* species,
Acinetobacter species, *Enterobacter* species, and *Candida* species. Endogenous
infection with coliform bacilli and sometimes with *Bacteroides* species and other
anaerobic non-sporing bacteria is a hazard in patients with abdominal wounds.
The reduction of gastric acid by the use of H_2-blockers may be followed by colonization of the stomach with Gram-negative bacilli. Aspiration of stomach
contents may lead to colonization of the oropharynx and the respiratory tract, and
possibly to bronchopneumonia. The use of sucralfate instead of H_2-blockers
appears to reduce the risk of colonization of the stomach, and consequently of
Gram-negative respiratory tract infection.

Staphylococcal infection may be transmitted by contact or by air, and epidemic
strains of MRSA are a particular hazard. Gram-negative bacilli, when not acquired
from the patient's own flora of skin, gut or upper respiratory tract, are most likely
to be acquired by contact, and from moist vectors such as solutions and medicaments, food, humidifiers of mechanical ventilators, etc. Airborne infection with
Gram-negative bacilli is a remote risk, except from aerosols produced by a contaminated nebulizer, or less commonly from removal of dressings (e.g. of burns) on
which heavily contaminated exudate has dried. Expectoration by patients with
tracheostomies or endotracheal tubes may cause heavy local contamination with
bronchial mucus, but the air of an intensive care unit has been found to be usually
free from *Pseudomonas aeruginosa,* even when several patients with respiratory
and urinary tract pseudomonas infection are in the ward. The suggestion that the
expired air of all patients undergoing artificial ventilation in the unit should be
filtered or exhausted to the exterior seems unnecessary.

CONTROL OF INFECTION – GENERAL ASPECTS

The general principles of aseptic care and hospital hygiene which are described in
Chapters 6 and 7 must be conscientiously applied, with certain additional precautions relating to special procedures of the intensive care unit (Craven and Steger,
1989).

DESIGN OF UNIT

Because of the need for quick and unimpaired access of staff to patients, it is
usually inappropriate for all of the patients to be in single-bed isolation rooms, but
one or two isolation rooms are required (e.g. in an 8-bed unit, there could be two
3-bed wards or divisions of a ward, and two isolation rooms). There should be
adequate space (e.g. 10–12 feet between bed centres) to allow easy access of staff
and equipment.

The isolation rooms should be suitable for use by either infected patients (*source
isolation*), or hypersusceptible patients who must be given maximum protection
against infection (*protective isolation*), or for combined source and protective
isolation (e.g. by plenum ventilation into the room and extraction of air, when
required, from the room to the outside of the hospital). It is probably desirable that

the open section of the unit should have mechanical ventilation with a turnover of air (e.g. 10 air changes/hour) sufficient to prevent a build-up of bacteria released by individuals in the unit, and to keep airborne bacteria at a low level. However, an intensive care unit may be reasonably safe without plenum ventilation, or with a degree of mechanical ventilation to provide maximum comfort.

FURNITURE AND FITTINGS

Floors and walls should be washable. Furniture should be reduced to a minimum. Monitoring equipment should be clear of the floor and easily moved and cleaned; suction apparatus and sphygmomanometers should be wall-mounted but detachable.

Sticky mats at the entrance to the unit have been shown to have no value in reducing contamination (Ayliffe *et al.*, 1967; Traore *et al.*, 1997).

CLEANING OF ENVIRONMENT

As in wards (see Chapter 6).

HANDLING OF PATIENTS

A high standard of aseptic care must be used by nurses, doctors, physiotherapists, radiographers, pathology technicians and others in handling intensive care patients. Hands should be washed with an antimicrobial detergent preparation, or preferably disinfected with 70% alcohol rubbed to dryness, which is rapid and effective. Plastic disposable (non-sterile) gloves should be worn for bronchial and oral toilet, and as many as possible of the procedures (e.g. oral toilet) should always be performed before 'dirty' procedures (e.g. taking rectal temperature).

Protective clothing (gowns or plastic aprons) should be worn when attending to a patient, but this is not necessary if there is no patient contact; all members of staff or visitors should wear a gown or apron used for that patient only. Overshoes, masks and disposable hats are unnecessary (see Chapter 11). Non-essential visiting should be discouraged, but relatives or close friends of the patient should be allowed to visit. They must have almost unrestricted access to prevent disorientation of the patient, which can cause severe psychological disturbance – one of the major problems for those who survive. Furthermore, there is good evidence that infection is more likely to be acquired from a member of the hospital staff who attends to other patients than from a (healthy) visitor who visits only one patient in the ward.

PROCEDURES

Tracheostomy and endotracheal intubation

The benefits of tracheostomy, by which exudates can be aspirated and mechanical ventilation established, are offset by the risks of infection. Colonization of the oral cavity and trachea, which may sometimes lead to the development of bronchopneumonia, can be caused by various organisms, but predominantly

Gram-negative bacilli introduced into the respiratory tract at the time of aspiration of exudate or during mechanical ventilation or humidification, or *Staphylococcus aureus* from the inspired air. Tracheostomy is used for patients who require long-term ventilation. However, most patients can be ventilated using endotracheal tubes. These may also be a channel of contamination, but they have the advantage of avoiding the need for an operation, with possible infection of the operation wound. There is usually no difficulty in re-intubating patients, and secretions can be aspirated as easily from an endotracheal tube as from a tracheostomy.

The control of infection in patients with a tracheostomy or endotracheal tube is difficult. When any patient in the unit has a multi-resistant Gram-negative infection (of the respiratory tract or of a wound), infection may spread to other patients in the unit. Care is needed during the removal of endotracheal tubes, and non-sterile plastic gloves should be worn. The most important procedure for reducing the spread of infection is handwashing between patients.

Intravenous catheters
See Chapter 7.

Ventilatory equipment
Prevention of infection from this source is very important. Various methods of decontamination are available (see Chapter 6). Of importance in the design of all modern lung ventilators is the ability either to isolate the ventilator completely from the patient by bacterial filters, or for the patient's circuit and humidifier to be easily removed for autoclaving, or both. It has been suggested that placing a filter between the patient and the circuit may reduce colonization of the ventilatory equipment and thus reduce the incidence of pneumonia, although conclusive evidence to support this hypothesis is lacking.

Urine drainage
A fluid balance is required as part of the management of patients in the intensive care unit. Drainage bags must be changed or emptied twice daily under aseptic conditions, and the urine collected for 24-hour analysis must not be stored at the bedside (see Chapter 7).

EQUIPMENT

All equipment used in intensive care units should be kept meticulously clean and dry. In a study on sources of infection, washing bowls used by patients in an intensive care unit were often found to be contaminated with *Pseudomonas aeruginosa* in residues of moisture. Individual bowls that have been heat disinfected or at least thoroughly washed and dried after use are desirable. Shaving brushes should be avoided, and electric razors used on one patient and then on another are also potential vectors of infection. An individual shaving kit is desirable. Chapter 6 gives information on disinfection of ventilators, nebulizers, humidifiers and suction equipment. Food mixers are also a potential source of infection. Water in flower vases is frequently contaminated with *Pseudomonas* species, although this is an unlikely source of infection. Storage of equipment in fluids should be avoided.

ANTIBIOTIC PROPHYLAXIS

Antibiotic prophylaxis should generally be avoided to reduce the risks of selecting multi-resistant opportunistic organisms. However, selective decontamination of the oropharynx and gastrointestinal tract with antibiotics has been used successfully in several studies, to prevent colonization with aerobic Gram-negative bacilli. One such regime includes applications of a paste containing polymyxin B, tobramycin and amphotericin B to the oral pharynx, the introduction of these agents into the stomach with a nasogastric tube and the systemic administration of cefotaxime (Van Saene et al., 1991). Respiratory infection has been shown to be significantly reduced by this regime. Other studies have shown similar results, although there is less evidence that mortality is reduced. Further studies over a longer time period are still required to determine the specific applications for this routine, and to determine whether selective decontamination will also select highly resistant strains.

BURNS AND OPEN TRAUMATIC WOUNDS (Ayliffe and Lawrence, 1985)

Burns are at first free or virtually free from bacteria, which have been killed by the heat, but soon the layer of dead tissue and exudate becomes heavily colonized by bacteria unless effective measures are taken to exclude them. In small superficial burns and in many deeper and more extensive burns the bacteria cause no apparent ill effects, although this depends on the types of bacteria present and on the patient's resistance. In more extensive burns, bacterial infection is the most important cause of illness and death.

Staphylococcus aureus is the most common isolate from burns in the UK, and *Acinetobacter* species are now isolated more frequently than *Pseudomonas aeruginosa* (Papini et al., 1995). *Streptococcus pyogenes,* when present, will usually cause the complete failure of skin grafts and delay healing. Today it rarely causes invasive infection, although it may cause fever. Of the other bacteria, *Pseudomonas aeruginosa* has proved to be the most important cause of septicaemia and toxaemia. It can also cause the failure of skin grafts, but to a smaller extent than *Streptococcus pyogenes*. Other Gram-negative bacilli (*Proteus* species, *Klebsiella* species, *Serratia* species, *Acinetobacter* species, etc.) and *Staphylococcus aureus* are usually less important pathogens, although they can occasionally cause septicaemia in severely burned patients. Methicillin-resistant *Staphylococcus aureus* (MRSA) is a common cause of colonization of burns. These strains are rare causes of clinical infection in most units in the UK (Settle, 1985), but some units, particularly in the USA, have had major infection problems (Crossley et al., 1979). Rarer pathogens include *Candida albicans* and other fungi, gas gangrene and tetanus bacilli and herpes virus.

Pseudomonas aeruginosa and other bacteria are usually acquired from the burns of other patients in the ward, transmitted on the hands of nurses, by various fomites and by air. Air is a less significant route, especially for Gram-negative bacilli, but it may be important if large dressings are changed in an open ward.

In addition to the burn, the urinary tract, respiratory tract and intravenous infusion sites are important portals of entry and sites of infection.

Open wounds resemble burns, but there is usually less necrotic tissue in which small numbers of bacteria can multiply. Contaminants acquired at the time of injury, including tetanus and gas-gangrene bacilli, are more likely to play a role in the infection of open wounds than of burns, but hospital-acquired infection (both exogenous and endogenous) is potentially more important than contamination at the time of injury.

DESIGN OF UNITS (Working Party of the British Burn Association and Hospital Infection Research Society, 1991)

A burns unit should if possible be self-contained with its own operating-theatre and intensive care facilities. It should preferably be part of a teaching or district general hospital with ready access to other specialist activities (e.g. renal dialysis).

The number of rooms and their bed content depends on the workload, but internal flexibility in room size is desirable. Single rooms should be available for isolation, and at least two of them should be equipped to intensive care standards. Wash hand-basins should be adjacent to all beds in the unit. Filtered air should be provided to isolation rooms and the dressing room and extracted to the exterior. Several options for ventilating rooms are available (Working Party Report, 1991). A window air extractor would be adequate for some single rooms, which can then be used for source isolation if required.

PREVENTION OF INFECTION

Mortality from sepsis and other causes has decreased in recent years, but infection is still a major problem.

The main requirements for reducing infection and mortality are as follows:
- adequate resuscitation (Nguyen *et al.*, 1996);
- early excision and grafting of burn (Papini *et al.*, 1995);
- use of topical antibacterial agents;
- routine microbiological surveillance;
- rapid and effective treatment of clinical infection;
- good aseptic techniques.

The bacterial flora of all burns should be examined on admission and at all changes of dressings for *Streptococcus pyogenes, Pseudomonas aeruginosa* and other common aerobic bacteria. If *Streptococcus pyogenes* is present, the patient must be treated with systemic penicillin, flucloxacillin or erythromycin (if penicillin allergic), and grafting operations must be postponed until the burn is free of this organism. Benzyl or phenoxymethyl penicillin are not suitable if *Staphylococcus aureus* is present because they are likely to be inactivated by penicillinase from other bacteria colonizing the same burn. Prophylaxis against infection of burns can be subdivided into two lines of defence (Lowbury, 1992).

The first line of defence
The first line of defence (i.e. methods of protecting the patient against microbial contaminants) includes the following:

1 primary excision (within 5 days, and preferably earlier) and skin grafting (only suitable for relatively small burns of full thickness) or on application of a dermal template (e.g. Integra);
2 antisepsis (i.e. application of antibacterial substances to the burn);
3 asepsis (Newsom, 1998).

Antisepsis
Local treatment with appropriate antimicrobial agents has been shown in controlled trials to protect burns against colonization by *Pseudomonas aeruginosa, Streptococcus pyogenes, Staphylococcus aureus* and other bacteria, and to reduce the septic consequences of infection, including skin graft failure and mortality. The qualities looked for in such prophylactic agents are effectiveness against all strains of significant burn pathogens, minimal local or systemic toxicity, and failure to select resistant variants in patients under treatment. There is no ideal preparation that fulfils all requirements. Silver sulphadiazine cream has been widely adopted as a standard prophylactic application, but a preponderant flora of sulphonamide-resistant Gram-negative bacilli has been found to emerge in one centre where silver sulphadiazine was in regular use for several years.

When silver sulphadiazine is rejected for such reasons, an alternative prophylactic application is required and can be made available by co-operation of the hospital pharmacy. In patients with extensive burns, silver nitrate compresses (0.5%) have proved highly effective, especially against *Pseudomonas aeruginosa* and *Proteus* species, but patients who receive this treatment need supplements of electrolytes by mouth and laboratory control of serum electrolytes to avoid imbalance. The method is not suitable for infants. A further disadvantage is the black staining of all items that come into contact with the silver solution (including walls). Silver sulphadiazine, when acceptable, is more suitable for smaller burns and for children and, although less active against *Pseudomonas aeruginosa* and *Proteus* species, it is more active against some other Gram-negative bacilli. Chlorhexidine 0.2% or cerium nitrate may be added to silver sulphadiazine or silver nitrate cream. For minor burns (especially those treated in out-patient clinics), a tulle gras containing 0.5% chlorhexidine ('Bactigras') has been found to be appropriate. Burns treated by the exposure method have a physical protective barrier against infection once a dry eschar has formed. This can be anticipated and supplemented by topical chemoprophylaxis with povidone-iodine (7.5%, with 0.75% available iodine), or with aqueous silver nitrate (0.5%) dabbed on three or four times a day for 6–8 days.

Antibiotics should preferably not be used for topical prophylaxis because of the risks of emergence of resistant organisms and of toxic or allergic effects in the patients (Lowbury, 1976). Monitoring of the sensitivity of burn flora is an important routine procedure in a burns unit. This should be performed at every dressing change or if the burns are exposed daily from the lumened area.

Asepsis

Dressing of burns in a ventilated dressing room, barrier nursing, source and protective isolation of patients and good ward hygiene contribute to control of infection (see Chapters 7 and 8). The dressing may be carried out in a single isolation room provided that the ventilation system and facilities are adequate. For patients with burns in hospital, a dressing technique with two nurses should be used if possible in a room with combined source and protective isolation (e.g. plenum ventilation with an exhaust-ventilated airlock). Exposure treatment, which is clinically desirable for many burns of the trunk and the face, provides some protection by the development of a dry eschar on which bacteria cannot grow (but which may cover a zone of heavy growth and suppuration). Exposure treatment is better than moist applications with no antibacterial activity.

The second line of defence

This consists of methods of preventing invasion of the tissues and bloodstream by bacteria growing on the burn. This includes: *antibiotic therapy, active and passive immunization* and *general supportive measures* (treatment of diabetes, anaemia, etc.). Systemic treatment of all *Streptococcus pyogenes* infections with an appropriate antibiotic protects all patients in the ward by eliminating reservoirs of infection during a major outbreak. In rare circumstances all patients in the ward, whether infected or not, may be treated prophylactically. Severely burned patients who have acquired heavy growths of *Pseudomonas aeruginosa* may be given protection with a systemic antipseudomonal agent (e.g. ceftazidime or a quinolone). A more promising procedure would be the use of a polyvalent *Pseudomonas* vaccine which has been found to give early protection and reduced mortality in patients with severe burns. Hyperimmune globulin prepared from immunized human volunteers has also proved valuable, but commercial preparations are not available. Prophylaxis against tetanus, by use of a 'boosting' dose of toxoid when the patient is known to be actively immune, or by means of antiserum (human antitetanus globulin) if there is no evidence of active immunity, should be given to all patients with burns who are admitted to hospital (see Chapter 15).

SPECIAL PROBLEMS OF STERILIZATION AND DISINFECTION

The principles of sterile supply outlined in Chapter 17 are relevant to patients with burns. The outside of electrical equipment, cardiac monitoring equipment, portable lights, diathermy and X-ray machines, suction apparatus and respiratory ventilators must be cleaned after use because of the possibilities of heavy contamination (e.g. with 70% alcohol).

The disinfection of respiratory ventilators and anaesthetic apparatus is described in Chapter 6. Water-circulating mattresses may be disinfected with a chlorine-releasing agent, and body temperature recorders may be disinfected with 70% alcohol. Mattress covers may be damaged by repeated application of phenolic disinfectants or by silver nitrate treatment of patients. Gram-negative bacilli are then likely to grow in the mattress. Mattresses should therefore be inspected regularly for damage.

Beds that provide air-support systems are sometimes used for the management of extensive injuries, including burns, or in the case of the patients who are at special risk of ulcer formation. One type of bed (the 'fluidized-bead bed') has a trough filled with silica beads and covered with a special sheet, through which air is pumped. Another type (the 'low-air-loss bed') is constructed from a series of inflatable cushions, air being continuously pumped through these, with pneumatic controls to vary the elevation.

The risk of dispersing bacteria into the environment from these beds, even when they are occupied by heavily infected patients, has been shown to be no greater than that from a standard hospital bed. If these beds are colonized with enterococci it has been suggested that the heat tolerance of this organism allows it to survive decontamination procedures. This has been identified as a risk factor for transmission of vancomycin-resistant enterococci. Otherwise, normal cleaning procedures (e.g. with a cloth moistened with a detergent solution) are generally adequate (Gould and Freeman, 1993; Bradley and Fraise, 1996). If the external surfaces are known to be contaminated, they should be cleansed with a chlorine-releasing agent, rinsed and allowed to dry. The air sacs of low-air-loss beds should be machine-washed at a temperature of 60°C (but this may be inadequate for ente-rococci). The advice of the manufacturer should be sought when internal ducting has become contaminated, and also with regard to appropriate agents for disin-fection (see Chapter 6).

Baths are a potential source of Gram-negative infection, particularly of *Pseudomonas aeruginosa*. Recirculating systems (e.g. jacuzzis, etc.) are difficult to clean and disinfect, and should not be used unless adequate disinfection is possible.

METHICILLIN-RESISTANT *STAPHYLOCOCCUS AUREUS*

Attempts at eradication of epidemic MRSA from a burns unit usually fail and are rarely cost-effective. However, the introduction of full control measures may be necessary if clinical infections are causing a problem, but closure of a large unit is rarely possible.

Large burns should be protected from colonization whenever possible, and particular care is required in the management of intravenous lines. Staff should preferably not work in other wards, and routine screening of staff should only be carried out if an eradication programme is indicated.

Screening and isolation of patients from other countries or hospitals with a known MRSA problem should be carried out if possible, but MRSA carriers should not be refused admission to a specialist burns unit if admission is clinically indi-cated.

HOMOGRAFTS AS VECTORS OF INFECTION

Homografts are potentially sources of infection with pathogenic bacteria; HIV can be transmitted in this way from a donor who is a carrier, and it is probable that other viruses (e.g. HBV, HCV and cytomegalovirus) can also be transmitted on skin homografts.

Homografts are now mainly processed in skin banks in the UK. Cadaver donors are screened for infections and grafts are stored as non-viable glycerolized skin or cryopreserved viable skin.

DERMATOLOGICAL WARDS

Most patients with skin diseases are not physically very 'ill', but their condition often causes them some mental stress. When it is considered necessary to use source isolation procedures, it is important that it should be explained to the patient that, with certain exceptions, the underlying skin condition (e.g. eczema or psoriasis) in itself is not infectious and will not spread to the rest of the family or to visitors. The risk is of the transfer of bacteria capable of causing infection in susceptible patients in hospital (e.g. patients undergoing surgery). Healthy people will not become infected from them even when in close contact. This does not apply to certain septic lesions (e.g. impetigo) where there is a definite risk of transfer to healthy subjects.

Patients in dermatological wards often have generalized desquamating lesions which are heavily colonized with *Staphylococcus aureus*. These patients are often heavy dispersers and cross-infection is frequent, but clinical sepsis is rarely caused by these staphylococci. However, such a patient admitted to a surgical ward may be responsible for widespread nasal colonization and wound sepsis. These strains of staphylococci are commonly resistant to two or more antibiotics, and MRSA is a particular hazard. Children admitted with clinically apparent staphylococcal infections (e.g. impetigo) not only spread infection, but cause similar septic lesions in other children and sometimes also pyogenic lesions in the staff. These strains are often resistant to penicillin only, and are initially acquired outside hospital. Some of these infections are caused by β-haemolytic streptococci (often associated with *Staphylococcus aureus*) and may similarly spread to other patients. Cross-infection with Gram-negative bacilli (e.g. *Pseudomonas aeruginosa* and *Proteus* species) is also common in dermatological wards, and these organisms are usually found in varicose ulcers, but clinical sepsis is unusual.

Candida infection may also occur, although there is little evidence of cross-infection. Patients with dermatophyte infections are not usually admitted to hospital, but the risk of cross-infection exists (e.g. *Tinea corporis* and *Tinea pedis*, which may not be clinically obvious). Transmission of *Tinea capitis* between children occurs readily in schools, and could spread similarly in paediatric wards.

The spread of virus infection is not a particular risk in dermatological wards.

CONTROL OF INFECTION

Staphylococcal infection in dermatology wards spreads both by contact and by air. Environmental contamination may be so heavy that prevention of cross-infection is difficult, but some potentially effective measures are possible, especially the following.

1 Children with clinical sepsis must be isolated in single rooms, whether in general or dermatological wards.

2 Patients with diffuse desquamating lesions should be kept in single rooms if admitted to general hospital wards.
3 General hospitals should where possible have wards kept solely for dermatological patients.
4 When isolation is required, it must be complete (i.e. patients should not leave the ward to visit other patients).

DRESSING TECHNIQUES

Open lesions (e.g. ulcers) and wounds should be treated as in a general surgical ward, using SSD packs and a no-touch technique. If possible, a special room should be provided for performing surgical techniques (e.g. biopsies). The dressing of patients with non-surgical lesions is rather different, as it is not necessarily an aseptic procedure.
1 Dressing rooms should be immediately adjacent to the bathroom and should have an extractor fan.
2 Couches in dressing rooms should be covered with paper covers which are changed between patients.
3 Dressing materials in contact with broken skin should have been sterilized.
4 Large bags should be provided for disposal of contaminated dressings.
5 Gloves or instruments should be used for performing dressing techniques whenever possible; creams and ointments should be applied when possible with a gloved hand. Staff should wash their hands thoroughly with soap or an antiseptic detergent preparation and water after handling each patient.
6 Staff should wear plastic, disposable aprons which should be discarded at the end of each dressing session.

ADDITIONAL PRECAUTIONS

1 Disposable toilet-seat covers and bath-mats may be of some value, and patients should be instructed in their use.
2 Floors should be cleaned with a vacuum-cleaner that is capable of removing skin scales.
3 Special attention should be paid to the disinfection of baths and wash-bowls after each use. In general, cleaning methods and techniques are similar to those recommended for rooms containing infected patients (see Chapter 6).

ANTIBIOTIC TREATMENT

Emergence of resistance is especially likely to occur in patients with skin disease because of the large populations of bacteria on the skin. Antibiotic treatment (especially topical treatment) should be avoided whenever possible, and other antimicrobial agents should be used if they are available or suitable (e.g. silver nitrate, chlorhexidine). Resistance emerges particularly readily to erythromycin, lincomycin (or clindamycin) and fusidic acid, and their use should be controlled.

Neomycin and bacitracin are useful topical antibiotics, although resistance of *Staphylococcus aureus* and hypersensitivity to neomycin are common. Gentamicin is a useful systemic antibiotic and should not be used topically in hospital. The combination of neomycin with chlorhexidine in a topical preparation may reduce the likelihood of resistance emerging. Mupirocin is particularly effective in removing *Staphylococcus aureus* from carriage sites and eczematous lesions. However, resistant strains are now emerging and its use should preferably be restricted to treatment of MRSA carriers. If applied to a skin lesion, its use (and that of other topical antibiotic agents) should be limited to a period of 7 days.

OINTMENTS AND OTHER MEDICAMENTS

As patients with widespread skin lesions are particularly susceptible to infection and large amounts of topical medicaments are often applied, the application must be free from pathogenic bacteria. Tubes should be used whenever possible for creams and ointments. Jars or bottles should be thoroughly cleaned (or preferably disinfected) and dried before refilling, and occasional bacterial checks should be made on preparations and distilled water in the pharmacy. Topical preparations supplied by manufacturers should also be checked, unless the manufacturer's system of preparation and testing is known to be satisfactory. In the wards, ointments or creams should be supplied for the individual patient, and if jars are used the ointment should never be removed with the fingers.

NEUROSURGERY DEPARTMENTS

The meninges are particularly susceptible to infection, and clinical infection may be caused through contamination occurring at operation or during a lumbar or ventricular puncture, by Gram-negative bacilli of low pathogenicity, as well as by the usual organisms causing wound infection. Infections caused by these opportunistic organisms (e.g. *Pseudomonas aeruginosa, Serratia marcescens* and flavobacteria) have occurred because of inadequate sterilization or maintenance of sterility of instruments or water applied topically. Organisms normally present on the skin (e.g. coagulase-negative staphylococci) which are usually of low pathogenicity may also cause low-grade infections, particularly in association with Spitz–Holter valves and other prostheses. *Staphylococcus aureus* is the commonest pathogen isolated from wound infections (Gantz and Godofsky, 1996). Infections may be transmitted on the hands of staff from infected patients or following the use of contaminated nailbrushes, hand-creams, soaps or detergents. Inadequate disinfection of the patient's skin pre-operatively, or use of contaminated shaving equipment, may also be followed by infection. With regard to other types of infection, neurosurgical units have the same problems as other departments, and some neurosurgical patients are in hospital for long periods. They may have indwelling catheters, and tracheostomy or endotracheal intubation is sometimes necessary. Patients with ear infection may be admitted to the unit. Unconscious patients are apt to acquire chest infections or bedsores. Although cerebral abscesses are usually endogenous in origin, hospital strains of Gram-negative bacilli and *Staphylococcus aureus* are likely to spread in the ward and be acquired in the nasal or intestinal flora, becoming a potential source of endogenous infection unless effective control measures are employed.

PREVENTION OF INFECTION

Isolation and barrier-nursing of infected patients, particularly patients with pseudomonas or multiresistant staphylococcal infection, are important measures in neurosurgical units. If possible, dressings of wounds exposing the meninges should be changed in the operating-theatre or, if not, in a plenum-ventilated dressing room. The patient's own single-bedded room, if the facilities are adequate, may be suitable for many of the routine procedures. Special wards are required for intensive care treatment, including patients with tracheostomies (see the section on intensive care units in Chapter 16). Other procedures (e.g. lumbar puncture and catheterization) may be performed in non-specialized wards. The relevant precautions are described elsewhere (see Chapter 7). Pre-operative shaving should be performed on the day of operation, to avoid the possibility that small scratches or excoriations which sometimes occur might become heavily colonized. Shaving of either head hair or pubic hair for vertebral angiography should be completed before disinfection of the scalp or skin. Shaving brushes should not be used. Razors should be sterilized or adequately disinfected and individual sterilized gauze swabs should be used to apply shaving cream. If shaving cream is used, it should contain an antiseptic which prevents the growth of organisms that might cause infection. A povidone-iodine shampoo or chlorhexidine detergent may also be used before shaving. Subsequent skin preparation in the operating-theatre is performed with 0.5% alcoholic chlorhexidine. Equipment for aseptic procedures should be autoclaved, and SSD packs supplied whenever possible, e.g. for lumbar puncture, catheterization, wound dressing and tracheostomy toilet. Particular care is required to avoid contamination of lotions. If aspiration of an effusion from a craniotomy wound is required, insert the needle through intact skin and not through the suture line. Organisms may enter the bloodstream from monitoring equipment and set up an infection at the operation site. This equipment should be regularly disinfected or sterilized, preferably by heat.

Antibiotic prophylaxis reduces the infection rate in craniotomy operations. Cloxicillin, a cephalosporin or vancomycin, with or without gentamicin, appear to be effective and are commonly given for 24 hours (Gantz and Godofsky, 1996).

OPHTHALMIC DEPARTMENTS

PROBLEMS OF INFECTION

The eye is particularly susceptible to infection with Gram-negative bacilli, fungi, adenoviruses and herpes simplex virus, organisms which are often or always resistant to antibiotics sometimes used for prophylaxis. Traumatic wounds and surgical operations increase or determine the risks of severe infection with these organisms.

EXTRA-OCULAR AND ORBITAL SURGERY

Control of infection in extra-ocular and orbital operations presents problems which are in general similar to those in any other branch of surgery. Many of these operations are performed for cosmetic reasons, so any unsightly scarring due to infection is a serious complication.

There are special considerations when implants are used in the orbit, either on the scleral surface to produce enfolding in retinal detachment surgery, or when nucleation implants are used to impart movement to an artificial eye. Any contamination during such operations carries a grave risk of inflammation and possible extrusion of the implant.

INTRA-OCULAR SURGERY

The greatest risks from contamination occur in intra-ocular operations, and also in patients who have corneal injuries or ulceration. The transparent ocular media have no direct blood circulation and are deficient in antibodies. However, they are well oxygenated and provide good culture media for exogenous micro-organisms (in particular, *Pseudomonas aeruginosa*).

CONTROL OF INFECTION

Pre-operative disinfection of the conjunctiva

1 Present practice is variable, and the value of disinfection remains uncertain, but antibiotic drops (e.g. 0.5% chloramphenicol, 0.3% ciprofloxacin or 5% cefuroxime) are usually instilled into the eye pre- and post-operatively. Some departments use sub-conjunctival cefuroxime or gentamicin post-operatively. Disinfectants are often not well tolerated, although 5% povidone-iodine has been used and is microbiologically effective. Pre-operative microbiological sampling is occasionally performed, but its value is limited and it may delay the operation unnecessarily.

2 With solutions, eyedrops and ointments the greatest risks of intra-ocular infection are associated with the use of contaminated fluids due to either inadequate sterilization or to recontamination through inadequate handling or multiple-use containers. Sterile drops without a preservative should be supplied for pre-operative use if such a preparation is available and discarded. A fresh supply of multi-dose drops is given post-operatively (Department of Health and Social Security, 1975).

3 In corneal grafts, the cornea is the only tissue from the eye which is transplanted. Donors should be tested for HIV, HCV and HBV.

Sterilization of instruments and appliances

Although autoclaving provides satisfactory sterilization, some instruments (e.g. cataract knives) may suffer damage to their delicate cutting edge if sterilized in this way. Some authorities accept sterilization by dry heat at 160°C (320°F) for 1 hour, or at lower temperatures for longer periods, as being satisfactory (Ophthalmic Society of the United Kingdom, 1973). As this method is much slower than autoclaving, a stock of sterile instruments must be maintained to replace an instrument at short notice (e.g. when an instrument is dropped or otherwise contaminated). Gamma-sterilized disposable knives and autoclaved diamond knives are now solving some of these problems.

The use of disposable equipment has a significant associated cost, and there is therefore a tendency to reuse single-use items. This practice is not endorsed by the Medical Devices Agency (MDA) of the Department of Health, although it can be acceptable if defined conditions are followed (Medical Devices Agency, 1995). Legal responsibility lies with the person reprocessing the item. Ethylene oxide has a particular application in the sterilization of cryothermy leads and other heat-labile items. As the gas must be allowed to escape from the sterilized pack for at least 24 hours before use of the equipment on patients, this method requires reserve supplies of essential apparatus to cover the 'turnover' of sterilization, especially where transport to another centre adds further delays.

New alternatives to ethylene oxide (e.g. gas plasma sterilization) are still being evaluated. Vitrectomy and other aspiration/infusion apparatus also require sterilization, as the vitreous provides an ideal nidus for colonization by micro-organisms.

The adjustment of the operating microscope and other equipment by the surgeon requires special precautions. The provision of dry sterile guards is usually considered satisfactory, and most microscopes can now be adjusted by the foot or by other methods that do not require direct handling by the surgeon. The equipment must be kept meticulously clean, as cleaning during the operation is not possible.

SURGICAL TECHNIQUE

During operations, instruments are held in such a way that the part which comes into contact with the eye is not touched either primarily or secondarily with the fingers that control them. This is a standard part of the discipline of the surgical team.

Instruments are more effectively controlled when they are regularly used with an operating microscope, which is also an effective mechanism for excluding foreign material from the operating area. Some surgeons prefer to use the ungloved hand, because of the finer control which they believe they can attain in this way. If it can be assumed that the hands are dry and never touch the operation area or the operating ends of instruments, this may involve little risk. Regular and repeated use of an effective detergent antiseptic (e.g. 4% chlorhexidine detergent ('Hibiscrub') or 0.5% alcoholic chlorhexidine) is a particularly important precaution if gloves are not worn. There may be a risk of infection from the ungloved hand through accidental contact or from dry epidermal scales which are likely to drop from the hands during the course of a long operation. Most surgeons now prefer to accept the slight disadvantage of wearing gloves, when this is weighed against the disastrous consequences of a post-operative infection. If the edges of the wound are carefully apposed, the wound is secure and there should be little risk of intra-ocular contamination from the exterior from about 48 hours after the operation.

WARDS

Dressing packs from the SSD are used, and also individual droppers, which are provided as single-use sterile containers. Multi-dose eyedrop bottles should not be used for more than 7 days. Eyedrops may be preserved with benzalkonium chloride (0.01% w/v) or, for short-term use by patients, with phenylmercuric nitrate or acetate (0.002% w/v) or chlorhexidine acetate (0.01% w/v).

OUT-PATIENTS

Multiple-use containers are used on patients other than those with external eye disease, and are discarded at the end of a clinic session. Multiple-use containers should be discarded after use on a single patient in external eye clinics and in casualty departments. Epidemics of adenovirus kerato-conjunctivitis have been associated with the use of inadequately decontaminated applanation tonometers (see p. 113).

CONTACT LENSES

Hard lenses are difficult to contaminate and simple hygiene is usually sufficient. However, they may be disinfected with benzalkonium chloride (0.01% w/v). This method is not suitable for soft lenses. Low-water-content soft lenses can be satisfactorily disinfected by heating to 80°C for 20 min daily. High-water-content lenses may be damaged by heating, and require chemical disinfection. Stabilized hydrogen peroxide (10 vols, 3%) is commonly used. This should be thoroughly washed off or preferably neutralized. Saline solutions used for storage should be changed daily.

EAR, NOSE AND THROAT (ENT) DEPARTMENTS

Patients in ENT departments may be divided into two groups with different problems of hospital-acquired infection. Short-stay patients who are admitted for operations such as tonsillectomy are vulnerable in the post-operative period to endemic hospital organisms, such as staphylococci, but also to β-haemolytic streptococci and other community-type organisms which are brought into hospital by patients. Viruses such as measles which are spread by droplet infection are also especially hazardous in the operative period.

Long-stay patients are usually suffering from a more severe illness, such as carcinoma of the larynx, where the tissues are more susceptible to infection and where, in addition, operative procedures such as tracheostomy provide an alternative route for colonization and ultimately infection by hospital strains of *Pseudomonas aeruginosa* and other Gram-negative bacilli. The mode of spread in these cases is usually by contact. Medical apparatus, such as suction tubing or ventilators, may also be important.

Apart from these, many patients with community-acquired infections may be admitted to the wards, further increasing the risks. These include patients with tonsillitis, quinsy or acute otitis media (caused by streptococci, pneumococci, haemophilus or staphylococci) and patients with chronic external otitis (often heavily colonized with Gram-negative bacilli, staphylococci, yeasts or fungi).

PREVENTION OF INFECTION

Isolation facilities are essential in ENT departments, both to isolate infected cases coming into hospital and to protect those that are particularly susceptible to infection. Long-stay patients with tracheostomy should ideally be nursed in separate rooms. Patients with streptococcal infections, if admitted at all, must be in a room separate from patients who require operations. Children admitted for tonsillectomy and found to be pyrexial are best isolated or, as is common practice, sent home. Patients with chronic ear disease do not generally merit isolation, although the organisms present are often highly resistant to antibiotics and care should be taken to prevent contact spread, particularly by fomites. However, most of these patients are treated as out-patients. Children and adults should preferably be in separate wards.

Operations on the ear, throat and sinuses require incision through colonized mucous membranes, and surface disinfection poses considerable difficulties. Some agents damage the membranes or may lead to fistula formation if they gain access to the middle ear. Patients who require operation on the middle ear may require intensive out-patient treatment of infection, if present. At the time of operation many surgeons use 1% aqueous cetrimide as a membrane disinfectant, but this agent has poor activity against *Pseudomonas aeruginosa*, and an alternative (e.g. an aqueous solution of iodine or iodophor) should be considered. Care of tracheostomy is described in the section on intensive care units. The hospital hygiene problems associated with ENT wards do not differ from those encountered in other wards. SSDs should be able to supply sterile apparatus for examination of patients and for minor procedures. Nasal and aural specula must be used on one patient only before being treated in SSD or decontaminated on site. Many units without immediate access to SSD may need to decontaminate these small items in the clinic or ward. This may be done by boiling in water for 5–10 min or, less desirably, by immersion for 5 min in 70% alcohol solution. Sterilization in a small autoclave is preferable (Medical Devices Agency, 1996, 1998). In each case the specula should be allowed to dry and be stored covered in the dry state. Tracheostomy tubes, suction catheters and similar apparatus must be supplied sterile either from SSD or in commercial pre-sterilized packs. Most laryngoscopes are capable of withstanding autoclave temperatures and should therefore be treated in this way. Fibre-optic bronchoscopes are usually disinfected with glutaraldehyde (see Chapter 6).

Operating microscopes pose some difficulties. Wiping with 70% ethyl alcohol is probably the most effective method of disinfection.

Particular risks to and from personnel in the department are similar to those in other wards, but emphasis should be placed on two infections. *Streptococcal disease* is especially hazardous in ENT departments, so staff with sore throats should be excluded. *Tuberculous laryngitis* can lead to dissemination of many tubercle bacilli into the air, so that a tuberculin test and routine checks by the occupational health department are mandatory for nurses and doctors working in the unit. Tuberculin-negative staff should not be employed (see Chapter 13).

PAEDIATRIC DEPARTMENTS

Richard George

SPECIAL PROBLEMS OF INFECTION

Many children are admitted to hospital with (or incubating) community-acquired infections. Some of these infections (e.g. respiratory virus infections, severe gastroenteritis and infected skin lesions) are difficult to keep under control and may spread rapidly. Children are also more susceptible than adults to community-acquired diseases, as many of them have not developed immunity to the common infectious fevers. Most children's wards also contain a few patients who are particularly susceptible, (e.g. those with blood disorders or receiving steroids). The increase in the use of invasive techniques has been associated with more infections, including the emergence of coagulase-negative staphylococci as pathogens. Patient discipline is understandably rather lax in children's departments, and care must be taken to avoid the escape of children from isolation cubicles, and also misguided generosity in the sharing of toys, dummies, etc.

The organisms which may be involved in cross-infection are many, including viruses such as respiratory syncytial virus (RSV), varicella zoster virus, gastroenteritis viruses such as rotavirus, bacteria such as Group A streptococci, enteropathogenic *E.coli, Campylobacter* species, fungi such as *Candida albicans,* dermatophytes that affect the scalp, and even skin or intestinal parasites (e.g. cryptosporidium). *Pseudomonas aeruginosa, Pseudomonas cepacia* and *Staphylococcus aureus* occasionally cross-infect children suffering from cystic fibrosis. Outbreaks of tuberculosis occasionally occur in paediatric wards. Infections are usually contracted from staff, but a parent whose child had 'closed' TB was implicated in one large outbreak. It is safest to isolate children with 'closed' TB, as well as 'open' TB, until the source is identified. Chapter 8 (on isolation and barrier nursing) is particularly relevant to paediatric departments, and procedures are suggested for the management of children admitted with community-acquired infections.

PREVENTION OF INFECTION (see also section on maternity departments)

The number of nursing staff and the quality of their training are major factors in controlling the spread of infection. Isolation facilities are needed for up to 50% of general paediatric cases, about 10% of routine surgical cases, and in specialist wards the figure depends on the types of patients admitted. Because of the risks of gastroenteritis, no more than four infants should be in any one room, and they should preferably be in cubicles with one or two cots only. Adequate washing facilities must be available in each cubicle, and each cubicle, should have its own weighing machine. Older children should not be in wards with adults. Each ward should have a playroom and a separate examination room. There should be beds available to allow some parents to sleep in the hospital. Screening the faeces of all children admitted to paediatric wards for the presence of *Salmonella* species has been found to be useful by some microbiologists, although it is generally not considered to be practicable or worthwhile.

Outbreaks of rotavirus and RSV infection are particularly common in paediatric wards (see also Chapter 9). Handwashing is important in the control of these infections. Rotavirus infection is associated with heavy environmental contamination, and the large numbers of organisms may be difficult to remove from the hands. The use of gloves is recommended when handling excreta or contaminated materials. An alcoholic handrub following handwashing is also effective. Prevention of RSV spread to staff is important and, in addition to handwashing, staff should be advised to avoid touching the nose and eyes. The use of goggles that cover the nose and eyes of staff has been associated with a reduction in infection in the USA, although the acceptability of this device remains uncertain.

The increase in intravenous site infections, often caused by coagulase-negative staphylococci, is mainly associated with central venous catheterization and parenteral feeding. Efficient skin disinfection and care of the site are important requirements (see Chapter 7).

There is evidence that frequent and prolonged visiting of their own children by parents does not have any significant effect on infection rates. However, it is useful to have a written policy for parents included in the hospital information booklet, stating that 'parents should consult the ward sister if they have any infection, however trivial, so as to protect other children within the unit whose resistance to infection is poor'. Similar provisos apply to visiting by siblings, but it is advisable to bar children with minor respiratory infections, as these may be prodromal signs of measles, etc. Parents should notify staff if a visitor to the hospital develops a transmissible infection within 7 days of visiting, or a patient within the week of discharge. This enables susceptible contacts to be traced. Gowns or plastic aprons should be worn by parents nursing children with gastroenteritis, and handwashing facilities must be available to them, together with instructions on how to avoid acquiring the infection. Visiting of children with dangerous infections, such as diphtheria, poliomyelitis and (for the first 48 hours) meningococcal meningitis should be restricted to parents, and preferably those who are immune, when this is possible. Visitors of infectious patients should avoid contact with other patients.

For information on preparation of feeds, see page 320; for treatment of incubators, suction equipment, thermometers and other equipment, see Chapter 6). Crockery and cutlery need only be domestically clean, but washing in a machine at 70–80°C (158–176°F) is preferable, and is essential on isolation wards.

TOILET ARRANGEMENTS

Because of the common occurrence of intestinal infections in children, special precautions are necessary for toilet areas and bedpan handling. The toilet areas require a high standard of domestic cleanliness, especially the toilet seat, which should be washed at least daily, and more frequently if this is necessary. Spraying the toilet seat and cistern handle with 70% alcohol or cleaning with hypochlorite solution (and rinsing) after each patient is useful during outbreaks of viral gastroenteritis, but attention to handwashing and use of paper towels is of greater importance. A steam or hot-water supply capable of destroying vegetative forms of bacteria should be fitted to bedpan washers (see Chapter 6).

LAUNDRY

Napkins are sealed in plastic or alginate bags for transport, and the bags may be labelled with the words 'used napkins', depending on the laundry policy (see Chapter 12). Disposable napkins are standard practice in developed countries.

PERSONNEL

Communicable diseases may be acquired from patients by staff if they are not immune, and may then in turn be passed on to patients and visitors. One of the most important of these is rubella. Staff of both sexes should be screened for immunity to rubella and be immunized if they are non-immune, because of the number of pregnant women who visit children in hospital. The acquisition of salmonella and shigella by nursing staff can have disastrous consequences, and most outbreaks of infection in hospital due to these organisms have been associated with the infection among the nursing staff. Herpes simplex infection in attendants may produce a variety of lesions and may cause severe infections in children. Staff with herpetic lesions should not handle babies.

SURVEILLANCE SYSTEMS

A list of patients with infection admitted to the ward or acquired in the ward is useful in the investigation of spread of infection. The infections which are most usefully recorded are those due to shigellae, rotavirus and other gastrointestinal pathogens, MRSA, group A streptococci, respiratory syncytial virus (RSV) and the common infectious diseases (particularly chicken-pox).

MATERNITY DEPARTMENTS

Richard George

As in paediatric departments, screening of staff of both sexes for immunity to rubella is recommended, with immunization of non-immune individuals.

RISKS OF INFECTION

In the maternity department there are three types of patients for whom there are special risks of infection. First, the antenatal patient is at particular risk only if the fetal membranes have ruptured, allowing access of organisms to the fetus and liquor amnii, an exception being exposure of non-immune patients to chicken-pox or B19 virus. Second, the postnatal patient has a large endometrial surface with thrombosed blood vessels which is vulnerable to invasion by many organisms. Wound infection may follow a Caesarean section. Third, there are the problems of the neonate, who has very little natural immunity to infection, having come from a sterile environment, and who is now encountering bacteria for the first time. Premature or damaged babies are particularly vulnerable to infection. The increased survival of low-birth-weight babies has been associated with additional problems of infection.

Almost any organism may give rise to dangerous disease in maternity departments, even those (e.g. coliforms, enterococci, group B streptococci, coagulase-negative staphylococci or bacteroides) which are often of low pathogenicity. *Streptococcus pyogenes* and *Clostridium perfringens* are particularly dangerous. The infant may be infected by organisms derived from the mother either *in utero* (e.g. cytomegalovirus, HBV, HIV, listeria, rubella, syphilis, toxoplasma, tuberculosis, VZ virus) or during delivery (e.g. chlamydial eye infections, gonococcal ophthalmia, salmonellosis), and may be highly infectious. Mothers known to be HBV or HIV carriers may from time to time be admitted for delivery, in which case special precautions are required (see Chapter 10). Colonization of the child with bacteria starts shortly after birth. The intestinal tract and often the throat are colonized by antibiotic-sensitive coliforms which may be rapidly replaced by resistant strains if the baby is treated with antibiotics. In susceptible infants, these may cause respiratory tract infection, meningitis and septicaemia. Within a few days of delivery, *Staphylococcus aureus* may be found, particularly in the flexures and on moist areas of skin (e.g. axillae, groin and napkin area) and on the umbilical stump. *Staphylococcus aureus* is found in the throat or nose of many newborn infants after a few days. The carriage of these organisms is usually inconsequential, but may be associated with minor skin pustules or eye infections. Severe forms of skin infection, such as bullous impetigo or staphylococcal 'scalded skin syndrome' (epidermolysis bullosa) sometimes occur when strains of staphylococcus, which produce exfoliation, spread within the hospital. Invasive disease, including septicaemia, osteomyelitis and pneumonia, sometimes occurs. Breast abscess may occur in the mother, sometimes weeks after she has been discharged. *Candida albicans* is also common, causing oral and skin infection, and can produce invasive disease in weaker babies.

The infant must be protected as far as is possible from acquiring a heavy load of pathogenic organisms, for in addition to the risk that it will develop an infection, it will in its turn disseminate these organisms into the environment. Poor standards of hygiene may be followed by heavy contamination. However, good hygiene lowers the risk. Infants are liable to get sticky eyes within a few days of birth. A variety of organisms may be isolated from these, and it seems likely that conjunctivitis is often of chemical origin, caused by the antiseptics used during labour. Gonococci, chlamydia, Group B streptococci, staphylococci, coliforms and other organisms should be excluded. Napkin rash is due to the action of bacteria (mainly coliforms) which produce ammonia and other substances which damage the wet skin. Spread of infection after delivery is mainly by contact, usually on attendants' hands, with some additional spread of Gram-negative bacilli by way of apparatus or disinfectants and, less commonly, of staphylococci in the air.

PREVENTION OF SPREAD

Isolation facilities are necessary for both mothers and babies. Maternal diseases that require isolation include puerperal sepsis, which may be due to *Streptococcus pyogenes* (Group A β-haemolytic streptococcus), gastrointestinal infections, breast abscesses and staphylococcal skin sepsis. Infected neonates should also be placed in isolation as soon as an infection is suspected. It may be necessary to separate infants from their mothers if the latter are infected, particularly in cases of maternal typhoid or shigella infections. Infant nurseries should be small, should preferably contain not more than four beds, and should be equipped with hand-washing basins. Overcrowding and staff shortages may be associated with cross-infection in the nursery. Cross-infection may also be reduced by rooming in (i.e. keeping the baby in the mother's room). If there are insufficient numbers of small rooms, cohort nursing is a particularly useful routine measure for prevention of infection or for ending an outbreak. Babies born over a period of 24 to 48 hours are kept in one nursery, and when all of these babies are discharged from hospital, the room is cleaned if necessary and another batch of babies is admitted. A nursery should be designed to allow cohort nursing in the event of an outbreak.

Babies born with gastroenteritis should be isolated immediately. If an infection is severe, or more than two cases occur, the ward should be closed to further admissions. The other infants should be screened and all carriers kept in one nursery. If possible, separate nurses should attend babies in the infected and non-infected nurseries. Nurses preparing feeds should not handle infected babies or their contacts.

As the main method of spread of infection is via attendants' hands, these require special care. Hands should be washed after any procedure involving handling of a baby or its immediate environment. Washing with soap and water is usually adequate, but an antiseptic preparation should be used for handwashing by staff in premature baby units and in outbreaks of infection. Povidone-iodine or chlorhex-idine-detergent preparations are equally suitable, but use of an alcoholic handrub (see Chapter 6) is as or more effective, and more convenient. In overcrowded nurs-eries and during outbreaks of staphylococcal infection, dusting the axillae, groin and umbilicus with hexachlorophane powder until discharge from hospital, but for no longer than 7 days, is a safe and effective method of reducing staphylococcal colonization (Allen *et al.*, 1994). Chlorhexidine bathing is also effective, and may be introduced during outbreaks of infection (see p. 186). Baths should be thor-oughly cleaned and disinfected between patients (see Chapter 6). Masks are unnecessary in nurseries. Gowns or aprons should be worn and changed regularly, but not necessarily after attending each baby. Separate gowns or aprons should be worn for handling babies in special-care units, but are not necessary if the baby is not removed from the incubator. Specific procedures that require standardization include napkin-changing and disposal, bottle-feeding, tube-feeding and bathing. Napkins should be disposed of into a bucket lined with a plastic bag which is sealed when full. Alginate or hot-water-soluble bags may also be used. The use of disposable napkins should be considered during outbreaks of infections, but are standard issue in most hospitals in developed countries. Separate sterile catheters should be used for each tube feed and discarded after use. If not disposable, catheters should be processed in the sterile services department (SSD) and auto-claved. If it is necessary to leave the tube *in situ* for feeding (e.g. nasal catheters), its use should be limited to essential times only.

Although the administration of antibiotics may be necessary as soon as infection of a neonate is suspected, the widespread use of chemoprophylaxis is not recom-mended. The use of antibiotics selects resistant strains of bacteria, including *Klebsiella* and *Enterobacter* species, *Pseudomonas aeruginosa* and *Serratia marcescens*. The prevalence of resistant bacteria (e.g. gentamicin-resistant organisms in nurseries) should be determined from time to time as a guide to the choice of antibiotics for treating undiagnosed infections arising in the unit.

The SSD can provide much of the equipment needed in maternity departments. Delivery packs, episiotomy sets, dressings and sterile sanitary pads are routine supplies in most hospitals. In addition, as far as possible the SSD should sterilize equipment for preparing special feeds on the wards, and the containers and teats and tube-feeding equipment for neonates. Cleaning and disinfection of incubators and suction equipment are also best performed in the SSD if it is conveniently near. If incubators must be processed in the maternity department, space must be set aside for this purpose and procedures similar to those used in the SSD (see Chapter 6) followed.

Disinfection of teats and bottles on wards should be avoided. (Milk kitchens and infant feeds are discussed below.)

The hazard of a major outbreak is much increased if one milk kitchen supplies feeds for all babies in a large unit.

The risks of infection spreading from workers in the unit to the patients are similar to those in other wards, but two special infections, namely herpes (facial lesions or herpetic whitlow of the fingers) and candida paronychia, are readily spread to neonates. Attendants with these lesions should therefore be excluded while they are infected.

Colonization of the genital tract with group B streptococci occurs in up to 40% of pregnant women. Many are carriers early in pregnancy, whilst others only become colonized immediately preterm, making screening logistically difficult. Antibiotics make little difference to the spontaneous loss of the carrier state. Not all babies become colonized from their mother, and less than 1% of these develop overt infection. For these reasons, we do not recommend routine screening. Group B streptococcal infection must be borne in mind in any sick neonate, particularly the low-birth-weight or premature infant, and in those with respiratory distress.

Some maternity units require nose and throat swabs from new members of staff before starting work, to exclude carriers of pathogenic staphylococci and strepto-cocci, but most units have abandoned these procedures without ill effect. However, the resurgence of MRSA may warrant selective screening of staff before employment in neonatal units. Other routine screening systems have been suggested, including that of mothers for carriage of *Salmonella* or *Shigella* species before admission to the unit. These suggestions followed the occurrence of several outbreaks of gastroenteritis in maternity departments, but are impractical as a routine procedure. *Salmonella* species may not be detected even if they are present. The organisms may be acquired after the faeces have been examined, and some infected patients are unbooked. Furthermore, most laboratories could not offer such a service without reducing their more essential services, and it is costly. However, if there is reason to suspect that a patient has a gastrointestinal infection or is a *Salmonella* or *Shigella* carrier, faeces must be examined and the patient must immediately be isolated. After delivery of a patient with enteric fever, careful follow-up of other patients in the unit is necessary.

Surveillance of infections is particularly important in neonatal units (staphylococcal infections, those due to Enterobacteriecae and other Gram-negative bacteria), so that immediate action may be taken to prevent extension of an outbreak.

MANAGEMENT OF DELIVERY OF MOTHERS WHO ARE CARRIERS OF HBV OR HIV

The recommended precautions are described in Chapter 10 (see also Working Party of the Royal College of Obstetricians and Gynaecologists, 1997).

PREPARATION OF INFANT FEEDS AND USE OF MILK KITCHENS

Milk is an excellent growth medium for most pathogenic or potentially pathogenic bacteria, and contamination of feeds is a particular hazard in neonatal nurseries. Although there is little published evidence that contaminated feeds have caused outbreaks of infection, it seems likely that such outbreaks have occurred more commonly than is reported. Many organisms, sometimes in large numbers, have been isolated from feeds (e.g. *Salmonella* species, enteropathogenic and other strains of *E.coli*, group A and other groups of β-haemolytic streptococci, *Candida albicans, Proteus* species, *Klebsiella* and *Pseudomonas* species, *Staphylococcus aureus* and many other organisms.

All feeds must be free from intestinal pathogens. The greatest risk is from these organisms, but other bacteria (e.g. *Proteus* and *Klebsiella* species), may cause infection if they are abundant.

Contamination of feed can occur due to faulty disinfection of bottles, teats, and dispensing and mixing equipment. Milk, water or other additives may be contaminated prior to use. Recontamination or additional contamination can occur at any time during the preparation process or when feeding the baby. This may be from the air, from the hands of preparation room or ward staff, or from the mother.

Usually the level of initial contamination of the feed is low, and the main hazard is storage at room temperature for a sufficient time to allow organisms to grow. An additional risk is caused by warming the feed in a contaminated sink or container immediately before administration. Newborn infants will usually accept a feed at room temperature and, if possible, warming before use should be avoided. If the feed is warmed, a special container should be used and kept for this purpose only. The container should be filled with boiled water, or with fresh water and boiled for

5 min. The bottle with intact teat cover should be placed in the container at body temperature, and the water level should be well below the neck of the bottle. After use the container should be immediately emptied, cleaned and dried.

PREFERRED METHODS

Commercially supplied pre-sterilized or, if locally produced, terminally sterilized or heat-disinfected feeds should be used in all maternity units. The choice between these two methods must be made on the basis of effectiveness, economy, availability of staff and space. When feeds are locally produced and sterilized or disinfected by heat, controls to ensure exposure of the feed for the required time at the correct temperature are necessary. Charts showing this information should be regularly inspected by the head of the department. Disinfection by heat, including pasteurization in a specially designed machine, is satisfactory if the processes are adequate. In these instances, bacteriological tests should also be performed at intervals (e.g. monthly). Commercially prepared presterilized feeds should be bacteriologically safe, provided that their control and testing process is satisfactory. Bottles and caps should be inspected before use for obvious damage, and if any doubt exists the bottle should be discarded. Commercially supplied presterilized feeds with the teat already attached to the bottle and adequately protected from contamination are preferable. Single-use teats packed separately are almost as satisfactory, if put on (preferably by the mother) immediately before giving the feed. If teats are used repeatedly, they should be thoroughly cleaned and autoclaved after each use.

OTHER METHODS

Chemical disinfection of bottles and teats (by hypochlorite) is only reliable if correctly performed, is more difficult to control than those methods already described, and is more susceptible to individual staff errors. The hypochlorite method of disinfection is only suitable for use in developing countries and at home. The risk of infection in well-controlled units using chemical methods is not very great provided that dispensing equipment involves taps which are taken apart and autoclaved after each use, and if disinfection is well supervised. Bottles and teats should be thoroughly cleaned before disinfection or sterilization by any method, but particularly prior to chemical disinfection. The disinfectant solution should be made up to the correct strength (hypochlorite – 125 ppm available chlorine). All equipment should be completely immersed, with removal of air bubbles, and should be left for at least the recommended time. Autoclaving of bottles and teats is preferable to chemical disinfection because of the greater reliability of the process. Boiling, correctly performed, should also be more reliable than a chemical method, but the boiling of bottles and teats in an open container is difficult to control and is not recommended.

PAEDIATRIC FEEDS

The recommendations are similar to those for maternity units. Commercially prepared feeds are often not suitable, as a number of babies may require special feeds. Arrangements for terminal sterilization, or autoclaving of bottles and teats, are still necessary in these units.

MILK KITCHEN AND STAFF (Burnett et al., 1989)

For hospitals where commercially prepared presterilized feeds are used, a clean store-room is all that is required. In units where feeds are prepared on site, a kitchen which is used only for preparation of feeds is required. In all milk kitchens, washing up of used bottles, teats and other equipment should be done in a room separate from that used for preparing feeds. A handwashing basin should be available immediately adjacent to the milk kitchen. Staff should be trained in techniques of feed preparation, and in personal hygiene. This training should include methods of preventing contamination (e.g. thorough cleaning of equipment, and the reduction of airborne and contact transfer by hands to a minimum). If possible, the preparation of feeds should be carried out by staff who are not handling babies, and should be supervised by a senior member of the nursing staff. After preparation, feeds (unless sterilized) should be placed in a refrigerator (at 4°C) preferably within 30 min and not after more than 60 min.

Non-sterile feeds should be discarded after 24 hours. Supplements should be added to the feed immediately before use.

HUMAN EXPRESSED BREAST MILK

Human milk contains antimicrobial factors which are believed to give premature infants some protection against infection. Some of these factors are heat-labile, although the inactivating effect of pasteurization on the antimicrobial factors at relatively low temperatures such as 63–65°C (145–149°F) is greatly reduced. Inadequately collected or stored milk may be heavily contaminated with potential pathogens such as *Klebsiella* species, *Pseudomonas aeruginosa* and *Staphylococcus aureus*. Milk from the mother fed to her own baby may be used unpasteurized but must be stored refrigerated. The Human Milk Banking Association of North America (1993a,b) Guidelines state that routine microbiological testing for administration to a mother's own infant is unnecessary, but they recommend freezing if it is not used within 48 hours.

To ensure milk of an acceptable microbiological standard, careful attention must be paid to hygienic methods of collection. These high standards are more easily achieved in hospital than in the home. Potential donors should have blood tests to exclude syphilis, HBV, HCV, and HIV infection, should not be excreting drugs in the milk, and should be able to produce sufficient milk to make collection worthwhile. They should be trained in aseptic practices and supplied with suitable equipment for disinfection. The home conditions should be hygienically acceptable. In addition, several samples should be tested microbiologically before the donor is accepted. Instructions on collection and storage should be clear and precise, and should include hand washing, care of the breast, and methods of cleaning, disinfection and storage of the pump. Whenever possible, sterilized equipment should be supplied. The first 5 mL of milk should be discarded and the remainder transferred to a sterile bottle which is labelled with the time of collection, the storage time and the temperature. It must be placed in a refrigerator as soon as possible at 4°C (39°F) and the temperature during transport should not be allowed to rise above 10°C (50°F). The time out of the refrigerator should not exceed 2 hours, and refrigerated transport or insulated containers may be required for transport.

Although samples are collected from infection-screened mothers, pasteurization is still advisable, but excessive heating should be avoided. Exposure at 63°C (149°F) and not less than 57°C for 30 min is recommended (Royal College of Paediatricians and Child Health Working Party, 1999). The process must be carefully controlled and temperatures checked with a thermometer initially and at regular intervals afterwards. Any bacterial growth is unacceptable. A standard volume of milk should be treated, and should be cooled rapidly. As well as temperature checks, microbiological tests should be made on setting up the process and at regular intervals afterwards. Milk should be deep-frozen (–9 to –18°C); 18°F) as quickly as possible after collection, and repeated thawing and freezing should be avoided.

MICROBIOLOGICAL STANDARDS

Some centres still feed raw 'donor' milk to infants, in which case microbiological tests of each sample are essential. As the numbers of organisms required to infect the infant – as well as the role of relatively non-pathogenic organisms – remain uncertain, suggested standards differ. The resistance of the recipient infant to infection is also variable, and the possible deleterious effect of pasteurization is uncertain. It is generally agreed that Gram-negative bacilli should be absent. Some authorities accept the presence of normal flora in raw milk up to 10^7/mL (Carroll *et al.*, 1979), whilst others have suggested total counts less than 10^3/mL (Williamson *et al.*, 1978) or 10^4/mL (Human Milk Banking Association of North America, 1993a, b).

We support the following standards.

1. Total counts of normal skin flora (coagulase-negative, staphylococci, diphtheroids or *Streptococcus viridans* should not exceed 10^5 colony-forming units (CFU)/mL (Royal College of Paediatricians and Child Health Working Party, 1999);
2. Enterobacteriaceae, pseudomonas, other Gram-negative bacilli, groupable streptococci, *Staphylococcus aureus* and other potential pathogens should be absent. Although there is no evidence of infection occurring from milk that complies with these standards, we believe that it is safer to pasteurize all donor breast milk before use.

UROLOGICAL UNITS

Urinary tract infection is the commonest type of acquired infection in hospitals. Many patients already have a urinary infection when they enter the unit, but instrumentation and operations on the urinary tract can lead to infection, either by introducing organisms into a previously uninfected tract, or by replacing the existing organisms with hospital strains which are more resistant to antibiotic therapy (Slade and Gillespie, 1985).

Although some patients acquire urinary tract infections without having had instrumentation, most infections follow catheterization, cystoscopy, drainage or more extensive operative procedures. In particular, the indwelling catheter can be hazardous and, if precautions are not taken to prevent contamination, the incidence of bladder infections in patients on continuous drainage approaches 100%, often in less than 1 week.

ROUTES OF CONTAMINATION AND CROSS-INFECTION

The entry of bacteria into the bladder may occur either through the lumen of the catheter or between the catheter and the wall of the urethra. Both routes are important, and every effort is needed to close both (Falkiner, 1993).

The organisms most likely to be found in urological patients with urinary tract infection vary. If there has not been any manipulation of the urinary tract, the organisms are usually *E.coli* or *Proteus mirabilis*, which are sensitive to many common antibiotics (e.g. sulphonamides, trimethoprim, ampicillin and nitrofurantoin). In hospital-acquired infections, *Klebsiella* species, indole-positive *Proteus* species, *Pseudomonas aeruginosa* and enterococci are more common. Less frequent are *Acinetobacter* species and *Providencia* species. These organisms are usually resistant to many antibiotics and may prove difficult to eradicate. They are likely to spread to other patients. The emergence of strains resistant to gentamicin, third-generation cephalosporins and quinolones is particularly worrying, as they limit the available treatment in a unit. These organisms are commonly associated with indwelling catheterization, and the mode of spread is thought to be mainly via the hands of staff. The management of catheterized patients is discussed in Chapter 7. However, some attention should be given to the environment (e.g. disinfection of bedpans and urinals by heat (not a tank of disinfectant), correct drying and stacking of wash-bowls, disinfection by heat or use of disposable containers for emptying urine bags and urine testing equipment, and adequate disinfection of baths, etc.).

Urine from patients with renal tuberculosis should be disposed of with care. The bottle used for collecting the urine must be disinfected, and the patient should have his or her own urine bottle. Collection of specimens for laboratory examination should be directly into a sterile universal container. The use of the urine bottle as an intermediary container often gives false-positive results because of failure to decontaminate the bottle between patients. Routine microbiological monitoring of the environment is not recommended. However, surveys of the microbial flora in the environment may be justified if there is evidence of cross-infection. Single-room isolation is not usually recommended for Gram-negative infections unless they are due to a multiresistant strain (Fryklund *et al.*, 1997). Restriction of certain antibiotics may also be desirable if multiresistant strains are frequently isolated.

REFERENCES

Allen, K.D., Ridgway, E.J. and Parsons, L.A. (1994) Hexachlorophane powder and neonatal infection. *Journal of Hospital Infection* 27, 29.

Ayliffe, G.A.J. and Lawrence, J.C. (eds) (1985) Symposium on Infection control in burns. *Journal of Hospital Infection*, 6 (Supplement B), 3.

Ayliffe, G.A.J., Collins, B.J., Lowbury, E.T.L. *et al.* (1967) Ward floors and other surfaces as reservoirs of hospital infection. *Journal of Hygiene* 65, 515.

Bradley, C.R. and Fraise, A.P. (1996) Heat and chemical resistance of enterococci. *Journal of Hospital Infection* 34, 191.

Burnett, I.A., Wardley, B.L. and Magee, J.T. (1989) The milk kitchen at Sheffield Children's Hospital before and after a review. *Journal of Hospital Infection* 13, 179.

Carroll, L., Osman, M., Davies, D.P. and McNeish, A.S. (1979) Bacteriological criteria for feeding raw milk to babies on neonatal units. *Lancet* ii, 732.

Craven, D.E. and Steger, K.A. (1989) Nosocomial pneumonia in the intubated patient. In Weber, D.J. and Rutala, W.A. (eds), Nosocomial infections: new issues and strategies for prevention. *Infectious Disease Clinics of North America*. Philadelphia, PA: W.B. Saunders, 843.

Crossley, K., Landesman, B. and Zaske, D. (1979) An outbreak of infection caused by epidemic strains resistant to methicillin and caminoglycosides. Two epidemiologic slides. *Journal of Infectious Diseases* 139, 280.

Department of Health and Social Security (1975) *Preservation of sterility in ophthalmic preparations in hospitals*. Health Service Circular. London: HMSO.

Falkiner, F.R. (1993) The insertion and management of indwelling catheters – minimizing the risk of infection. *Journal of Hospital Infection* 25, 79.

Fryklund, B., Haeggman, S. and Burman, L.G. (1997) Transmission of urinary bacterial strains between patients with indwelling catheters – nursing in the same room and in separate rooms compared. *Journal of Hospital Infection* 36, 147.

Gantz, N.M. and Godofsky, E.W. (1996) Nosocomial central nervous system infections. In Mayhall, C.G. (ed.), *Hospital epidemiology and infection control*. Baltimore, MD: Williams & Wilkins, 246.

Gould, F.H. and Freeman, R. (1993) Nosocomial infection with microsphere beads. *Lancet* 342, 241.

Human Milk Banking Association of North America (1993a) *Guidelines for the establishment and operation of a Donor Human Milk Bank*. Hartford, CT: HMBA North America.

Human Milk Banking Association of North America (1993b) *Recommendations for collection, storage and handling of a mother's milk for her own infant in the hospital setting*. Hartford, CT: HMBA North America.

Lowbury, E.J.L. (1976) Prophylaxis and treatment for infection of burns. *British Journal of Hospital Medicine* 16, 566.

Lowbury, E.J.L. (1992) Special problems in hospital antisepsis. In Russell, A.D., Hugo, W.B. and Ayliffe, G.A.J. *Principles and practice of disinfection, preservation and sterilization*, 2nd edn. Oxford: Blackwell Scientific Publications, 310.

Medical Devices Agency (1995) *The reuse of medical devices supplied for single use only.* London: Department of Health.

Medical Devices Agency (1996) *The purchase, operation and maintenance of benchtop sterilizers.* London: Department of Health.

Medical Devices Agency (1998) *The validation and periodic testing of benchtop vacuum steam sterilizers.* London: Department of Health.

Ophthalmic Society of the United Kingdom (1973) The sterilization of surgical instruments. *Transactions of the Ophthalmic Society of the UK* 92, 539.

Newsom, S.W.B. (1998) Special problems in hospital antisepsis. In Russell, A.D., Hugo, W.B. and Ayliffe, G.A.J. *Principles and practice of disinfection, preservation and sterilization.* 3rd edn Oxford: Blackwell Science, 416.

Nguyen, T.T., Gilpin, D.A., Meyer, N.A. *et al.* (1996) Current treatment of severely burned patients. *Annals of Surgery* 223, 14.

Papini, R.P.G., Wilson, A.P.R., Steer, J.A. *et al.* (1995) Wound management in burn centres in the UK. *British Journal of Surgery* 82, 505.

Royal College of Paediatricians and Child Health Working Party (1999) *Guidelines for the establishment of human milk banks in the UK.* London: Royal College of Paediatrics and Child Health.

Settle, J. (1985) Infection in burns. *Journal of Hospital Infection*, 6 **(Supplement B),** 19.

Slade, N. and Gillespie, W.A. (1985) *The urinary tract and the catheter: infection and other problems.* Chichester: John Wiley & Sons.

Traore, O., Eschapasse, D. and Laveran, H. (1997) A bacteriological study of a contamination control tacky mat. *Journal of Hospital Infection* 36, 158.

van Saene, H.K.F., Stoutenbeek, L.P. and Hart, CA. (1991) Selective decontamination of the digestive tract (SSD) in intensive care patients: a critical evaluation of the clinical bacteriological and epidemiological benefits. *Journal of Hospital Infection* 18, 261.

Williamson, S., Hewitt, J.H. and Finucane, E. (1978) Organisation of a bank of raw and pasteurised human milk for neonatal intensive care. *British Medical Journal* 1, 393.

Working Party of the British Burn Association and Hospital Infection Research Society (1991) Principles of design of burns unit; report of a working party of the British Burn Association and Hospital Infection Research Society. *Journal of Hospital Infection* 19, 63.

Working Party of the Royal College of Obstetricians and Gynaecologists (1997) *HIV infection in maternity care and gynaecology.* London: Royal College of Obstetricians and Gynaecologists Press.

chapter 17

SPECIAL WARDS AND DEPARTMENTS. II

OUT-PATIENTS AND ACCIDENT AND EMERGENCY DEPARTMENTS

As many of the patients who attend out-patient departments have recently been in hospital wards, their wounds and other lesions may be infected with antibiotic-resistant Gram-negative bacilli and *Staphylococcus aureus* (e.g. MRSA) which they acquired in hospital. Patients with skin diseases may have been treated with a variety of antibiotics, and are also likely to be carrying antibiotic-resistant strains. The risk of cross-infection with Gram-negative bacilli and *Staphylococcus aureus* in out-patient or casualty departments is less than that in wards but, owing to the large number of patients attending out-patient departments, there is a high risk of spread of community-acquired infections (e.g. measles, influenza, etc.). The consequences could be severe if a case of undiagnosed Lassa fever is brought into the department, and staff must inform the microbiologist, CCDC or infectious disease physician if such an infection is suspected.

Many patients are also particularly susceptible to infection (e.g. those with immunodeficiency diseases), and they may come into close contact with infected patients. The range of surgical procedures performed in out-patient theatres is increasing, and clean operations may alternate with incisions of abscesses. Diagnostic procedures (e.g. endoscopy) are also now more frequently performed in out-patient departments, and it is important that infection control procedures are followed appropriately.

PREVENTION OF INFECTION

Surgical procedures should, when possible, be performed in a mechanically ventilated operating-theatre, and aseptic and cleaning techniques should correspond to those used in the main operating-theatres (see Chapter 10). These recommendations are particularly applicable to the types of operation which previously required admission to hospital for several days, although the wearing of masks and caps is not essential for incision of abscesses. The risk of airborne spread of infection after drainage of abscesses to patients subsequently undergoing operations in the same operating room is not great, especially if the theatre is mechanically ventilated, but precautions against contact spread, (e.g. adequate cleaning of operating tables) are necessary. The general principles of prevention of infection are similar to those which apply in other areas in the hospital, and a few reliable techniques will reduce the risk to a minimum. Accident departments may be associated with considerable blood spillage from injured individuals. Wearing of gloves and a plastic apron for handling wounds is advised. Facilities for minor surgery and for dressing wounds should be adequate, with rooms for laying up of trolleys and disposal of contaminated dressings and linen.

Sufficient handwashing basins and disposable paper towels should be provided for the staff. Handwashing by the staff between handling patients and before and after procedures is one of the most important measures. Wearing of a gown or plastic apron when handling infected patients, and covering of couches with paper or a cleanable plastic material when examining potentially infected patients are also useful measures. Linen should be changed after use on an infected patient, and at least daily. Gowns for patients to wear during examination should preferably be disposable, but owing to expense and as the risk of transfer of infection is usually not great, it may be necessary to use gowns for a whole morning or afternoon session. A separate gown should be provided for patients with infections or with a skin disease in which heavy skin colonization by potential pathogens is likely. Some segregation of patients is also advisable. In particular, hypersusceptible patients should not be mixed with those who are likely to be infected (e.g. chronic bronchitis cases with leukaemics, or dermatological cases with surgical cases). A separate clinic for patients with varicose ulcers may also be advisable.

Facilities should be provided for examination of patients with communicable diseases. A room which can be adequately decontaminated is required for isolation of cases of suspected viral haemorrhagic fever and other dangerous or highly transmissible infections, and a routine for management of these cases must be available (see Chapter 9). Plentiful supplies of specula and other instruments (either disposable or provided by the SSD) should be available in the departments. If disposable equipment is not available, such equipment should be sterilized in a small benchtop autoclave. Disinfection by chemicals or by boiling should be avoided if possible. Although disinfection by immersion of a clean instrument in 70% alcohol, with or without 0.5% chlorhexidine for 10 min (not for vaginal specula), or by boiling in water for 5 min, is effective (against vegetative organisms and most viruses), it should rarely be necessary to do without proper sterilization. Non-disposable instruments and needles should be stored in a dry state and not in chemical disinfectants. They should be disinfected by heat immediately before use or, if possible, sterilized in the SSD and supplied in packs. A routine for disinfection of endoscopes and other instruments which are heat-labile and of emergency equipment should be known and always followed in the department (see Chapter 6). The use of 2% glutaraldehyde should be avoided if possible, except for disinfection of endoscopes. If used, adequate safety precautions are required (p. 84).

RADIOLOGY AND RADIOTHERAPY DEPARTMENTS

RADIOGRAPHY

Patients are brought to this department from all parts of the hospital and from the community. Patients arriving from different wards may be responsible for the spread of infection between wards. The radiographers also visit patients in the wards and may transmit infection on their hands or clothing, or on equipment. The principles of control are similar to those which apply in other areas of the hospital. The staff should be informed of any patient with communicable disease sent to their department, or if an X-ray is required on such a patient in the ward. Radiological procedures involving the gastrointestinal tract require precautions, particularly for *Clostridium difficile* infection or colonization, which can spread by contact to other patients in the radiography department as well as in wards. Respiratory tuberculosis may also require special precautions (see Chapter 8). In the ward, the radiographers should follow the recommended barrier-nursing routine, paying particular attention to handwashing and gowning techniques. Similar procedures may be necessary if the patient is brought to their department, and it may be necessary to cover the X-ray table with disposable paper, or to disinfect it after use. X-ray equipment is not an important source of infection, and routine cleaning with a detergent, then allowing it to dry, will usually be sufficient. Cleaning the equipment between patients is not necessary except if a patient is known to be infected. Disinfection by wiping with 70% alcohol is quick and fairly effective, and it may be necessary after X-raying an infected patient, or if the equipment is taken into the operating-theatre. Wiping with other disinfectant solutions is rarely necessary. (For cleaning of the environment, see Chapter 7.)

Many procedures involving aseptic techniques are now performed in the X-ray department, and facilities should be adequate, including a handwashing basin. The room used for such procedures should be well ventilated and unnecessary equipment should be excluded. It should, if possible, be reserved for procedures involving aseptic techniques. As few people as possible should be in the room during the procedure, particularly if a catheter remains *in situ*. Good surgical techniques are as necessary for these procedures as they are in operating-theatres. Instruments and dressings should be supplied by the SSD. The use of patients' gowns is described in the section on out-patient departments.

RADIOTHERAPY

Patients treated in this department may be particularly susceptible to infection, (e.g. immunosuppressed patients, or those with low natural immunity). If in general wards, these patients, depending on their degree of immunosuppression, should be nursed in single-bed cubicles with protective isolation precautions (see Chapter 8). Special skills are often necessary when nursing these patients, and suitably trained staff should be available. Other patients may be sources of infection. Isolation of these patients and techniques to prevent contact infection (e.g. handwashing and wearing of plastic gowns) are necessary. The protection of examination couches and provision of patients' gowns are discussed above (see section on out-patient and casualty departments). The equipment used is often difficult to sterilize or disinfect. Whenever possible it should be autoclaved and supplied in packs by the SSD. If the equipment is heat-labile, ethylene oxide or low-temperature steam and formaldehyde treatment in the SSD is preferable to chemical solutions.

Immersion in 70% alcohol (with or without 0.5% chlorhexidine) for 5–10 min will be appropriate for most other purposes, but great care is necessary when drying after immersion in alcohol if the equipment is likely to contact mucous membranes or the conjunctiva (see Chapter 6). For rapid disinfection of surfaces of larger items of equipment, wiping with 70% alcohol is satisfactory, and is preferable to the use of aqueous disinfectants.

It is essential that radiotherapy staff are trained in aseptic techniques and control of infection, and that the system for warning the radiological department of infection hazards is effective. This applies particularly to patients with or at high risk of bloodborne infection, in order to ensure that appropriate precautions are taken.

PHYSIOTHERAPY DEPARTMENTS

Physiotherapists treat many ill or infected patients and move from one patient to another and from ward to ward. Infected wounds are exposed during certain treatments. Patients are also handled, and the opportunities for contact transfer of infection are therefore high. Patients attend the physiotherapy department from all parts of the hospital and also from the community. Infection from patients with wounds or skin lesions may readily be transferred on couches, equipment, other fomites and on the hands of the staff. Treatment with wax or water baths and in hydrotherapy units may aid the spread of infection. Fungal infection of the feet may be spread in the gymnasium, particularly if patients exercise with bare feet or wear communal shoes.

PREVENTION OF INFECTION

The physiotherapy department should be informed of patients known to have a communicable disease or hospital infection which could spread to other patients, and appropriate precautions should be taken. Open pulmonary tuberculosis requires particular care. Meticulous care in handwashing before and after handling any patient, and wearing a plastic apron when treating an infected patient, are both important. This applies both to wards and to the physiotherapy department. Infected wounds should be effectively sealed whenever possible with an impermeable dressing during treatment, and contaminated dressings should only be handled with forceps or plastic gloves. The department should have adequate facilities for dressing wounds and lesions, a comprehensive SSD supply and an effective disposal system for contaminated linen and dressings. Recommended aseptic dressing techniques should be used. Other facilities are described in the sections on wards and out-patient departments but, in particular, treatment couches should be covered with paper or cleaned after each infected patient. Bedding should be changed after use by an infected patient and at least daily. Physiotherapists should also be aware of universal precautions and techniques for source and protective isolation.

The skin of the hands of patients undergoing paraffin wax treatment should be inspected, and any patients with an infected lesion should not be treated until the lesion has healed. If this is not possible, they should wear polythene gloves. Patients should wash their hands before and after treatment, and used wax should be heated to disinfect it before being returned to the wax bath.

THE HYDROTHERAPY UNIT

THE HYDROTHERAPY POOL

A variety of infections have been attributed to hydrotherapy and recreational pools. These include skin infections and otitis externa caused by *Pseudomonas aeruginosa*, and more recently legionella infection. Dermatophyte infections of the feet are acquired from the area surrounding the pool. Good hygienic standards are required, particularly in the pools used by hospital patients. A senior physiotherapist trained in hydrotherapy and pool management should be in charge and responsible for daily maintenance. A daily log should be kept of cleanliness, bathing load, pH and chlorine concentration and temperature. The physiotherapist should collaborate with the engineer and microbiologist to ensure that the correct conditions are maintained (Public Health Laboratory Service, 1990; Penny, 1991; Dadswell, 1999). If any health problems occur they should be reported immediately to the infection control team or occupational health physician. Clean footwear should be worn in the pool area.

The following are some of the important measures required.

1 Patients should be adequately prepared (e.g. by emptying of bladder, ensuring safe bladder drainage, and bowel evacuation of incontinent patients before entering the pool).
2 Patients' feet and skin should be inspected for infected lesions.
3 Patients should take showers both before entering the water and after leaving it.
4 Everyone entering the water must step through a footbath containing a hypochlorite or a iodophor solution. Use of a mycostatic powder after bathing might be of some value.
5 Patients should use the same swimsuit for the duration of their course of treatment, and the suit should be laundered after each attendance.
6 The water is continually circulating and is tested daily for adequacy of chlorination. Residual chlorine levels should be maintained at 1.5–3.00 mg/L (ppm). Periodically, bacteriological tests of the water should be performed.
7 Contamination of the poolside with urine or faeces should be cleaned immediately with a solution containing 1000 ppm of free chlorine. 'Shock' chlorination of the pool (2 to 5-fold higher than normal levels) may be required after heavy faecal pollution.
8 Floors should be washed down each evening with pool water, and at least weekly with a solution containing 200 mg/L available chlorine.

THE GYMNASIUM

1 All patients should be inspected for skin infections, especially those of the feet (e.g. athlete's foot).

2 Patients should be issued with a pair of shorts which are kept by them for the course of treatment and sent to the hospital laundry on completion of treatment.
3 Staff should wear special training shoes which are kept only for the gymnasium.
4 Patients should preferably wear their own or disinfected gym shoes when entering the gymnasium.
5 The gymnasium, patient toilet and changing-room floors should be cleaned each evening.
6 Equipment should be washed at regular intervals.
7 Patients should be encouraged to take a shower after their classes, and should be supplied with towels.

TRAINING

Physiotherapists should be trained in aseptic methods and control of infection.

PHARMACEUTICAL DEPARTMENTS

The pharmaceutical department issues medicinal products, disinfectants and other related preparations to wards and departments and sometimes to other hospitals. It has an important responsibility for preventing hospital infection caused by the use of contaminated supplies of these products. In addition, the department has an important role in monitoring and implementing antibiotic and disinfectant policies in collaboration with the infection control team. A back-up service of drug information is also provided.

Sterile medicinal products for injection into blood or for instillation into tissues or viscera which are normally sterile must be provided. Although sterility is not essential for preparations which are ingested or applied to surfaces which have a normal microbial flora (e.g. skin, mouth, vagina), pathogens must be excluded and large numbers of any micro-organisms must be avoided in these products. Contamination may occur due to inadequate sterilization of preparations that are required to be sterile, or to the subsequent acquisition of micro-organisms by sterilized or aseptically prepared medicaments through inadequate storage or handling. Safeguards to prevent contamination by either of these channels are necessary. Aqueous solutions which may allow bacterial growth during storage represent a special hazard. Unlike human tissues, pharmaceutical preparations cannot protect themselves against small numbers of bacteria, so the degree of environmental cleanliness in areas where aseptic dispensing is performed must be very high. Areas where fluids are being prepared for sterilization do not demand such a high standard of environmental cleanliness as those used for aseptic preparation of medicaments which are not to be sterilized. Nevertheless, strict measures are currently in force as an insurance policy against unforeseen hazards.

STERILE PHARMACEUTICAL PRODUCTS

Sterile medicinal products and pharmaceutical preparations are produced in departments that have specialized facilities. Sterile production units should concentrate on non-commercially available preparations (e.g. sterile topical and irrigation solutions). Hospital pharmacies that produce sterile preparations are manufacturers in terms of the law, and therefore need to meet various legislative standards. They are expected by the Medicines Control Agency to attain similar standards to those in industry, and they require licensing. Where possible, licensed commercially available products should be used. Details of the requirements to produce sterile pharmaceuticals are set out in the *Guide to good manufacturing practice* (Anon, 1977), Anon. (1993) and also Underwood (1999). These guidelines provide information on personnel and training, documentation, work-flow systems, changing-rooms, clean room standards, preparation and filling rooms, sterilizing and product quarantine areas. Equipment should be designed, located and maintained to suit the processes and products. For example, autoclaves should have planned operational and maintenance programmes as recommended in HTM 2010 (Department of Health, 1994a).

Sterile pharmaceuticals are also prepared as a dispensing service for named patients. This service is available for injections, creams, powders and sterile products (e.g. for parenteral nutrition) required for treatment of patients without delay. Licensing is not required for this service. Isolators are now commonly used instead of laminar-flow cabinets for these procedures. Positive-pressure units are used for non-hazardous products, whereas negative-pressure units are used for cytotoxic drugs and radiochemicals. Guidelines are available on the operation of isolators (e.g. monitoring, room environments) (Department of Health, 1994b; Lee and Midcalf, 1994; NHS Quality Control Committee, 1995) (and 1998 appendix). The guidelines require routine microbiological monitoring which is not generally related to risks of infection to patients, and requires careful evaluation.

Pharmaceutical production now has quality control built into its procedures, so that the quality, safety and efficacy of the manufactured product is assured. Final product analysis and testing of samples for sterility completes the quality control procedure before the product is released for use in the hospital, although most aseptically produced products have short storage lives and/or are individualized for specific patients. Product testing is not usually required in these instances. However, sterility testing of samples must not be regarded as providing guarantees of sterility – nothing short of tests on the whole batch could provide that. It can, of course, provide evidence of gross or moderate contamination, but as bacteria can grow rapidly from very small numbers in many solutions, the value of sample testing, although cumulative, is uncertain, and the main emphasis in producing sterile pharmaceuticals must rely on other criteria.

Whenever possible, pharmaceutical preparations are supplied in unit-dose packs, to minimize bacterial contamination of the preparations. For example, eyedrops may be supplied in single-dose applicator packs, tablets in unit-dose strip packs, injections in single-dose glass containers, and oral mixtures in small-volume containers for use by a single patient. As pharmaceuticals are good media for bacterial growth, opened containers should be exposed for a minimal period of time. As a rough guide, injections should be administered at once and any residue discarded, oral mixtures may be kept for up to 10–14 days after opening, whilst tablets can be kept for a longer time period, if they are properly stored for an indefinite period, or until the activity of the drug diminishes or alters. A practicable storage time of 28 days for tablets has been suggested.

WORK OF THE PHARMACEUTICAL DEPARTMENT

The work in pharmaceutical departments is segregated into a number of specialized areas. Sterile products are manufactured in controlled production areas. Those terminally sterilized by heating in an autoclave are prepared in clean rooms, although this practice is now uncommon as commercial products are mainly used. Thermolabile preparations are produced in aseptic rooms which have a very high standard of cleanliness. The prepacking of tablets takes place in rooms provided with dust-extraction facilities to minimize contamination. Oral mixtures and ointments are prepared in manufacturing areas maintained to the requisite standards (Anon., 1977; Underwood, 1999).

It is of utmost importance that an efficient work-flow pattern should be achieved in manufacturing areas so that every product is subjected to the full quality assurance procedures before it is released from quarantine for administration to patients.

The work flow in the pharmacy should not permit intermingling of 'dirty' returned containers from wards with 'clean' supplies to be issued to the wards. Reuse of containers was an economical part of the pharmaceutical service, and such containers must be thoroughly washed and dried prior to recycling. However, reprocessing is now not considered to be cost-effective in many countries. Containers which are damaged or which cannot be satisfactorily cleaned and disinfected or sterilized are destroyed. Staff are provided with the appropriate clean clothes, suitable for the purpose, which are worn only in specific areas in the pharmacy department, and the staff must observe a high standard of personal hygiene.

STORAGE AND HANDLING

Pharmaceutical products require special conditions of storage and handling. Directions on storage (e.g. in a refrigerator or protected from light) should be noted and adhered to. Ampoules and vials should be kept in their outer containers or wrappings to protect them, as far as possible, from external contamination.

Parenteral solutions
Ampoules (or vials). The contents of the opened ampoule or vial must be withdrawn into a syringe immediately, and any surplus discarded, although this is now considered to be a potentially dangerous practice, and pre-filled syringes are used if possible. Ampoules of solution for intrathecal injections should be sterilized by autoclaving inside a sealed container. Some solutions are not thermostable, and these will not withstand this process, so before subjecting injections to this procedure the pharmacist's advice must be sought.

Multidose vials. The cap or diaphragm must be swabbed with an antiseptic solution that acts rapidly (e.g. ethyl alcohol (70%) or a spirit-impregnated swab –

available in sachets) of the type commonly used for preparing the skin before injection.

On no account should an injectable solution be transferred to a gallipot before it is drawn into a syringe. This increases the risk of contamination and also introduces the more dangerous risk of administering the wrong injection.

The contents of multidose containers do not keep indefinitely, and must be inspected routinely for opalescence before use. Such containers must not be held over for subsequent use after a clinic.

Rubber-capped vials of dry powder for preparing injections. The cap should be swabbed with an antiseptic solution (e.g. ethyl alcohol (70%) or a spirit-impregnated swab) before injecting the vehicle into the vial. Most of these are intended for single doses, but some may be used for several doses provided that the solution is stable enough to retain its potency, and that it is used within 24 hours of being reconstituted. The pharmacist will give advice on specific preparations.

Intravenous infusion solutions and emulsions (see Chapter 7).

Topical preparations

Many chlorhexidine or chlorhexidine/cetrimide ('Savlon') solutions are available in sterilized sachets (e.g. 'Savlodil' or 'Hibidil') for immediate use or for dilution immediately before use. Alternatively, antiseptic solutions may be issued in clean and disinfected bottles with preservatives if required (e.g. isopropanol 7% w/v). Such solutions need to be diluted as appropriate.

Bladder irrigation solutions

These should be isotonic and pyrogen-free. Commercially available solutions, usually in 1- or 3-L plastic containers, are now normally used, although solutions may be prepared in a hospital pharmacy if facilities are available. Preparations of BCG are sometimes used for bladder tumours. Preparation must take place in a safety cabinet to protect staff. It is also important that a separate cabinet or isolator is used for the preparation of intravenous cytotoxic chemotherapeutic agents.

Irrigation solutions for the eye, wounds and body cavities

These are sterile solutions diluted ready for use, and they should be used on one occasion only.

STERILE SERVICES DEPARTMENTS (SSD)

The function of the SSD is to supply a range of sterilized or disinfected items to operating-theatres, wards, other units and health-care establishments (e.g. community health centres). The manager, advised by the infection control team, is responsible for monitoring all decontamination processes, and for ensuring that all protocols for the handling and processing of equipment meet the required standards. Records must be kept of tests of efficacy of sterilizers and of all sterilization cycles and decontaminating processes. These records must be related to packs issued to users (Institute of Sterile Services Management, 1998a, b). The SSD is also responsible for the safe and effective processing of reusable medical equipment, preventing any risk of transfer of infection or other risk to patients or staff. The responsibility for reuse of expensive 'high-risk' single-use items (e.g. cardiac catheters) is ultimately that of the user, with advice on processing and packaging from the infection control team and the SSD manager. This practice for 'single-use' high-risk items is rarely endorsed by government agencies in developed countries. Reprocessing of low-risk single-use items is more often carried out if it is cost-effective and the process conforms to recommended protocols (e.g. Medical Devices Agency, 1995). As the hospital and processor as well as the user may also be legally responsible for the safety of reprocessing, it is advisable, particularly for single-use items, for decisions on whether an item is suitable for reprocessing and what is an appropriate protocol to be taken by a reprocessing committee (Working Party of the Central Sterilizing Club, 1999) (see also Chapter 2).

The SSD must develop good communications with the users (i.e. medical and nursing staff), and should remain a clinical service as well as an efficient distribution and cost-effective processing unit. The manager should be a member of relevant committees (e.g. theatre users, reprocessing of single-use items and control of infection).

Central supply services were developed in the USA, and the first purpose-built civilian central sterile supply department (CSSD) in the UK was opened in Belfast in 1958. Since then there have been many developments, including the addition of independent sections or units, such as a theatre sterile supply unit (TSSU) and a hospital sterilization and disinfection unit (HSDU). The latter unit processes items of medical equipment (e.g. respiratory ventilators, suction pumps and respiratory circuits and infant incubators). Periodic maintenance and instrument calibration may be carried out (e.g. by medical engineers either in the unit or in an adjacent area). This should be done after decontamination and before the items are returned for use. Processing of respiratory ventilators is now infrequently required, as they are protected by filters. Babies' incubators are usually processed in a room in the clinical area. The requirement for a specialized HSDU has therefore decreased, but it is important that staff who carry out reprocessing in other parts of the hospital are trained by the SSD.

The present SSDs have rationalized their function and now obtain a large range of sterile procedure packs, dressings and single-use supplementary instruments from commercial sources.

With the introduction of consumer legislation, recent EC Directives and loss of crown immunity, departments should operate good manufacturing practices which should be in accordance with existing guidelines and practices, such as those produced by the Institute of Sterile Supplies Management (1989, 1998a, b) and the Medical Devices Directorate (1993, 1996, 1999). The European Medical Devices Directive 93/42/EEC indicates that an SSD which supplies products to another organization (e.g. another hospital or health-care establishment) is considered to be a manufacturer of the product and should fulfil the requirements of the Directive. If the product is approved under the Directive, it can be labelled with the CE mark. Although most of the recommendations of the GMP and other standard documents are acceptable, some of them are rather excessive in terms of microbiological requirements, especially routine sampling (Atfield, 1991) – for example, in rooms used for packing instruments and dressings which will subsequently be sterilized. However, packs should be assembled in a room which is as clean and dust free as is reasonably practicable. Inadequate cleaning of instruments could be associated with a much greater bioburden on an instrument than exposure to unfiltered air. Appropriately controlled conditions are necessary to meet the European Directive, but these are not defined. However, quality systems to meet the Directive are available (BS EN 46001, BS EN 46002, British Standards Institution, 1976).

Manufacturers are legally responsible for providing directions on the decontamination of reusable equipment (Medical Devices Directorate, 1993, 1996, 1999). However, the final decision should be made by the infection control team (e.g. immersion of items in 2% glutaraldehyde for 10 hours as recommended by some manufacturers for sterilization is obviously not practicable).

DESIGN OF DEPARTMENTS AND WORK FLOW

The design features for an SSD are described in NHS Estates (1992). The design provides for two distinct flow lines:
1 for routine processing of surgical instruments/utensils; and
2 for medical equipment.

The typical work flow for surgical instruments and utensils is as follows:
1 sorting, washing, heat disinfection and drying;
2 inspection, setting trays and assembling packs;
3 sterilization;
4 transfer to sterile goods store;
5 distribution to wards and other units.

The work flow should be in one direction only, and all stages of the decontamination process should be documented (Medical Devices Directorate, 1993, 1996, 1999).

Other medical equipment is similarly treated, but may require stripping down to component parts before cleaning, reassembling and checking after processing.

COLLECTION AND RETURN OF USED EQUIPMENT TO THE SSD

Equipment should be effectively contained so that there is no risk to personnel during transport to the SSD. Single-use items should be correctly disposed of by the user, especially sharps (e.g. needles and blades), and not returned with reprocessable equipment. Delicate items must be well protected. Body fluids in suction bottles or hollow-ware should preferably be discarded by the user. Used surgical instruments are commonly returned in sets in their original trays or metal boxes, and are checked before processing. The reception area in the SSD should be separate from clean areas and have readily cleanable surfaces.

PROCESSING PROCEDURES FOR USED EQUIPMENT

Sterile services staff (and most other health service staff) have become increasingly concerned about the hazard of acquiring HBV and HIV infection, despite the extremely low risk. However, staff must assume that there is a possibility of infection from any used item that is returned to the SSD. The risk can be reduced by wearing gloves (household), visors and plastic aprons when handling all items, particularly those that are bloodstained, and exercising care when handling sharp instruments. Any existing cuts or damaged skin on the hands should be covered with a waterproof dressing, and the hands should be thoroughly washed after removal of gloves. All staff handling potentially contaminated instruments or equipment should be immunized against hepatitis B.

Known high-risk equipment should be decontaminated as soon as possible after receipt with minimal handling. All returned items that require cleaning should be disinfected by heat after cleaning (see also Chapter 6). Forceps and scissors require opening before washing in a machine to ensure penetration of the joints with cleaning agent and hot water. Some items (e.g. tubes or some items contaminated with secretions which have been subject to prolonged drying) may still require washing by hand. Chemical disinfection may be ineffective before cleaning and will thus give a false sense of security. Autoclaving before cleaning will coagulate protein, making it difficult to remove during subsequent washing. A washer-disinfector commissioned and monitored in accordance with BS2745 (British Standards Institution, 1993) is desirable, but cleaning by hand or in an ultrasonic machine should be a safe procedure if it is carried out by trained staff wearing the correct protective clothing. The choice of methods for dealing with contaminated items must be made by the manager in association with the ICT. Washer-disinfectors are also of considerable value for processing anaesthetic and respiratory equipment, as the items can then be dried and packaged without further treatment.

Routine decontamination procedures should be sufficient for equipment from high-infection risk patients, but it may be advisable for SSD managers to be informed of any unusual hazard.

TESTING OF WASHER-DISINFECTORS AND STERILIZERS

If washer-disinfectors are to be used for the decontamination of high-risk items, agreement should be reached with the ICT on what is an acceptable process. Cleaning efficacy and time/temperature parameters should be checked when commissioning washer-disinfectors and at periodic intervals (BS2745, HTM 2030, Department of Health, 1995; see also Chapter 5). Routine microbiological testing other than possibly during commissioning should be unnecessary if the process is well controlled and monitored. Sterilizers should be routinely monitored according to HTM 2020 (Department of Health, 1994a) and the Medical Devices Directorate (1993, 1996, 1999).

QUALITY SYSTEMS AND AUDIT

Fulfilling the requirements for good manufacturing practice and conducting internal audits by SSD managers, possibly with a member of the ICT, will provide evidence of a quality service. However, external assessment and audit by a certification body is being increasingly required for evidence of conformation with quality standards for

BS EN ISO 9002 (British Standards Institution, 1994) quality systems model, for quality assurance in productions, installations, servicing and EN46002 (specification for application of EN ISO 9002 to the manufacture of medical devices) and other regulations and requirements to comply with the Directive for Medical Devices. External assessment is not required if products are not sold to other establishments.

RETURNING EQUIPMENT FOR SERVICING OR REPAIR

It is a requirement of the Department of Health that certificates are issued stating that equipment returned for servicing or repair is microbiologically safe (Department of Health, 1991). However, it is not always possible to ensure that the internal surfaces of some items of equipment have been adequately decontaminated. It may also be necessary to return equipment that has not been decontaminated due to failure in use (e.g. an endoscope with a blocked channel). In these circumstances, a note should be attached to the returned equipment indicating safe methods of handling and suitable decontamination methods.

All single-use components should be removed and discarded as clinical waste. Non-disposable components should be cleaned and preferably autoclaved (if heat tolerant) or disinfected in a washing-machine. If this is not possible, immersion in a disinfectant such as 70% ethanol, a solution of a chlorine-releasing agent (1000 ppm available chlorine) or a peroxygen compound is acceptable provided that it is effective against the probable contaminating organisms and compatible with the surface (see Chapters 5 and 6 for choice of disinfectants and advantages and disadvantages of these agents).

Following immersion, items should be thoroughly rinsed and dried. If there are difficulties in decontaminating the internal surfaces, all external surfaces should be cleaned before returning an item to the manufacturer. Maintenance staff should be provided with suitable protective clothing, disinfectants and decontamination equipment. They should also be trained in handling and disinfection procedures.

WARDS OF PSYCHIATRIC, GERIATRIC AND MENTALLY HANDICAPPED PATIENTS

Many of these patients who would formerly have been hospitalized are now cared for in the community. However, some of them will always require long-term hospital treatment.

They are often incapable of understanding the principles of personal hygiene or of carrying out normal hygienic procedures, and some may be incontinent of faeces or urine, or both. In addition, the elderly are particularly susceptible to infection. Effective isolation of these patients in single rooms may be difficult to maintain, and can often have adverse psychological effects. Gastrointestinal and skin infections or infestations, pulmonary tuberculosis, influenza, hepatitis A and hepatitis B are likely to spread in these units.

Methods of control are similar in principle to those used in other wards, and are described elsewhere in the book, but there are special problems. Surveillance and immediate action are particularly important. New patients who are thought to have infections should be admitted to a special ward and screened for skin infection and infestation and for pulmonary tuberculosis as appropriate, faeces should be examined if there is a history of diarrhoea, and swabs should be taken from superficial lesions.

Food poisoning is a particular hazard in these wards, and should be considered in any outbreak of diarrhoea and vomiting. Ward staff should inform the ICN of cases of diarrhoea which are probably of infective origin, particularly if there is more than one case. Patients with diarrhoea should be isolated, and if more than one case of a salmonella or shigella infection occurs in a ward, the faeces of other patients and staff should be examined. However, outbreaks of diarrhoea of viral origin are common and usually self-limiting, and isolation of all patients may be impracticable. Hygienic measures, particularly handwashing of both patients and staff and disinfection of toilet seats, etc., should be reinforced. It may be necessary to restrict admissions until the ward is clear of infection.

Outbreaks of hepatitis A can occur in units for children with mental handicaps. In the event of such an outbreak, screening for antibody in patients and staff and the administration of gamma-globulin to uninfected patients may be required, in addition to improvements in hygiene. Hepatitis A vaccine may be considered for staff in these units. Hepatitis B can also be a problem in units for the mentally handicapped and for drug addicts, and staff should be advised to be vaccinated. Particular care is required in psychiatric units with violent or unpredictable patients with known or suspected HBV, HCV or HIV infection, particularly when taking blood samples.

Pulmonary tuberculosis is sometimes detected in a patient who has been in the ward for a long period. Patient contacts and staff should have a chest X-ray, which should be repeated after 3 months. Staff should be checked for previous tuberculin test results and BCG administration by the occupational health department.

Outbreaks of influenza tend to have a high mortality rate in geriatric wards, and annual vaccination of patients and staff is advisable. The administration of a pneumococcal vaccine should also be considered for geriatric patients.

Patients with long-term catheterization are likely to have urine infected or colonized with antibiotic-resistant Gram-negative bacilli, which could be a cross-infection hazard if transferred to an acute surgical ward. Removal of the catheter and use of incontinence pads should be considered whenever possible. Pressure sores and varicose ulcers may similarly be colonized with antibiotic-resistant organisms. If the lesion is colonized with MRSA, the patient's medical notes should be marked appropriately and, if the patient is transferred to another hospital, the infection control department of that hospital should be informed. MRSA are rarely responsible for clinical problems in geriatric wards, but they could be if transferred to an acute surgical unit. Scabies may also spread in these units, and if several cases have occurred it may be advisable to treat all patients and staff.

Skin infections should be treated promptly, particularly if caused by β-haemolytic streptococci of group A. If there is an outbreak of skin sepsis, all patients and staff should use antiseptic soaps or detergents for all washing and bathing. Staff should maintain as high a standard of hygiene as possible, including washing hands (both of patients and their own) before eating, and regular cleaning of toilets and baths. The use of communal towels and flannels should be avoided. Floors, walls and furniture should be washable. Although carpets may seem desirable in such units, these are difficult to keep clean and maintain, and should generally be avoided if contamination from incontinent patients is frequent (see Chapter 6). It is desirable for patients to wear clothes that can be disinfected by heat. If psychological considerations require that patients wear their own clothes, which are often heat labile, it must be recognized that some risk of infection exists.

PATHOLOGY LABORATORIES

Reports of outbreaks of laboratory-acquired infection and the introduction of the Health and Safety at Work Act (1974) and Health Services Commission (1988) have been followed by the publication of guidelines from several committees and other publications. As new evidence emerges, these guidelines continue to be modified (Health Services Advisory Committee, 1991a; Department of Health, 1998; Collins and Kennedy, 1999).

The Advisory Committee on Dangerous Pathogens has classified organisms into four hazard and containment categories (Advisory Committee on Dangerous Pathogens, 1995). Category 1 includes agents unlikely to cause human disease, and requires no special precautions. Category 2 includes most organisms isolated in clinical laboratories, and requires good microbiological practice. Category 3 includes organisms of special risk to laboratory workers (e.g. *Salmonella typhi*, *Mycobacterium tuberculosis*), and requires special containment facilities. Category 4 includes organisms that are extremely hazardous to laboratory workers and which may cause serious epidemic disease (e.g. Lassa, Ebola and Marburg viruses), which require particularly stringent containment. It is recognized that Category 3 organisms may be isolated in routine laboratories, and on identification subsequent work on them must be carried out in the appropriate containment category. Modified requirements are adequate for handling samples from patients with hepatitis B or HIV antibody, but work in a cabinet may be preferred. These viruses are transferred by contact with blood and not by the airborne route.

The recommendations in these codes and guidelines are extensive and demand much from the laboratory worker and also from those who design or direct laboratories. They comprise all the sensible and feasible precautions which need to be taken in diagnostic clinical (and research) laboratories, although no code of practice can prevent infections due to negligence or poor technique of the laboratory worker. Everyone who works in a pathology department must develop habits of safe and careful technique. However, precautions against laboratory-acquired infection should be reasonable and, whenever possible, based on scientific or clinical evidence. Rituals should be discouraged. For example, ventilated rooms cannot be expected to influence the transmission of bloodborne infections such as HBV or HIV or organisms transferred by the faecal–oral route such as *Salmonella typhi*.

SPECIAL RISKS OF INFECTION

There are several ways in which the pathology department may be involved in the spread of infection in hospital. Patients are at risk from infection carried from the laboratory by laboratory staff collecting specimens in wards or out-patient departments, and may also be infected by procedures performed by the technician involving transfer of microbes from one patient to another. Laboratory staff are at risk both from patients and from specimens of biological material and cultures examined in the laboratory. This last involvement (i.e. risk to laboratory staff from biological specimens) is in practice the most likely to have serious consequences. Many risks are well known and precautions are taken to prevent spread, but infections can also arise from unsuspected sources, (e.g. a request form contaminated by faeces and handled by clerical staff, or serum containing HBV examined in the biochemistry department).

There are many routes by which infections are acquired in pathology departments (e.g. infected aerosols or sprays generated when pipetting or pouring liquids in the laboratory may be inhaled by workers, or HBV or HIV may enter through skin abrasions). Tuberculosis and hepatitis B have been particularly important in hospital and laboratory infections in the UK, but hepatitis B has been acquired less in microbiological than in biochemical and haematological laboratories. In recent years such infections have become less frequent as a result of better training in safe working. There is no evidence that HIV has been transferred to laboratory workers from clinical samples, but despite the very low risk of transmission, HIV infection is such a dangerous infection that particular care is necessary. In general, it is not usually a specimen which is already known to be infective that causes an infection, but one which is not suspected of being dangerous. Some areas (e.g. animal houses, tuberculosis laboratories and hospital mortuaries) are especially hazardous and require special precautions.

PREVENTION OF INFECTION

Methods of collecting specimens while minimizing infection risks are described in Chapter 7. All samples should be handled with care (e.g. transported in sealed plastic bags and handled with disposable gloves), as the diagnosis may not be known until laboratory tests have been completed. However, many laboratories still label high-risk specimens (containing category 3 pathogens) as 'biohazard' or 'danger of infection', although this should not be necessary. Specimens must be received in an area used exclusively for the purpose. The general office can be used if the reception area is separated from the clerical area. Staff handling specimens should be adequately trained. A handwash basin with pedal or elbow taps should be readily available, as well as appropriate materials and disinfectants for cleaning up any spillage, and a container for disposal of spillage.

Laboratory staff visiting the wards should be trained in barrier-nursing techniques, and must follow carefully the instructions for handling infected patients.

TRANSPORT OF SPECIMENS

Attention should be given to the containers used to transport specimens from patient areas to laboratories. The specimen containers should be leak-proof, robust, and transported in trays or boxes which will hold the specimens upright. Some laboratories seal all specimens in plastic bags with a pocket to keep the forms free from contamination. Simple, clear rules need to be formulated for staff who are involved in transporting specimens. The Code of Practice (Health Services Advisory Committee, 1991a) recommends that metal boxes used for transporting specimens should be autoclaved weekly. Staff involved in the transport of specimens should be trained to cope with spillage.

PROCEDURES WITHIN THE LABORATORY

Details of hazards and their avoidance are given in several publications (for example, Collins and Kennedy, 1999). When handling specimens, particular attention should be given to centrifuges and other possible sources of infective aerosols. Infected materials (e.g. slides and pipettes) should be discarded into jars containing a phenolic or chlorine-releasing disinfectant which is replaced daily (see Chapters 5 and 6). Plastic pipettes should be used whenever possible to reduce the hazards of trauma when handling. The elimination of unnecessary glassware is one of the most important measures for reducing risks of blood-borne infection. Plastic petri dishes involve problems of disposal. If possible, they should be made safe before removal from the laboratory, and this is best achieved by autoclaving in a suitable container or in stainless steel buckets. The resultant lumps of polyethylene can be handled by the refuse collectors, but should be kept in sealed plastic bags. Difficulties have arisen when plates have been discarded without treatment and subsequently appear on local refuse sites. Incineration, preferably on site, without prior autoclaving is acceptable provided that the waste is effectively contained during transport. Incineration of plastic plates in bulk may lead to an unacceptable level of smoke pollution. Used glass petri dishes should be autoclaved by trained staff before being handled by domestics. Other glass containers (e.g. bijou bottles containing infective material) should be similarly autoclaved before leaving the laboratory, whether they are going to be reprocessed or disposed of.

Care is needed during selection of the container for autoclaving. Failure to remove air from bags or buckets is likely to cause failure of decontamination. Various designs of containers have been suggested, as well as autoclave modifications (Public Health Laboratory Service Subcommittee, 1981; Oates *et al.*, 1983). Sterilizing temperatures are usually recommended, but are rarely required to achieve adequate decontamination, unless the work of the laboratory involves spore-bearing organisms that are hazardous to workers (e.g. *Bacillus anthracis*, *Clostridium tetani* or *Clostridium botulinum*). It is important that temperatures in the coolest part of the load are regularly checked with thermocouples.

IMMUNIZATION OF LABORATORY STAFF

Infections against which immunization should be offered to laboratory staff include tuberculosis, poliomyelitis and tetanus. Female staff should also be offered rubella vaccination, preferably after testing the immune state. None of these procedures is mandatory, except for BCG protection of tuberculin-negative staff, who must be excluded from work with material that contains or is likely to contain tubercle bacilli until conversion has taken place (British Thoracic Society, 1990). Other protective measures should be strongly encouraged to all staff on joining the laboratory (see Chapter 15).

The hepatitis B vaccine should be offered to all laboratory staff who handle clinical specimens, and may be a condition of employment if the member of staff is involved in invasive procedures.

TRAINING AND INSTRUCTIONS FOR STAFF

Training of staff in aseptic procedures and in methods of handling infected material is part of the routine education in microbiology departments. In most hospitals the various branches of pathology recruit their own staff and, as multi-disciplinary training is now rare, there is often no opportunity for biochemists or technicians to acquire experience in microbiology departments. In these cases, some basic instruction should be given on methods of spread of infection, aseptic procedures and handling of potentially infected biological or toxic materials. The Code of Practice and other relevant documents should be readily available for consultation. The COSHH regulations apply to micro-organisms as well as to toxic chemicals, and each laboratory should produce its own Safety Code which includes the most important rules.

PRECAUTIONS AGAINST LABORATORY INFECTION

The following is an example of such information given to laboratory staff:

Any specimen entering the laboratory may be infectious, and some will certainly contain the agents that cause HBV, HCV and HIV infection, typhoid, tuberculosis and other infections. Your own and your family's safety, and that of your colleagues, depend on observing the following instructions.

General

There must be no smoking, no eating and no drinking in the laboratory. Keep your bench clean and tidy.

Wash your hands thoroughly on leaving the laboratory before taking food or drink or handling personal possessions, after handling specimens, after changing tubing or dialysers or diluters in the auto-analysers, and if you think you have contaminated them, thoroughly wash with soap and water. If contamination with bacterial cultures has occurred, and in 'high-risk' laboratories, use an antiseptic handwashing method. Thorough application of 70% alcohol after washing is particularly effective.

Handwashing

This is your most important safeguard. Wear gloves when handling high-risk specimens (or when cleaning up spillage). Wash hands after removing gloves.

Cuts and abrasions

Wash well in running water. Cover with waterproof protective dressing. If you splash your eye with serum or a culture, wash it thoroughly with saline or tap water. Report to the laboratory manager or their deputy at once, and enter the incident in the accident book (needlestick injuries must be entered and immediately reported).

Spilt specimens – treatment of contaminated area, floor or other surfaces

Swab with plenty of a 2% clear soluble phenolic solution on the areas of contamination, or with a chlorine-releasing agent containing 10 000 ppm available chlorine when cleaning up blood or organic materials that possibly contain viruses; 1000 ppm is adequate for small amounts of spillage or routine cleaning. Rinse well, particularly if a metal surface is involved. Thoroughly covering the spillage with a chlorine-releasing or peroxygen powder or granules before removal with paper towels is also effective. Do not use a chlorine-releasing powder or granules for large amounts of spillage, as excessive amounts of chlorine may be released. Wear gloves when handling contaminated materials or disinfectants.

Pipettes

Avoid mouth suction. Use automatic pipettes, rubber bulbs or teats. Discard all Pasteur pipettes and graduated pipettes into enough clear soluble phenolic (2%) or a chlorine-releasing solution – 0.25% (2500 ppm available chlorine) – to cover them completely. It is preferable to use a jar with a screw lid.

Other equipment

Mastic tubes, pilot tubes and other plastic disposables should be incinerated. Slides should be autoclaved in the discard jars in which they have been placed. Syringes and needles should be discarded into an approved container (see Chapter 7).

Centrifuging

Use only closed centrifuges, with wind-shields if possible, and preferably with sealed buckets which should be opened only within a protective exhaust cabinet if dangerous pathogens are involved.

Swab out the centrifuge bowl with a clear soluble phenolic or, for virus infections, 70% alcohol after washing. Wear disposable gloves.

If a breakage occurs, autoclave the bucket and its contents. Swab the bowl as described above.

White coats

A plentiful supply of white coats is necessary. Coats must be changed immediately if they become contaminated, all coats should be treated as infected linen in the laundry, and coats known to be contaminated with particularly hazardous pathogens should be autoclaved in the laboratory autoclave. Fully protective coats should be worn when handling Category 3 pathogens.

Do not wear your laboratory coat to visit the wards.

Do not wear *any* white coat to visit the coffee room or toilet.

INFECTIONS IN CONTAINMENT CATEGORY 3 – LABORATORIES

As this containment category is required for handling sputum specimens that may contain *Mycobacterium tuberculosis*, most large laboratories will now have this facility. The room will contain a cabinet with exhaust ventilation that is filtered before discharge, usually to the outside. The cabinet and system should be disinfected with formalin both routinely and before maintenance, and air flows should be regularly checked. Gloves should be worn for all manipulations, and staff must be adequately trained in order to avoid a false sense of security when using a cabinet. Careful work on an open bench may often be safer, particularly if one is working with viruses such as HBV or HIV, which do not spread in the air. It is therefore recommended that for the clinical examination of samples containing HBV or HIV, the work may be carried out at a defined work station which allows sufficient seclusion to avoid inoculation accidents.

A fully protective gown or plastic apron and a visor should be worn, as well as disposable gloves, for more dangerous manipulations. Staff must be adequately trained in the use of aseptic measures in addition to provision of this protective clothing, otherwise a false sense of security may lead to simple errors which would not arise if gloves were not being worn.

Fungi

Cultures of fungi that cause communicable systemic infection (e.g. *Histoplasma*) should be processed in a ventilated cabinet, as recommended for tubercle bacilli.

POST-MORTEM ROOM AND MORTUARY (see also Health Services Advisory Committee, 1991b)

The dead body, whether previously infected or not, may be a source of infection, and mortuary and post-mortem staff are at risk. As in the ward, bacteria may spread by air or by contact, but there are special hazards when a post-mortem examination is being performed. Contaminated aerosols or splashes may be released through squeezing sponges, cutting tissues such as the lung or incising abscesses, and the sawing of bones may also release small contaminated chips into the air. Cutting or pricking a finger with a contaminated instrument or ragged bone edge is one of the commonest modes of infection. Although most organisms in the dead body are unlikely to infect healthy individuals with intact skin, there are some specific hazards. Tubercle bacilli may be spread in large numbers in aerosols. Salmonella, shigella and other intestinal pathogens may be transmitted from the intestinal tract. Following a break in the skin of the operator, large numbers of *Staphylococcus aureus* or *Streptococcus pyogenes* may be introduced, and unless treatment with appropriate antibiotics is given promptly, these may cause a severe local infection and sometimes septicaemia. HBV, HCV or HIV introduced by a cut or needle-prick are a major potential hazard. The conjunctiva may be infected by splashes or aerosols, and a severe local infection may follow. Bloodborne viruses may also enter the body by this route (see Chapter 10).

PREVENTION OF INFECTION

The risks of infection are not high if adequate precautions are taken. Cleanliness of the mortuary, refrigerator and post-mortem room, as well as good personal hygiene of members of staff, are essential. The post-mortem room should be mechanically ventilated and designed so that cleaning can be readily achieved. Fly-proofing arrangements in the mortuary and post-mortem room should be efficient. A shower, with soap and towels supplied, should be available for the post-mortem room staff. When performing post-mortem examinations, the pathologist and mortuary technicians should completely change their outer clothing, and a disposable plastic apron, disposable gloves and rubber boots should be worn. Clean white trousers, vests and jackets should be supplied daily if possible, or at least several times a week or if they become contaminated. Visitors to the post-mortem room who are not going to be in close contact with the body should wear a gown and overshoes. A wash-basin with disposable paper towels, soap and an antiseptic handwashing preparation (povidone-iodine or chlorhexidine detergent, or 70% ethanol) should be available in the post-mortem room.

Staff should wash their hands thoroughly after handling any contaminated surface or material, irrespective of whether gloves are worn, and always on leaving the post-mortem room. If the hands are likely to have become contaminated, they should also be washed before handling case-notes or any other clean items.

If the skin or eye is splashed, it should be thoroughly washed. An eyewash bottle containing sterile saline should be available. Any cut or finger-prick should be immediately reported to the pathologist, after thorough washing under running water and application of an antiseptic (e.g. 0.5% alcoholic or aqueous chlorhexidine or 1% iodine in 70% alcohol). All pre-existing cuts or open lesions on the hands should be covered with a waterproof dressing. Open injuries, other than minor ones, should be treated in the casualty department.

Instruments should be routinely cleaned before disinfection, as the presence of organic matter may protect the organisms from the disinfectant. Boiling in water or immersion in 2% 'Stericol' or other phenolics for 10 min are less satisfactory alternatives to autoclaving, but if properly carried out are safe procedures. A small washer-disinfector would be preferable, as washing by hand would be avoided. After treatment with a disinfectant, all instruments should be rinsed and dried. Immersion in a chlorine-releasing solution (1000 ppm available chlorine) rather than a phenolic is advised after a post-mortem on a patient with an HBV or HIV infection, although autoclaving or treatment in a washer-disinfector would be preferable. For disinfection and cleaning of instruments and the room used at autopsies of patients with infections caused by the agents of the transmissible spongiform encephalopathies, see below. The room and other equipment should be thoroughly cleaned after use with a phenolic disinfectant (e.g. 2% 'Stericol'), or with a chlorine-releasing agent (1000 ppm available chlorine) if HBV, HCV, HIV infection or poliomyelitis was diagnosed in the patient before death. If chlorine-releasing agents are used on metal surfaces, they should be immediately rinsed in order to avoid corrosion.

Linen should be sent in a sealed bag and treated as 'infected' by the laundry. Dressings, waste materials and body tissues should be sealed in plastic bags and treated as clinical waste.

Special precautions should be taken with certain infections. In post-mortem examinations of patients with untreated pulmonary tuberculosis, filter-type masks should be worn by operators. Post-mortems on patients with known or suspected HBV, HCV or HIV infection should be avoided unless absolutely essential (for general precautions, see Chapter 10). Special care is necessary to avoid cuts and needle-pricks.

Viruses that cause spongiform encephalopathy (e.g. Creutzfeldt–Jakob disease) and other slow virus infections are relatively resistant to heat and are also resistant to most chemical disinfectants, especially aldehydes. The environment should be disinfected with a strong chlorine-releasing solution (containing 0.25% available chlorine), and blood should be mopped up with a solution containing 1% (10 000 ppm) available chlorine or following the application of a chlorine-releasing powder. If the skin is contaminated, wash thoroughly with soap and water and apply 2 M sodium hydroxide for 10 min. Instruments should be autoclaved at 134°C for 18 min (e.g. six 3-min cycles) after thorough washing (see also Chapter 6). Immersion in 2 M sodium hydroxide is a possible alternative if autoclaving is not possible (see p. 114).

Formaldehyde used for the preservation of tissues is an effective antimicrobial agent. Thorough penetration should be ensured before handling, particularly if lesions are caused by potentially dangerous infections (e.g. tuberculosis, typhoid or hepatitis). It is ineffective against prions.

It is most important that the mortuary staff and undertakers should be informed about the bodies of patients who have died or were suffering from a communicable disease. These should be enclosed in a plastic bag, and it would be useful to attach a warning label to them in the ward. Training of mortuary staff in prevention of infection is also necessary. Immunization should be offered as for laboratory staff.

RENAL DIALYSIS

The general considerations with regard to hospital infection apply to dialysis and transplant units, but there are special hazards.

Bloodborne viruses (HBV, HCV and HIV)

Patients suffering from chronic renal failure may show few physical signs when infected with HBV, but become long-term carriers. This virus is often present in high titre, and transfer of infection to staff and other patients is a particular hazard. Blood transfusion is now a rare source of infection of HBV in most countries, as transfusion blood is usually screened. Blood is frequently screened for HCV and HIV, but this is more variable in countries with limited resources. Spread of HIV has not been reported in renal units. Spread of bloodborne viruses can also occur through shared and inadequately decontaminated equipment.

Dialysis machines

The dialysis fluid used for haemodialysis does not need to be sterile, but a heavy growth of bacteria leads to risks both of infection and of changes in the chemical composition of the fluid which may be associated with endotoxins crossing the membrane. Gram-negative bacilli (e.g. *Pseudomonas, Acinetobacter, Aeromonas* and *Serratia* species and non-tuberculous mycobacteria (e.g. *Mycobacterium chelonae*) can grow in dialysis machines and cause septicaemia and pyrogenic reactions.

Vascular access site, catheter exit site and peritoneal infections

Staphylococcus aureus and *Staphylococcus epidermidis* are the commonest causes of infection, but Gram-negative bacilli (e.g. *E. coli* and *Pseudomonas aeruginosa*) can cause peritonitis. In addition to local sepsis and peritonitis, bacteraemia and endocarditis are also possible complications.

PREVENTION OF INFECTION

Viral infections

These are discussed in more detail in Chapter 10 (see also Department of Health and Social Security, 1972). Patients should be screened for HBV (and possibly HCV) on admission to the dialysis programme. Screening for HIV remains controversial, as it is not necessary as an infection control measure. Patients and staff should be immunized against hepatitis B if they are not already immune. Routine surveillance for HBV is important for susceptible patients (e.g. 3-monthly) and staff (6-monthly), but it is not necessary for control of HCV and HIV infection (Favero *et al.*, 1996). However, units will decide on their own screening and surveillance requirements.

Universal precautions should be practised. For example, gloves and disposable aprons should be routinely used when handling blood and other body fluids or contaminated equipment, or for clearing spillage. These should be changed between patients, and hands should be washed after removing gloves and apron. Eye protection is necessary if splashing of blood is likely. The safe disposal of sharps, waste and linen is described in the appropriate chapters. Source isolation and use of dedicated dialysis machines are still often advised for patients in the acute stages of HBV infection, or if they are carrying the 'e' antigen. However, effective universal precautions should enable all carriers of HBV, HCV and HIV to be treated similarly to other patients in the unit.

Bacterial infections

Meticulous attention should be paid to all aspects of environmental hygiene and to aseptic techniques. There is evidence that staphylococcal carriers are more likely to acquire clinical infections than non-carriers (Yu *et al.*, 1986). Treatment of nasal carriers with mupirocin in varying regimes has been shown to reduce nasal carriage considerably and to reduce infection rates significantly, including bacteraemias (Hudson, 1994). Continuous treatment with mupirocin appears to be more effective than an initial course plus a repeat course if a recurrence of carriage occurs (Boelaert *et al.*, 1989). However, resistance to mupirocin has emerged (Eltringham, 1997) and many chronic staphylococcal carriers do not develop sepsis. It may be preferable to restrict nasal prophylaxis to those who develop repeated infections. The use of other less effective agents (e.g. neomycin, bacitracin, chlorhexidine) may be preferred for long-term prophylaxis (see Chapter 9).

SUBCUTANEOUS ARTERIOVENOUS FISTULAE

The subcutaneous fistula has a great advantage over the external shunt in that there is no open wound once post-operative healing has occurred. The technique for management is as follows.

1 A wide area of the arm is cleaned with 0.5% chlorhexidine in 70% ethyl alcohol. It is essential that this preliminary skin preparation should be very thorough, in order to avoid the introduction of bacteria directly into the bloodstream.

2 Local anaesthesia is usually necessary in view of the wide bore of the needle to be inserted. Lignocaine (2%) in 2-mL ampoules is recommended for this purpose.

3 It is desirable to avoid inserting the needle through the identical point of insertion made during the preceding dialysis, where a small infected clot or scab may have formed.

4 The fistula needle is strapped into position after reinsertion into the fistula sites, but no dressing is necessary.

5 Haemorrhage after withdrawal of the needle can occur, and severe blood loss can be troublesome if adequate steps are not taken. To prevent this, a protamine-soaked or other haemostatic swab is placed over the site and held in place firmly for 10 min. This is replaced by a sterile gauze square, and firmly bandaged for 2 hours.

EXTERNAL ARTERIOVENOUS SHUNTS AND VENOUS CANNULAE

The basic bacteriological problem presented by the external access device can be stated simply – it is how to avoid infection in a permanently open wound containing a foreign body. This obviously presents considerable difficulties. However, prevention of infection at the access site is of major importance if suppuration is to be avoided. This may lead to destruction and abandonment of an important site when the number of sites is strictly limited, and to the risk of septic emboli and fatal septicaemia.

In view of these considerations, the care of the access site must be seen to begin in the wider context of general hygiene and ward cleanliness, and the measures used to control cross-infection in the general hospital ward situation should be applied even more rigorously to the renal unit.

Routine care of access site

The main object is to prevent introduction of pathogens. This is achieved by observance of strict aseptic principles in the dressing and handling of the access site, by an occlusive dressing, and by keeping the site dry at all times as far as possible.

TRAINING FOR HOME DIALYSIS

Although it is important that home dialysis patients should be trained to be self-sufficient, it is valuable in most circumstances for the spouse, relative or friend who may help the patient to be fully instructed in both the principles and practice of access-site care, bearing in mind that both they and the patient find the technique completely foreign and the aseptic precautions without apparent reason. Experience suggests that teaching is best done by example. At the same time, the dangers of autogenous infection must be stressed in order to encourage the highest standards of personal hygiene.

INFECTION IN THE ACCESS SITE

If there is clinical evidence of infection at the site, a swab is taken for bacteriological examination, and swabs of nose, throat, axilla and groin are also taken. If the clinical condition warrants antibiotic therapy pending the bacteriological report, antistaphylococcal drugs (e.g. flucloxacillin or an initial dose of vancomycin) are started. Treatment is reviewed and altered if necessary on receipt of the bacteriological report. If possible, antibiotics that may accumulate to toxic levels in renal failure should be avoided (see Chapter 13).

Treatment is continued until there is bacteriological evidence of clearance. Carrier sites are treated as outlined above if they are found to carry pathogens.

The maintenance of an infection-free access site depends on rigorous attention to basic aseptic principles, keeping the site dry, prevention of colonization of carrier sites by pathogens, and a high level of personal and environmental hygiene.

ACUTE AND INTERMITTENT DIALYSIS

Peritoneal dialysis may be used for the treatment of acute renal failure, usually via a semi-rigid catheter inserted percutaneously into the abdomen followed by fairly rapid (e.g. hourly) exchanges of dialysis fluid, often with automated control of inflow and outflow using a suitable design of peritoneal dialysis machine. Such a procedure can also be applied intermittently to patients with chronic renal failure using a more permanent form of peritoneal access. Sterile pyrogen-free solutions and sterile cannulae and tubing are required for this procedure. Abdominal drainage should be through a closed system.

Adequate skin preparation and stringent aseptic techniques are required for insertion of the peritoneal cannula. A suture should be placed around the catheter and tied so that the latter cannot be pushed freely in and out by the staff attendant, and the site should be covered by a simple gauze dressing.

Manual methods often include the use of a water bath or sink for warming the bottles of dialysate before use. This water is likely to become contaminated with Gram-negative bacilli, including *Pseudomonas* species. The water should be changed frequently.

Automated systems for peritoneal dialysis usually include adequate instructions for sterilization.

Parts of the system that are likely to be in contact with dialysate must either be pre-sterilized disposable items or be autoclaved (see below).

Routine addition of prophylactic antibiotics to peritoneal dialysis fluid is not recommended. It is desirable to send samples to the laboratory every 24 hours for culture.

Peritoneal dialysis for chronic renal failure requires the use of a permanent indwelling silicone rubber peritoneal catheter. Such a catheter is plugged between use except when continuous dialysis is practised. The insertion and care of these catheters closely resembles the care of external arteriovenous shunts or cannulae. Whenever connections or disconnections are made, rigorous aseptic or no-touch techniques must be used. Peritonitis remains a common and serious complication of chronic peritoneal dialysis.

CONTINUOUS AMBULATORY PERITONEAL DIALYSIS (CAPD)

The technique of continuous ambulatory peritoneal dialysis (CAPD) utilizes plastic bags of dialysate which are changed by the patient several times daily. Patients must be taught to avoid contaminating the connections during these changes. Several types of connecting systems for CAPD are in use, and the manufacturer's instructions for each pattern should be followed. Various methods are available to reduce contamination of the line (e.g. flushing with hypochlorites and use of disinfectant-impregnated cuffs) (Anon., 1991; Ludlam, 1991), as well as systems using UV light and local heat application. Spraying with 70% ethanol is also effective. Systems are available which can be safely operated by blind patients. A type of connection is recommended which, while secure between bag changes, is easily undone by the patient with little risk of touching the parts that come into contact with dialysate. The catheter connection is usually changed periodically by the staff of the 'parent unit' using full aseptic precautions.

The major hazard of peritoneal dialysis is of course peritonitis. Infection in CAPD is most commonly by skin organisms, particularly *Staphylococcus epidermidis*. There is no doubt that meticulous attention to detail, including catheter care and avoidance of wetting the exit site, greatly reduces the incidence of infection. Peritonitis, often indicated by cloudy dialysis effluent and abdominal pain, requires antibiotic therapy – which is often added to the peritoneal dialysis fluid. Whilst awaiting positive cultures, a broad-spectrum antibiotic regime, including drugs active against *Staphylococcus epidermidis*, is usually instituted. Gram-negative and particularly fungal infections usually require temporary removal of the peritoneal catheter.

DISINFECTION OF EQUIPMENT AND MATERIALS

These should be single-use, autoclaved or heat treated whenever possible. Equipment should be capable of being easily dismantled to enable thorough cleaning. *Dialysers* are now relatively inexpensive and should be single-use if possible. Reprocessing may be necessary in some countries, but should be limited to one patient and a restricted number of uses (e.g. three). When reuse is contemplated, the dialyser (with or without blood lines) is thoroughly washed to remove all traces of blood. Disinfection with formaldehyde or glutaraldehyde is now rarely used, owing to their potential toxicity and sensitization properties. Alternatives are the chlorine-releasing agents, chlorine dioxide, peracetic acid and hydrogen peroxide. Disinfectants may damage the membranes and equipment components. Any new agent should be used according to the manufacturer's recommendations (see also Chapters 5 and 6).

Dialysis machines

Heat disinfection is preferable after physical cleaning. Chemical methods of disinfection should be used according to the manufacturer's instructions as described above. Peracetic acid is a sterilant over a short time period, and is relatively non-corrosive at in-use concentrations. Care is particularly necessary with pressure gauges which might have blind channels in which bacteria can grow, or which might become contaminated with blood, and are difficult to clean.

Appropriate treatment for water used to dilute the dialysate concentrate (e.g. reverse osmosis or ultrafiltration) should be instituted and monitored (Favero *et al.*, 1996). (For other aspects of environmental equipment, skin and hand disinfection, see Chapter 7.)

REFERENCES

Advisory Committee on Dangerous Pathogens (1995) *Categorisation of biological agents according to hazard and categories of containment*, 4th edn. London: HMSO.

Anon. (1977) *Guide to good manufacturing practice*. London: HMSO.

Anon. (1991) Editorial. Prevention of peritonitis in CAPD. *Lancet* 1, 22.

Anon. (1993) *Rules and guidance for pharmaceutical manufacturers*. London: HMSO.

Atfield, R.D. (1991) Hospital hygiene – a continuing assessment: a microbiological view of sterile services production. *Journal of Hospital Infection* 18 (Supplement A), 524.

Boelaert, J.R., De Smedt, R.A., De Baere, Y.A. *et al.* (1989) The influence of calcium mupirocin nasal ointment on the incidence of *Staphylococcus aureus* infections in haemodialysis. *Nephrology, Dialysis and Transplantation* 4, 278.

British Standards Institute (1976) *Environmental cleanliness in enclosed spaces. BS 5295: Parts 1, 2 5c 3*. London: British Standards Institute.

British Standards Institute (1993) *BS2745. Washer disinfectors Parts 1–3*. London: British Standards Institute.

British Standards Institute (1994) Quality systems: model for quality assurance in production, installation and servicing. BS EN ISO 9002. London: British Standards Institute.

British Thoracic Society (1990) Subcommittee of the Joint Tuberculosis Committee of the British Thoracic Society. Control and prevention of tuberculosis in Britain: an updated code of practice. *British Medical Journal* 300, 995.

Collins, C.H. and Kennedy, I.D.A. (1999) *Laboratory-acquired infections. History, incidence, causes and preventions*, 4th edn. Oxford: Butterworth Heinemann.

Dadswell, J.V. (1999) Recreational and hydrotherapy pools. In Russell, A.D., Hugo, W.B. and Ayliffe, G.A.J. (eds), *Principles and practice of disinfection, preservation and sterilization*, 3rd edn. Oxford: Blackwell Science, 446–53.

Department of Health (1991) *Decontamination of equipment, prior to inspections, service or repair*. London: HMSO.

Department of Health (1994a) *Health Technical Memorandum No. 2010. Sterilizers*. London: Department of Health.

Department of Health (1994b) *Aseptic dispensing for NHS patients*. London: Department of Health.

Department of Health (1995) *Health Technical Memorandum No. 2030*. London: Department of Health.

Department of Health (1998) *UK Health Departments guidance for clinical health care workers. Protection against infections with blood-borne viruses*. London: Department of Health.

Department of Health and Social Security (1972) *Rosenheim Advisory Group. Hepatitis and the treatment of chronic renal failure*. London: HMSO.

Eltringham, I. (1997) Mupirocin resistance and methicillin-resistant *Staphylococcus aureus* (MRSA). *Journal of Hospital Infection* 35, 1.

Favero, M.S., Alter, M.J. and Bland, L.A. (1996) Control of infections associated with hemodialysis. In Mayhall, G.I. (ed.), *Hospital epidemiology and infection control*. Baltimore, MD: Williams and Wilkins, 693.

Health Services Advisory Committee (1991a) *Safe working and the prevention of infection in clinical laboratories – model rules for staff and visitors*. London: HMSO.

Health Services Advisory Committee (1991b) *Safe working and the prevention of infection in the mortuary and post-mortem room*. London: HMSO.

Health Services Commission (1988) *Control of substances hazardous to health. Approved code of practice*. London: HMSO.

Hudson, I.R.B. (1994) The efficacy of intranasal mupirocin in the prevention of staphylococcal infections: a review of recent experience. *Journal of Hospital Infection* 27, 81.

Institute of Sterile Services Management (1989) *Guide to good manufacturing practice for national health sterile services departments*. London: Institute of Sterile Services Management.

Institute of Sterile Services Management (1998a) *Quality standards and recommended practices*. London: Institute of Sterile Services Management.

Institute of Sterile Services Management (1998b) *Sterile services resource manual*. London: Institute of Sterile Services Management.

Lee, M. and Midcalf, B. (1994) *Isolators for pharmaceutical applications*. London: HMSO.

Ludlam, H.A. (1991) Infectious consequences of continuous ambulatory peritoneal dialysis. *Journal of Hospital Infection* 18 (**Supplement A**), 34.

Medical Devices Agency (1995) *The reuse of medical devices supplied for single use only*. London: Department of Health.

Medical Devices Agency (1993, 1996, 1999) *Sterilization, disinfection and cleaning of medical equipment*. London: HMSO.

NHS Estates (1992) *Hospital Building Note No. 13. Hospital sterilization and disinfection unit*. London: NHS Estates.

NHS Quality Control Committee (1995) *Quality assurance of aseptic preparation services*, 2nd edn. London: NHS Quality Control Committee.

Oates, K., Deverill, C.E.A., Phelps, M. and Collins, B.J. (1983) Development of a laboratory autoclave system. *Journal of Hospital Infection* 4, 181.

Penny, P.T. (1991) Hydrotherapy pools of the future – the avoidance of health problems. *Journal of Hospital Infection* 18 (**Supplement A**), 535.

Public Health Laboratory Service (1990) *Report: hygiene for hydrotherapy pools*. London: Public Health Laboratory Service.

Public Health Laboratory Services Subcommittee (1981) Specifications for laboratory autoclaves. *Journal of Hospital Infection* 2, 377.

Underwood, E. (1999) Good manufacturing practice. In Russell, A.D., Hugo, W.B. and Ayliffe, G.A.J. *Principles and practice of disinfection, preservation and sterilization*, 3rd edn. Oxford: Blackwell Science, 374.

Working Party of the Central Sterilizing Club (1999) Reprocessing of single-use medical devices in hospitals. *Zeutral Sterilisation* 7, 37.

Yu, V.L., Goetz, A., Wagener, M. *et al.* (1986) *Staphylococcus aureus* nasal carriage and infection in patients on hemodialysis. *New England Journal of Medicine* 315, 91.

chapter 18

INFECTION CONTROL IN THE COMMUNITY

Section 1:
Administration, surveillance and control measures

Iain Blair

INTRODUCTION

The community can be defined as all environments that are outside hospital. This includes nursing and residential homes, hostels, day-care centres, schools, colleges and nurseries, factories, offices and other workplaces, leisure centres, hotels, restaurants, shops, cinemas, theatres and other places of entertainment, open spaces and communal areas, transport, and finally people's own homes and gardens. Patients are discharged earlier from hospital than in former times, and continuity of care is important. Hospital-acquired infection will often emerge in the community.

THE HISTORY OF COMMUNICABLE DISEASE CONTROL

In Britain before the eighteenth century the population was largely rural and the principal infectious diseases (e.g. smallpox, plague and leprosy) were controlled by a strategy of segregation and quarantine.

Rapid industrialization and urbanization in the early nineteenth century led to major problems with infections associated with overcrowding and poor ventilation and sanitation such as tuberculosis, typhus, typhoid, measles and scarlet fever.

In 1842 Edwin Chadwick's report on the Sanitary Conditions of the Labouring Population of Great Britain was published. This developed Chadwick's sanitary idea that disease is caused by foul air from filth, waste and poor ventilation. He proposed that there should be a local board of health in every district with responsibility for sanitary improvement, and that this would comprise a proper drainage system backed by a supply of running water.

Chadwick's report led to a Royal Commission which in turn led to the first Public Health Act of 1848. This allowed the setting up of local boards of health and the appointment of local Medical Officers of Health (MOH). A central General Board of Health was also set up, but this was not a success and was abolished in 1853.

A Royal Sanitary Commission made recommendations in 1871 and a central public health department was created the same year. The 1872 Public Health Act set up local sanitary authorities and the Act of 1875 consolidated existing sanitary law. This meant that in effect there was a national public health service for the first time. At local level the MOH had responsibility for housing, sanitation and infectious diseases. These arrangements continued until the turn of the century.

World War I saw the establishment of tuberculosis (TB), venereal diseases (VD) and maternity and child welfare services. The Ministry of Health was set up in 1919.

By the early 1900s, the MOH was responsible for the traditional environmental services of water and sewage disposal, food hygiene, housing, control of infectious disease, maternity and child welfare services (including midwives and health visitors), TB and VD clinics, the school medical service and the administration of the municipal hospitals.

The MOH held this position for 20 years until the formation of the National Health Service (NHS) in 1948, when local authorities were largely bypassed by the creation of a national rather than local authority-controlled health service. The NHS had a tripartite structure. Hospitals were under the control of hospital boards, executive councils had responsibility for general practitioner services, and local health authorities took charge of personal health services.

In 1974, the tripartite structure was integrated into a single administrative framework with a central department, regional, area and district health authorities. The public health departments of the local authorities vanished along with the MOH. Environmental services departments remained, staffed by environmental health officers (EHOs), who had been first appointed with the title of sanitary inspectors under the Public Health Act of 1872, but who were now no longer under direct medical supervision. Medical input to local authority departments came from staff employed by the community medicine departments of the new health authorities.

Further changes have taken place since that time. In 1982, area health authorities were abolished, and in the mid-1980s general management was introduced. Starting in 1992, NHS trusts were set up and in 1996 health authorities and family health service authorities merged and regional health authorities were abolished. Since the 1980s, the role of local authorities in the promotion of health has to some extent re-emerged, influenced by developments such as the World Health Organisation Health For All and Healthy Cities Programmes and, more recently, with Our Healthier Nation, Agenda 21 and the United Kingdom Environmental Health Action Plan.

ADMINISTRATIVE ARRANGEMENTS FOR THE CONTROL OF INFECTION IN THE COMMUNITY IN ENGLAND AND WALES

Communicable disease control in the community is a complex activity which relies on co-operation and collaboration between many different agencies and individuals. The individuals and organizations listed in Table 18.1 are a source of surveillance data, they diagnose and treat infections, implement control of infection measures, take action to prevent infections, give advice and enforce legislation. In turn they require information, advice, practical assistance and training (see also Chapter 2).

HEALTH AUTHORITIES

In England and Wales there are 105 health authorities serving populations which vary in size from 200 000 to 1 000 000. Health authorities are public bodies appointed by and accountable to the Secretary of State for Health. They are

Table 18.1 Staff responsible for infection control

Health authority	CCDC
	Community Infection Control Nurse
Hospitals	Medical microbiologist
	Infection Control Doctor
	Infection Control Nurse
	Infectious disease specialist
	TB specialist
	Genito-urinary medicine specialist
Community Trusts	Health visitors
	District nurses
	School health nurses and doctors
	TB nurse advisors
Local Authority Departments	
Environmental Health	Environmental health officers
Education	Teachers
Social Services	Social workers, home carers, residential home managers, safety managers
Local public health laboratory	Medical microbiologist
Public Health Laboratory Service	Medical microbiologist
Communicable Disease Surveillance Centre	Consultant epidemiologist
Primary care	General practitioners, practice nurses and other practice staff
Private nursing homes and residential homes	Managers, nursing staff, carers
Occupational health departments	Occupational health doctors and nurses
Day nurseries	Managers, nursery nurses
General public	Citizens (newspapers, radio, TV)

responsible for assessing the health needs of their resident population and purchasing an appropriate range, quantity and quality of services to meet those needs.

Health authorities, in collaboration with other agencies, protect public health by controlling communicable disease and infection and managing the human health aspects of other environmental hazards. They also ensure that there are adequate infection control arrangements within local hospitals and within the community, including general practice.

GENERAL PRACTITIONERS

General practitioners provide care, including diagnosis and treatment, for patients with infection. They notify cases of infection to the Consultant for Communicable Disease Control (CCDC). As a result of changes introduced by the new Labour Government in 1997, GPs and other primary care staff are forming Primary Care Groups (PCGs) which will have control over resources to commission services for local patients and contribute to the health authority's Health Improvement Programme (HImP), a partnership of local agencies to improve and promote public health.

HOSPITAL AND COMMUNITY TRUSTS

NHS health-care providers are run as non-profit-making trusts, and include acute hospitals and trusts providing health care in the community.

Hospital trusts have contracts with the local health authorities which will require satisfactory infection control arrangements, including allowing the CCDC and EHOs access to patients and clinical records. Contracts should also detail the range of tests offered by the microbiology laboratory and the arrangements for reporting positive results to the CCDC.

Within community trusts, infection control arrangements will vary. They should have an infection control doctor (ICD) and infection control team (ICT) cover. They may employ a community infection control nurse or, by agreement, receive a service from the CCDC and his or her team. Community nurses are employed by community trusts and work alongside general practitioners, usually as members of a primary health care team. They are a source of information about infection problems within the community, and in turn need access to infection control advice. This may be provided by the community infection control nurse, the CCDC or the hospital infection control team.

THE CCDC

Each health authority appoints a Consultant for Communicable Disease Control (CCDC) within its department of public health. The CCDC is responsible for the surveillance, prevention and control of communicable disease and infection within the health authority boundaries (see also Chapter 2). The CCDC usually has administrative support and may employ a scientist and a community infection control nurse.

The CCDC is a source of advice on all aspects of the control and prevention of infection, and has full responsibility for infection control in the community. Through contracts and professional collaboration with the ICT and ICD, the CCDC will ensure that there are effective arrangements for infection control in hospitals and community trusts. He or she will be a member of the local hospital infection control committee and will co-operate with the ICT and outbreak control group in the investigation and management of outbreaks of infection in hospitals.

The key tasks of the CCDC include securing the support of hospitals in implementing infection control within the community, ensuring that surveillance data and information are communicated to those who need to know, ensuring compliance with statutory requirements, following Department of Health and other relevant guidelines, and ensuring that residential homes, nursing homes and schools have access to infection control advice and assistance.

The CCDC will usually establish a District Infection Control Committee to review and advise on district-wide infection control strategies and policies, encourage collaboration between different providers, purchasers, local authorities and other agencies, and to assist the CCDC in his or her work.

LOCAL GOVERNMENT

Local government in England and Wales is based on democratically elected councils. This system has developed over many years and the councils are accountable to the residents that they serve. They are not directly accountable to central government, but exercise their responsibilities within a broad legal framework. They are funded both by central government and by locally raised revenue – the council tax.

There are 39 county councils, whose functions include police and fire services, education, social services, waste disposal, civil defence, highways, consumer protection and planning.

There are around 400 district councils, whose functions include environmental health, housing, planning, refuse collection, cemeteries and crematoria, markets and fairs, licensing activities and leisure and recreation. The district councils covering the large cities and London boroughs also perform county council functions.

Councils consist of elected members or councillors, and exercise their powers through committees, sub-committees or delegation to salaried officers. Officers acting on behalf of a council must ensure that the powers and responsibilities they exercise have been lawfully delegated to them by the elected members. Often legislation requires that the council must exercise its power through a specific officer, usually referred to as the proper officer. For some public health legislation the proper officer would be the CCDC.

Councils arrange themselves in a series of functional departments controlled by elected councillors and salaried officers. These departments include environmental health, education, social services, housing and leisure.

Environmental health departments

The responsibilities of environmental health departments include food safety, air quality, noise, waste, health and safety, water quality, port health controls at air and sea ports, refuse collection and pest control.

Environmental health officers

Environmental health officers (EHOs) are typically university graduates who have completed a period of practical training. EHOs investigate outbreaks of food and waterborne infections, advise on and enforce food safety legislation, routinely inspect food premises, investigate complaints and provide food hygiene training. They liaise with a wide range of other professionals, including the CCDC, general practitioners, teachers, microbiologists and veterinarians.

THE PUBLIC HEALTH LABORATORY SERVICE

The Public Health Laboratory Service (PHLS) began as the Emergency Public Health Laboratory Service (EPHLS) in the late 1930s when war was imminent and it was feared that the destruction of homes and the disruption of water and food supplies and sewage disposal would lead to epidemics of infectious disease. In the event there were no major epidemics and no breakdown of health services.

However, it was clear that a nationally organized network of laboratories was of great benefit to health authorities and to the medical officers of health of local government authorities. At the end of the war, the EPHLS was placed on a permanent footing with the formation of the PHLS. The aim of the PHLS is to protect the population from infection.

The modern PHLS consists of a network of some 50 public health laboratories organized into nine regional groups, together with two national centres, namely the Central Public Health Laboratory and the Communicable Disease Surveillance Centre (CDSC).

The PHLS provides information and advice to government departments to support the development of policies for the prevention and control of communicable disease.

Nearly all of the public health laboratories are based in NHS Trust Hospitals where they provide clinical diagnostic microbiological services to their host Trusts and local GPs. In addition, they undertake public health microbiology, including the testing of food, water, milk and environmental samples for local environmental health departments, and the investigation of clinical specimens from outbreaks. There are structured programmes for the microbiological surveillance of food and water.

The Central Public Health Laboratory (CPHL) is the major UK reference centre for microbiology, offering specialized tests and identification of unusual or difficult organisms and epidemiological typing.

The CDSC was set up within the PHLS in 1977, becoming the main surveillance centre, collecting, analysing and disseminating data on the occurrence and spread of communicable disease, and responding rapidly to national outbreaks or international threats of infection. The CDSC includes a regional services division which provides regional epidemiological services to the NHS Executive under contract (see below). The CDSC also provides advice and support to CCDCs, conducts national surveillance, produces the weekly *Communicable Disease Report (CDR)*, and provides training and teaching in communicable disease control.

The CPHL and CDSC play a leading role in the international surveillance and prevention of communicable disease.

THE DEPARTMENT OF HEALTH

In addition to its general responsibility for the provision of health services and social services, the Department of Health (DoH) has specific responsibility for public health, communicable disease surveillance and control, and the microbiological safety of food, water and the environment. The DoH makes policy, drafts legislation and issues guidance on legislation.

The DoH should be informed of any serious incident or outbreak of infection, and will co-ordinate the national response to any hazard, including food, medical supplies or drugs. This may include issuing appropriate hazard warning notices.

THE NATIONAL HEALTH SERVICE EXECUTIVE

The National Health Service Executive (NHSE) is a government executive agency with overall responsibility for ensuring that health services are available at local level. Regional offices of the NHS Executive provide support for the control of communicable disease through a contract for regional epidemiology services with the PHLS, and should be informed of significant incidents or outbreaks of infection in hospitals or the community.

THE HEALTH EDUCATION AUTHORITY

The Health Education Authority is the statutory body responsible for health education in England. It carries out public health education and health campaigns.

HEALTH AND SAFETY COMMISSION AND EXECUTIVE

The Health and Safety Commission (HSC) and Health and Safety Executive (HSE) are statutory bodies whose aims are to protect those at work and those who may be affected by any work-related activity (see also Chapter 2). In particular, the HSE is the enforcement agency for the Health and Safety at Work Act 1974, the Control of Substances Hazardous to Health (COSHH) Regulations 1994 and the Management of Health and Safety at Work (MHSW) Regulations 1994.

The COSHH regulations require employers to assess the risk of infection for their employees and others (e.g. waste-disposal workers, engineers and members of the public). The MHSW regulations require an assessment of risks to health, provision of health surveillance if appropriate, and provision of information for employees.

The Reporting of Incidents, Diseases and Dangerous Occurrences Regulations 1985 (RIDDOR) require employers to report acute illness requiring medical treatment where there is reason to believe that this resulted from exposure to a pathogen or infected material.

OCCUPATIONAL HEALTH SERVICES

Occupational Health Services advise managers and employees about the effect of work on health and the effect of health on work. They devise risk management programmes to ensure that the hazards which staff face during their work are minimized (see Chapter 15).

SURVEILLANCE IN THE COMMUNITY

The effective management of infectious disease depends on good surveillance. This is true whether infection occurs in hospital or in the community. Surveillance has been defined as the continuing scrutiny of all aspects of the occurrence and spread of a disease through the systematic collection, collation and analysis of data and the prompt dissemination of the resulting information to those who need to know so that action can result (see also Chapter 3). Surveillance has been described as information for action. To allow effective control, surveillance systems should be ongoing, practicable, consistent, timely, and of adequate accuracy and completeness.

THE PURPOSE OF SURVEILLANCE

1 Surveillance allows individual cases of infection to be identified so that action can be taken to prevent spread.
2 Surveillance measures the incidence of infectious disease. Changes in incidence may signal an outbreak which may need further investigation and the introduction of special control measures.
3 Surveillance tracks changes in the occurrence and risk factors of infectious disease. This allows existing control measures to be evaluated and additional measures to be introduced, if necessary, targeted at particular sections of the population. If new control measures are introduced, continuing surveillance will allow their effectiveness to be measured. For example, routine surveillance of vaccine-preventable infections allows the effectiveness of immunization programmes to be assessed. A fall in the incidence of an infection may allow existing control measures to be relaxed.
4 Surveillance allows the emergence of new infections of public health importance to be detected. It allows the epidemiology of these infections to be described, and will produce hypotheses about aetiology and risk factors.
5 Surveillance will indicate which sections of the populations are at increased risk of infection as a result of environmental or behavioural factors. This allows specific interventions to be targeted at those groups.

THE PRINCIPLES OF SURVEILLANCE

A good surveillance system consists of the following key steps.

There should be a case definition which includes clinical and/or microbiological criteria. For example, *food poisoning is defined as disease of an infectious or toxic nature caused by or thought to be caused by the consumption of food or water* (Chief Medical Officer, 1992). Case definitions have been published by the Public Health Medicine and Environmental Group and the Centers for Disease Control and Prevention.

Cases of infection are identified from a variety of sources, including reports from clinicians and laboratories. The case or an informant, who may be a relative, friend or medical or nursing attendant, is contacted by a member of the communicable disease control team by telephone, visit or letter, depending on the degree of urgency. A data-set is collected for each case. The data that is collected depends on the nature of the infection. For all infections the following minimum data set is collected: *name, date of birth, sex, address, ethnic group, place of work, occupation, name of GP, recent travel, immunization history, date of illness, clinical description of illness.*

For foodborne infections, food histories and food preferences may be recorded. For infections that are spread from person to person, the names and addresses of contacts may be requested, and for infections with an environmental source (e.g. Legionnaires' disease), places visited and routes taken may be recorded. For some infections where intervention is required, additional data is collected. For example, in the case of group C meningococcal infection, the names of close household contacts may be recorded so that chemoprophylaxis and immunization may be offered.

For rare or novel infections, or if there is a need to find out more about the epidemiology, an enhanced data-set may be collected or there may be a request for laboratory data to confirm the diagnosis. An example of this is the serological confirmation of clinical reports of measles, mumps and rubella using salivary antibody testing.

Some infections may be subject to an analytical study. In these circumstances, a detailed data-set will be collected and the cases may be matched with controls from whom a similar data-set is requested. Examples include the UK national case–control studies of hepatitis A infection, salmonella infection, campylobacter infection and verocytotoxin-producing *E. coli* infection.

Data is recorded on specially designed data-collection forms and collated in a computerized database.

One of the first uses of the data is to ensure that the cases satisfy the case definition. The database then allows analysis of the data and the production of summary statistics, including frequency counts and rates, if suitable denominators are available. This permits the epidemiology of the infection to be described in terms of person, place and time.

Local data can be shared and merged to produce data-sets at national or even international level.

Interpretation of the data and summary statistics yields information on trends and risk factors which is then disseminated so that action can be taken.

Dissemination can take place in a variety of ways, including local and national newsletters, the Internet and World Wide Web, electronic bulletin boards such as Epinet™, letters from the Chief Medical Officer and journals such as *Mortality and Morbidity Weekly Report* (MMWR), *Weekly Epidemiological Record* (WER), the *Communicable Disease Report* (CDR) and *Euro Surveillance*, a bilingual European Community disease bulletin.

There should be continuing surveillance to evaluate the effect of interventions.

SOURCES OF SURVEILLANCE DATA

A number of different data sources are available for the surveillance of infectious diseases. It is helpful to refer to the infectious disease pyramid (see Figure 18.1). Many cases of infection are subclinical. These cases can only be detected by serological surveys. Clinical infection that does not lead to a medical consultation can be measured by population surveys. Cases that are seen by a doctor may be reported via a primary care-reporting scheme or statutory notification system. Cases that are investigated by laboratory tests may be detected by a laboratory-reporting system, and those that are admitted to hospital will be detected by the hospital information system. Finally, the small proportion of infections that result in death will be detected by the death notification system.

When designing a surveillance system it is important to ensure that the most appropriate data source is utilized. For example, it is not sensible to rely on laboratory reports for the surveillance of pertussis which is only rarely diagnosed by the laboratory. In England and Wales the main routine data-collecting systems are as follows.

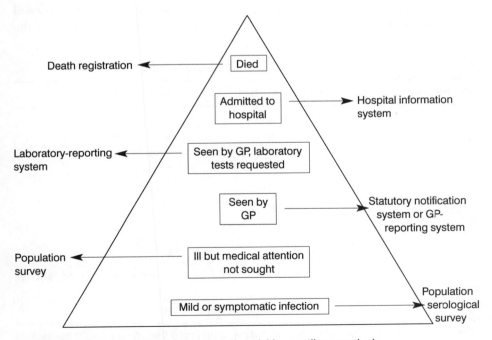

Figure 18.1 The infectious disease pyramid and available surveillance methods

STATUTORY NOTIFICATIONS OF INFECTIOUS DISEASE

The current list of notifiable infectious diseases is shown in Table 18.2. Any clinician who suspects these diagnoses is required to notify the proper officer of the local authority, who is usually the CCDC. The proper officer sends a return to the Office of National Statistics (ONS) every week. These are published weekly in the *Communicable Disease Report (CDR)*. There are also quarterly reports, and annual archives can be found on the PHLS website www.phls.co.uk, such as the *ONS Population and Health Monitor*. Statutory notifications are an important way of monitoring trends in infectious diseases, such as measles and whooping cough, for which the diagnosis is rarely confirmed by laboratory tests.

LABORATORY REPORTING SYSTEM

Public health laboratories, hospital laboratories and private laboratories should be able to offer a full diagnostic service for all common pathogenic micro-organisms. If the laboratory is unable to carry out this work, then specimens are forwarded to a suitable reference laboratory. Medical microbiologists ensure that any results of clinical significance are notified to the requesting clinician.

Micro-organisms of public health significance are also notified to the CCDC in accordance with previously agreed arrangements. This should be covered by a written policy. Typical arrangements for reporting to the CCDC are shown in Table 18.3. The method of reporting will vary depending on the urgency with which public health action is required. Increasingly, electronic reporting using Cosurv™ computer hardware and software (Henry, 1996) is being recommended, but telephone, facsimile and letter reporting are alternatives.

Reports are also sent to the CDSC either electronically or on specially designed forms. This data is collated and analysed, and is reported regularly in the

Table 18.2 Statutorily notifiable infectious diseases in England and Wales

Very rare infections	Rare infections	Common infections
Anthrax	Leptospirosis	Food poisoning[a]
Leprosy	Yellow fever	Viral hepatitis
Typhus[a]	Cholera[a]	Whooping cough
Relapsing fever[a]	Diphtheria	Tuberculosis
Plague[a]	Poliomyelitis	Malaria
Smallpox[a]	Typhoid fever	Meningitis
Viral haemorrhagic fever	Paratyphoid fever	Ophthalmia neonatorum
	Rabies	Measles
	Tetanus	Mumps
	Encephalitis	Dysentery (amoebic and bacillary)
		Rubella
		Scarlet fever

[a] Diseases that are notifiable under Section 10 of the Public Health (Control of Disease) Act 1984. The remainder are notifiable under the Public Health (Infectious Diseases) Regulations 1988.

Table 18.3 Newly diagnosed episodes of communicable and respiratory diseases reported to the Royal College of General Practitioners Birmingham Research Unit

Intestinal infectious diseases	Acute otitis media
Scarlet fever	Common cold
Whooping cough	Influenza-like illness
Meningitis/encephalitis	Sore throat/tonsillitis
Measles	Acute sinusitis
Rubella	Laryngitis and tracheitis
Chicken-pox	Epidemic influenza
Herpes zoster	Pneumonia and pneumonitis
Mumps	Acute bronchitis
Infective mononucleosis	Pleurisy
Infective hepatitis	Acute asthmatic episode
Scabies	Allergic rhinitis

Communicable Disease Report and is also available on request. Although the data is usually of high quality, it is limited to infections for which there is a suitable laboratory test. Infections which are easy to diagnose clinically tend to be inadequately covered. Trends are difficult to interpret as the data is sensitive to changes in testing or reporting by laboratories. In addition, denominators are not usually available, as neither the number of specimens tested nor the population at risk is known with certainty.

REPORTING FROM GENERAL PRACTICE

In both England and Wales there are systems which collect clinical data on initial consultations from a limited number of volunteer general practices. The data can be related to a defined population so that rates can be calculated for a selection of common diseases which are not notifiable, for which laboratory confirmation is not usually obtained, and which do not usually result in admission to hospital. These are listed in Table 18.3. The data is published by CDSC and is available on the Internet. About 70 general practices participate in the scheme, covering a population of 600 000. This population is too small for the surveillance of less common diseases, and may not be representative of the country as a whole.

HOSPITAL DATA

Data is available from district and regional information systems on infectious diseases that result in admission to hospital. This is a useful source of data on more severe diseases that are likely to result in admission to hospital (e.g. brucellosis and meningitis).

SEXUALLY TRANSMITTED DISEASES

Form KC60 records the number of initial contacts by diagnosis and sex, and is sent quarterly by all genito-urinary medicine (GUM) clinics to the Department of

Health. Male patients who are thought to have acquired their infections through homosexual contact and age group are recorded for selected infections. As clinics do not service defined catchment populations, this data is of limited use below regional or national level.

DEATH CERTIFICATION AND REGISTRATION

Mortality data on communicable diseases are of limited use because communicable diseases rarely cause death. Exceptions to this are deaths due to influenza and AIDS.

INTERNATIONAL SURVEILLANCE

Communicable disease surveillance in Europe was given considerable impetus by the World Health Organization (WHO) programme Health for All, which was first agreed in 1984. The programme includes targets such as the elimination of measles, polio, congenital rubella, diphtheria, congenital syphilis and malaria from member countries by the year 2000. Surveillance of communicable disease is undertaken by individual European countries, and collation of data from these countries is carried out on behalf of the WHO regional office for Europe in Copenhagen by WHO collaborating centres or WHO/European Community surveillance projects. Surveillance is undertaken for foodborne infections, rabies, travel-associated legionellosis, AIDS and HIV infection, influenza, tuberculosis and meningitis.

There are several European surveillance publications, including the *Rabies Bulletin of Europe*, *Tubercle and Lung Disease* and *World Health Statistics* (Healing, 1992).

OTHER SOURCES OF DATA

1 CDSC co-ordinates a national surveillance scheme for general outbreaks of infectious intestinal disease. These are outbreaks affecting members of more than one private residence or residents of an institution. They are distinct from family outbreaks, which affect members of the same private residence only. When an outbreak is over, the CCDC or lead investigator is asked to complete a structured questionnaire. The output from this scheme is reported regularly in the CDR.

2 The Medical Officers of Schools Association reports weekly to the CDSC illness in children in approximately 55 boarding-schools in England and Wales. This is useful in the surveillance of influenza.

3 The surveillance unit of the College of Paediatrics and Child Health (formerly the British Paediatric Association Surveillance Unit) co-ordinates surveillance of uncommon paediatric conditions. A reporting card listing 12–14 conditions is sent each month to consultant paediatricians in the UK. They indicate if they have seen a case that month and return the card. An investigator then contacts the paediatrician for further information. Conditions of infective origin that are under surveillance include AIDS/HIV

in childhood, congenital rubella, subacute sclerosing panencephalitis, congenital syphilis and *Haemophilus influenzae* type b (Hib) infection (Guy and Lynn,1996).

4 Cases of HIV and AIDS infection in England and Wales are reported to the CDSC on a structured report form by clinicians participating in a voluntary confidential reporting system. The form requests demographic, behavioural and clinical data.

5 Active surveillance of selected occupationally acquired infections is carried out by the Occupational Disease Intelligence Network (ODIN) at the Centre for Occupational Health, Manchester.

6 The CDSC has carried out surveillance of childhood immunization uptake since 1987 (Begg *et al.*, 1989). The results are reported regularly in the *CDR*.

7 CCDCs and local EHOs develop an informal surveillance network which receives reports from a wide range of individuals and agencies, including complaints from members of the public and reports from community and hospital medical and nursing staff.

CONTROL MEASURES FOR COMMUNITY INFECTION

The effective control of any infection in the community requires a detailed knowledge of its epidemiology, clinical features and immunology, including symptoms, signs, diagnosis, causative organism, incidence, prevalence, trends, reservoir, mode of transmission, incubation period and communicable period. Useful summaries are available (Benenson, 1995; Mandell *et al.*, 1995) (see also Chapter 8).

To prevent the spread of infection, measures can be taken to control the source of infection and the route of transmission, and susceptible individuals can be offered protection with antibiotics or immunization.

These measures are directed at the individual or case, his or her contacts, the environment and the wider community. The control measures that are adopted should be of proven effectiveness. If not, they should at least be rational. As in hospital infection control, there can be no place for infection control rituals.

PERSONAL

For surveillance purposes the case is contacted by visit, telephone or letter and details are recorded on a specially designed case-report form. Diagnostic samples may be requested (e.g. faecal samples in the case of suspected gastro-intestinal infections).

An assessment is made of the risk that the case may spread infection. Guidelines are available to aid this risk assessment. For example, with regard to gastrointestinal infections the case may be assigned to one of four risk groups, namely food-handler, health or social care worker, child aged less than 5 years or older child or adult with low standards of personal hygiene (Working Party of the PHLS

Salmonella Committee, 1995). Factors such as type of employment, availability of sanitary facilities and standards of personal hygiene should be taken into account. The risk assessment will help to determine the control measures that are needed.

1 The case may be isolated until he or she is no longer infectious. The extent of this isolation will vary. Usually isolation at home will be sufficient. However, strict isolation for highly infectious or virulent infections that spread by the airborne route as well as by direct contact may necessitate admission to a secure infectious diseases unit. It may be necessary to exclude infectious cases from school or work. The case may be kept under surveillance, examined clinically or undergo laboratory investigations.

2 The case may be treated to reduce the communicable period.

3 The case, his or her family and household contacts and medical and nursing attendants may be advised to follow certain precautions to reduce the risk of transmission. Precautions that are advised to prevent transmission of bloodborne pathogens include advice not to share personal items, careful use and disposal of needles and other sharp instruments, careful disposal of clinical waste, practice of safe sex and careful attention to blood spillages. Enteric precautions for gastro-intestinal infections may include the use of gloves and gowns, sanitary disposal of faeces and babies' nappies, attention to personal hygiene (including handwashing), regular cleaning and use of appropriate disinfectants. The case may be advised to restrict contact with young children and others who may be particularly susceptible to infection. He or she may also be advised not to prepare food for other household members.

Advice should be reinforced by written material such as leaflets, or a video may be provided. Legal powers are available, but are rarely used.

Public health law

The Public Health (Control of Disease) Act 1984 and the Public Health (Infectious Diseases) Regulations 1988 give local authorities wide-ranging powers to control communicable disease. Local government authorities exercise these powers in one of two ways, either by direct action or through the proper officer. The proper officer is an officer appointed by the local authority for a particular purpose. For communicable disease control issues, the proper officer is usually the CCDC.

Some powers, such as those which deal with the notification of diseases, are purely administrative. However, there are powers to control objects, premises and people. This includes sale of infected articles, preventing infected people from using public transport, cleaning and disinfection of premises, excluding people from work and school, offering immunization, compulsory examination, removal to hospital and detention in hospital, and obtaining information from house-holders and schools in order to prevent the spread of disease.

There are four pieces of legislation concerned with diseases which can be trans-mitted sexually. The Venereal Disease Act 1917 makes treatment and advertising treatment for STDs other than by designated clinics an offence. The National Health Service (Venereal Diseases) Regulations 1974 and the National Health

Service Trusts (Venereal Diseases) Directions 1991 give limited confidentiality to patients, and the AIDS (Control) Act 1987 requires information about AIDS to be sent to the Secretary of State.

There are public health regulations covering aircraft, ships and international trains which pass through the Channel Tunnel. These deal with infectious individuals or infectious animals or material on board.

CONTACTS

Contacts of a case of infectious disease may be at risk of acquiring infection themselves, or they may risk spreading infection to others. It is important to have a definition of a contact and to conduct a risk assessment.

For example, a contact of a case of gastrointestinal infection is someone who has been exposed to the excreta of a case. With regard to typhoid, this definition would be extended to those exposed to the same source as the case, such as those who were on the same visit abroad. A contact of a case of meningococcal infection is someone who has spent a night under the same roof as the case in the 7 days before onset or who has had mouth-kissing contact (PHLS Meningococcal Infections Working Group, 1995).

Contacts may be subjected to clinical or laboratory examination. For example, in the case of diphtheria they may be offered advice, placed under surveillance or offered prophylaxis with antibiotics or immunization. In some circumstances, contacts may be excluded from school or work. Legal powers are also available.

ENVIRONMENT

In some circumstances it may be appropriate to investigate the environment of a case of infection. This may involve inspection and laboratory investigation of a home or workplace. Examples include foodborne infections, gastrointestinal infections and Legionnaires' disease. There are legal powers to control the environment, including powers to seize, destroy and prohibit the use of certain objects. This may be necessary in the event of infection caused by a contaminated foodstuff. It may also be appropriate to advise on cleaning and disinfection.

COMMUNITY

The occurrence of cases of infection will have an effect on the wider community. For example, a case of Legionnaires' disease or tuberculosis may generate considerable anxiety in the work-force. In schools, meningitis and hepatitis B will have a similar effect on staff, pupils and parents. Scabies in day-care centres and headlice in schools are other examples.

It is helpful to keep all sections of the community informed about cases of infection. This can be done by letter or public meeting. In some circumstances it may be appropriate to set up a telephone advice line. In addition, it can be helpful to inform local newspapers, radio, television and politicians.

All sections of the community have information needs with regard to the prevention and control of infectious disease. Advice is available from a range of health professionals. This can be reinforced by leaflets, videos and through the media.

In community settings such as schools, nursing homes, residential homes and primary care it is helpful to make available written guidelines on infection control in the form of a manual or handbook. These materials can subsequently form the basis for training and audit in infection control.

PREVENTION OF INFECTIOUS DISEASE

Activity to prevent infection can be directed either at the host or at the environment.

HOST

Risk behaviour may be changed by health education campaigns. These may be national or local, and may be aimed at the general population or targeted at those who are particularly at risk.

Infections that have been the subject of national health education campaigns include HIV infection, STDs, salmonella, listeria, and *E. coli* VTEC infection. For example, the Chief Medical Officer has given the following food safety advice:

Avoid eating raw eggs or uncooked dishes made from eggs. Pregnant women, the elderly, the sick, babies and toddlers should only eat eggs that have been cooked until both the yolk and the white are solid. To avoid listeriosis, pregnant women and those people with decreased resistance to infection are advised to avoid eating soft ripe cheeses such as brie, camembert and blue vein varieties, and to avoid eating pâté. These groups are also advised to reheat cook-chilled meals and ready-to-eat poultry until piping hot, rather than eat them cold. Beefburgers should be cooked thoroughly throughout until the juices run clear and there are no pink bits inside.

Health services offer diagnosis, screening, treatment, prophylaxis and immunization. Examples include routine and selective immunization, services for tuberculosis screening and treatment for newly arrived immigrants, and services for STDs.

ENVIRONMENT

Local authority environmental health departments have responsibilities and legal powers to ensure that supplies of food and water are wholesome and will not harm health, and that there are adequate arrangements for the disposal of sewage, waste collection and disposal and pest control.

Over 99% of the population in the UK receives mains water supplies. These supplies are provided by private water companies in England and Wales. The quality of these supplies is very high, and all of them are safe to drink. Regulations require that water supplies must not contain any element, organism or substance at a concentration which would be detrimental to public health. There are legally enforceable standards for 55 different parameters. Water companies are legally obliged to test samples of the water that they supply and to report the results to the

Drinking Water Inspectorate, which since privatization has monitored quality on behalf of the government.

The Food Safety Act 1990 provides a framework for a range of food hygiene regulations which govern the activity of food businesses and implement European Community (EC) directives. The enforcement of food law is usually the responsibility of local authorities. There are statutory codes of practice which provide guidance.

The 1990 Act contains definitions of contaminated food and provides for a registration system for food businesses. There is also a requirement for hygiene training for food handlers. The Act gives EHOs powers to inspect any stage of food production, manufacturing and distribution, and to take samples for testing. EHOs can issue warnings or improvement notices, or initiate prosecutions. Regular routine inspection of food businesses is used to achieve agreed standards. The giving of advice forms a large part of this activity. The system for the inspection of food premises is based on an assessment of risk, with high-risk businesses being inspected more frequently than lower-risk premises. These inspections are an EC requirement, and the results of inspections are published regularly. The Food Safety Act 1990 Code of Practice No. 6 requires that incidents of illness and contamination of food products should be reported by the local authority to the appropriate central government department.

The Food Safety (General Food Hygiene) Regulations 1995 apply to all types of food businesses – from a hot-dog van to a five-star restaurant. They do not apply to food cooked at home for private consumption. They require food businesses to identify all steps which are critical to food safety, and to ensure that adequate safety controls are in place, maintained and reviewed. This is the formal system known as hazard analysis and critical control points (HACCP) (see also p. 250). EHOs advise businesses on how to approach HACCP. However, ultimately it is the responsibility of the food business to ensure compliance. In some cases enforcement officers may need to take action to avoid any risk to the consumer. Guidance notes and explanatory booklets are available.

The 1995 Regulations changed the arrangements governing food handlers' fitness to work (Department of Health Expert Working Party, 1995). The aim of the changes is to prevent the introduction of infection into the food business workplace by advising staff of their obligation to report to management any infectious or potentially infectious conditions, and to immediately leave the workplace if they should have such a condition. The conditions are diarrhoea and vomiting, gastrointestinal infections, enteric fever and infected lesions of the skin, eyes, ears and mouth. Before returning to work following illness due to gastrointestinal infection, there should have been no vomiting for 48 hours, a normal bowel habit for 48 hours, and good hygienic practices, particularly hand washing.

Some EC food hygiene directives require medical certification of employees in selected food businesses. The view in the UK is that there is no evidence that medical certification prevents the spread of infection from infected food handlers, as it only provides information about a prospective employee's health status at one point in time.

Other regulations include the Food Safety (Temperature Control) Regulations 1995, which detail the temperatures at which particular types of food should be stored before consumption (see p. 248). There are also a range of product-specific regulations covering fresh meat, wild game, minced meat and shellfish, aimed at dairies, meat processors or wholesale fish markets.

The government and local authorities conduct publicity campaigns about food safety and food hygiene which are aimed at food businesses and the general public.

The Meat Hygiene Service is an executive agency of the Ministry of Agriculture, Fisheries and Food, and has responsibility for hygiene and animal welfare inspection and enforcement in slaughterhouses and meat-cutting plants.

There is a comprehensive food surveillance programme with over 140 000 analyses performed each year for a wide range of food contaminants. The annual EC co-ordinated food control programmes require member states to carry out inspection and sampling of specified categories of food items, (e.g. refrigerated salads for *Listeria*). The government plans to set up a new independent Food Standards Agency in April 2000 charged with protecting public health in relation to food with powers to act at all points in the food chain.

MANAGING INFECTIOUS DISEASE INCIDENTS AND OUTBREAKS

An infectious disease incident may be defined in one of the following ways:
- two or more individuals with the same disease or symptoms or the same organism isolated from a diagnostic sample, who are linked through common exposure, personal characteristics, time or location;
- a higher than expected rate of infection compared to the usual background rate for a particular place and time;
- a single case of a particular rare or serious disease (e.g. diphtheria, rabies, viral haemorrhagic fever or poliomyelitis);
- a suspected, anticipated or actual event involving microbial or chemical contamination of food or water.

The first two of these categories may also be described as an outbreak. The control of an outbreak of infectious disease depends on early detection followed by a rapid structured investigation to uncover the source of infection and the route of transmission. This is followed by the application of appropriate control measures to prevent further cases.

Outbreaks of infectious disease in the community are usually investigated and managed by an informal team consisting of the CCDC, a medical microbiologist from the local hospital or public health laboratory, and an EHO from the local authority.

If the outbreak affects a large number of people, if it is a serious infection, if it affects a wide geographical area or if there is significant public or political interest, then consideration should be given to convening an outbreak control team to oversee the management of the episode (see p. 22). A written outbreak control plan detailing the steps that should be taken is an essential requirement (PHLS Working Group, 1993; Department of Health Working Group, 1994).

DETECTION

An outbreak will be recognized by case reports, complaints, or as a result of routine surveillance.

SYSTEMATIC INVESTIGATION

A systematic approach to the investigation of an outbreak consists of the following stages:
- establishing that a problem exists;
- confirming the diagnosis;
- immediate control measures;
- case-finding;
- collection of data;
- descriptive epidemiology;
- generating a hypothesis;
- testing the hypothesis.

Often several of these stages will be occurring simultaneously.

Establishing that a problem exists
A report of an outbreak of infection may be mistaken. It may result from increased clinical or laboratory detection of cases, changes in the size of the at-risk population or false-positive laboratory tests.

Confirming the diagnosis
Cases can be diagnosed either clinically or by laboratory investigations. At an early stage it is important to produce and adhere to a clear case definition. This is particularly important with regard to previously unrecognized diseases in which proper definitions are needed before epidemiological studies can proceed.

Immediate control measures
Control measures involve either controlling the source of infection, interrupting transmission or protecting those at risk.

Case finding
In an episode of infection, the cases that are first noticed may only be a small proportion of the total population affected, and may not be representative of that population. Efforts must be made to search for additional cases. This allows the extent of the incident to be quantified, it provides a more accurate picture of the range of illness that people have experienced, it enables individual cases to be treated and control measures to be taken, and it provides subjects for further descriptive and analytical epidemiology.

There are several ways of searching for additional cases:
- statutory notifications of infectious disease;
- requests for laboratory tests and reports of positive results;

- people attending their GPs, or the local accident and emergency department;
- hospital in-patients and out-patients;
- reports from the occupational health departments of large local businesses;
- reports from schools of absenteeism and illness;
- household enquiries;
- appeals through television, radio and local newspapers;
- screening tests applied to communities and population subgroups.

Collection of data

A set of data is collected from each of the cases. This includes the case's name, age, sex, address, occupation, name of GP, details of any recent travel, immunization history, date of illness and clinical description of illness.

Data should also be collected about exposure to possible sources of the infection. In the case of a foodborne infection, this would include a recent food history. In the case of infection spread by person-to-person contact, the case would be questioned about contact with other affected individuals. In the case of an infection spread by the airborne route, cases would be questioned about places they had visited.

It is preferable to collect this data by administering a detailed semi-structured questionnaire in a face-to-face interview. This allows the interviewer to ask probing questions which may sometimes uncover previously unsuspected associations between cases. Telephone interviews or self-completion questionnaires are less helpful at this stage of an investigation.

Descriptive epidemiology

Cases are described by the three epidemiological parameters of time, place and person. The description of cases by person includes clinical features, age, sex, occupation, social class, ethnic group, food history, travel history and leisure activities. The description of cases by place includes their home address and work address. The description of cases by time involves plotting the epidemic curve, a frequency distribution of date or time of onset. This may allow the incubation period to be estimated which, together with the clinical features, may give some clues about the causative organism (Table 18.4). The incubation period should be related to events that may have occurred in the environment of the cases and which may indicate possible sources of infection.

Generating a hypothesis

A detailed epidemiological description of typical cases may well provide the investigators with a hypothesis regarding the source of infection or the route of transmission. A description of atypical cases may also be helpful.

Testing the hypothesis

Finding that consumption of a particular food, visiting a particular place or being involved in a certain activity is occurring frequently among cases is only a first step. These risk factors may also be common among those individuals who have not been ill. To confirm an association between a risk factor and disease, further

Table 18.4 Clinical features of the main types of foodborne illnesses

Usual incubation time	Typical symptoms	Possible cause
Gastrointestinal disease		
Short		
1–14 hours	Vomiting, diarrhoea	*Bacillus subtilis*
1–5 hours	Vomiting, nausea	*Bacillus cereus*
2–6 hours	Vomiting, abdominal cramps, diarrhoea	*Staphylococcus aureus*
2–14 hours	Vomiting, abdominal cramps, diarrhoea	*Bacillus licheniformis*
Intermediate		
8–18 hours	Diarrhoea, abdominal pain	*Clostridium perfringens*
8–16 hours	Diarrhoea, abdominal pain	*Bacillus cereus*
Long		
12–48 hours	Diarrhoea, fever, abdominal pain lasting several days	*Salmonella*
12–24 hours	Nausea, vomiting, diarrhoea lasting 1–2 days	Small round structured virus
12–24 hours	Diarrhoea, abdominal pain	*Vibrio parahaemolyticus*
1–2 days	Diarrhoea plus special features (e.g. bloody diarrhoea, bloody urine)	*E.coli*
2–5 days	Diarrhoea (sometimes bloody) abdominal pain, fever	*Campylobacter*
Non-gastrointestinal disease		
13–36 hours	Weakness, double vision, swallowing difficulty, dry mouth	Botulism
12–20 days	Fever and other general signs of infection	*Salmonella typhi*
2–4 weeks	Jaundice, malaise	Hepatitis A

microbiological or environmental investigations may be required, or an analytical epidemiological study may be needed – this can be either a cohort study or a case–control study.

Case–control study. A case–control study compares exposure in individuals who are ill (the cases) with exposure in those who are not ill (the controls). Case–control studies are most useful when the affected population cannot be accurately defined. Controls can be selected from a GP's practice list, from the health authority patient register, from the laboratory that reported the case, from individuals nominated by the case or from neighbours selected at random from nearby houses.

Cohort study. The cohort study is a type of natural experiment in which a proportion of a population is exposed to a factor, while the remainder is not exposed. The incidence or attack rate of infection among exposed individuals is compared with the rate among unexposed individuals. For example, following a food poisoning outbreak at a social gathering, thought to be due to consumption of contaminated chocolate mousse, the cohort (all those who attended) is divided into those who ate the mousse (the exposed individuals) and those who did not (the unexposed individuals).

Collecting the data. A set of data is collected from both cases and controls or from the exposed and unexposed individuals within the cohort. To avoid any bias, the data must be collected from each subject in exactly the same way. Usually this is done by questionnaire. Unlike the hypothesis-generating questionnaire, the questionnaire for an analytical study is often shorter, more structured and uses mostly closed questions. It may be administered at interview or by telephone, or it may be a self-completion postal questionnaire. Questionnaires should be piloted before use. If several interviewers are to be used, they should be adequately briefed and provided with instructions to ensure that the questionnaire is administered in a consistent way.

Analysis. In both cohort and case–control studies initial analysis is by a 2 × 2 table. In cohort studies, the ratio of incidence in exposed to incidence in unexposed individuals is calculated. This is the relative risk. In case–control studies, the odds of exposure in the cases are compared with the odds of exposure in the controls. This is the odds ratio which approximates the relative risk.

Confidence intervals for these estimates can be calculated and tests of statistical significance applied. Computer programs which will perform these calculations are freely available (Dean *et al.*, 1994).

Section 2:
Hygienic and aseptic techniques (Public Health Medicine Environmental Group, 1996)

Hospital nursing procedures are based on the known availability of equipment, linen, sterile supplies, lotions and antibiotics (all at no direct cost to the patients), which are delivered to the ward or unit. The environment is controlled by the hospital authorities. The community nurse keeps such supplies and equipment as can be carried in the nursing bag or in her or his car, or which the patient can buy or loan. As a guest in the home, the community nurse has limited control over the environment, and laundry and refuse must be dealt with in the home by the patient or their relatives.

Changing patterns of hospital care have influenced domiciliary practice (e.g. early discharge of post-operative patients possibly with infected wounds or urine, or developing an infection shortly after leaving hospital), more minor surgery performed by general practitioners, early discharge of mothers who are sometimes carriers of HBV, HIV or *Salmonella typhi*, or babies carrying hospital-acquired organisms, use of disposable sharps and single-use packs (often bought on prescription, not supplied by an SSD), disposal of used dressings from discharging wounds in the absence of coal-burning fires, and disposal of colostomy bags and their contents). Special laundry and refuse collection services are sometimes but not always available, and may be expensive. Equipment supplied on loan may be difficult to disinfect adequately (e.g. commodes with fabric-covered seats). In addition, family practitioners will have their own views on methods of treatment, both in the home and in health centres or group practices. Community nurses and family practitioners are often more aware than their colleagues in hospital of the cost to the patient of procedures or treatments which they may recommend.

However, the patient at home has certain advantages over the patient in hospital. They are isolated and 'barrier-nursed' in their own home, and care is given by a limited number of trained nurses who tend to use the same methods.

The structure of the community nursing service is such that it is difficult to lay down procedures which can be universally applied. It is therefore important for community nurses to be able to apply principles of hygiene and asepsis wherever the patient may be, even in an isolated farm supplied with well water, or a caravan with no water supply.

The use of equipment which cannot be readily dried and which is used repeatedly should be avoided. This will include cotton hand towels, dish cloths for wiping surfaces, and soap dishes. Paper towels should be used for drying hands, or alternatively a freshly laundered towel. Paper towels should be used to clean and dry work surfaces. Soap should be stored dry. Failing this, washing-up liquid containing a preservative can be used. In either case, running water should be used, rather than static water in a washing bowl. Provided that the hands are physically clean, an alcoholic hand disinfectant containing an emollient which is rubbed on to the skin until it is dry is effective, and should be particularly useful in domiciliary practice. The addition of an emollient is necessary to prevent chapped hands in winter. Alcoholic wipes can also be useful for disinfecting hands and surfaces.

Sterile packs should ideally be supplied by a SSD. Although this is not always possible, SSD managers may be able to supply special packs to meet specific nursing requirements. However, there is a possible problem in Europe, in that an SSD supplying sterilized items to a different hospital or unit is considered to be a manufacturer, and must now comply with the Medical Devices Directorate, which requires industrial standards of production. For this reason, many SSDs will no longer supply health centres.

Disposable gloves are convenient for performing dressing techniques. Plastic bags, subsequently inverted and sealed, are useful for removing dressings. Dressing packs containing these items are available.

Although not microbiologically desirable, disposable insulin syringes may be re-used on the same patient for a limited period (e.g. 1 week) without increasing the risk of infection, and injections may be given without disinfecting the skin with alcohol. However, the skin must be kept clean. All needles should be discarded into an approved container (British Medical Association, 1990).

Disinfectants are seldom required for inanimate surfaces in the home. Washing with soap or detergent and water and thorough drying will usually be adequate, even when a sterile pack is to be opened on the surface. Sterile water or saline should be used for aseptic procedures. Sachets containing antiseptics (e.g. 'Savlodil') for cleaning dirty wounds are convenient.

Notes on the use of disinfectants can be found in Chapter 5. Metal instruments, generally scissors or forceps, may need to be disinfected in the home (Hoffman *et al.*,

1988; British Medical Association, 1989). Although boiling is effective in killing *Staphylococcus aureus* and other non-sporing bacteria and most viruses, instruments should preferably be supplied in sterilized packs. Scissors not used for aseptic procedures should be washed, dried and then wiped thoroughly with an alcohol-impregnated swab. A disposable plastic cover may be used for thermometers, or alternatively the thermometer can be disinfected by wiping with an alcohol-impregnated swab. Inexpensive portable autoclaves are now available and should be used in health centres. Diaphragms and rings used in family planning clinics can usually be boiled for 5–10 min after thorough washing (complete immersion is important). Immersion in a hypochlorite or other chlorine-releasing solution (1000 ppm available chlorine) for 30 min is a less desirable alternative. Disposable or autoclavable items are preferred (Working Party of the Royal College of Obstetricians and Gynaecologists, 1997). The new legal requirements for processing medical devices, which include surgical instruments, should apply to general practitioner surgeries involved in minor operations. Although infection risks are usually low, safe standards should still be used and should include a policy for testing and maintenance of autoclaves (Medical Devices Agency, 1996). A porous-load bench-top autoclave is necessary if instruments are wrapped or have a lumen. The Medical Devices Agency (1998) has produced a policy for validation and periodic testing of these porous-load autoclaves. This may not be easily carried out in a general practitioner surgery.

A disposable plastic apron should be worn to protect the nurse's uniform. The apron should be longer than those normally used in hospitals, because working heights tend to be lower than the waist area. The apron should be discarded after use.

The early discharge of mothers who are carriers of *Salmonella typhi*, HBV or HIV presents particular problems for community midwives. Salmonella carriers should be vigilant about their personal hygiene, especially with regard to handwashing before food preparation and after using the toilet. Simple isolation methods (e.g. handwashing and wearing of aprons) are described in Chapter 8, and are equally applicable in the home.

If an outbreak of gastroenteritis occurs, handwashing under running water is again the most important measure. Toilet seats, chamber pots, etc., should be washed frequently with a reliable disinfectant, but disinfectants are unnecessary for routine use in the home. Many disinfectants sold to the public are mainly of use as a deodorant, and should not be required if cleaning and drying is satisfactory. Linen from patients with hepatitis or intestinal infection can usually be laundered in the home at the highest temperature the material will withstand, provided that care is taken when handling the used linen. Cotton or cotton/polyester fabrics should be ironed when dry, using the heat of the iron to destroy any surviving pathogens. Nylon fabrics should be thoroughly dried, preferably out of doors, and stored dry for 48 hours before reuse. Disposal of clinical waste can be a problem. The risk of spread of infection from dressings, incontinence pads and disposable napkins is small. These items can be sealed in a plastic bag and safely discarded with domestic waste, but this may be unacceptable to waste handlers. A special collection service for clinical waste can be arranged if necessary. Community nurses should not be expected to carry clinical waste in their cars.

Outbreaks of boils or other superficial sepsis in a family may be caused by strains of *Staphylococcus aureus* brought home from a hospital. Patients should be treated with antibacterial nose creams and antiseptic baths (see Chapter 8). It may be necessary to sample and treat all members of the family (Leigh, 1979). Bed linen and underclothes should be laundered at as high a temperature as possible soon after treatment has commenced, and this procedure should be repeated after completion of treatment.

Epidemic strains of MRSA are present in many acute hospitals throughout the world. These are often transferred to nursing homes for the long-term care of the community (Fraise *et al.*, 1997; see also Chapter 9). Residents in these establishments are usually only colonized (e.g. nose, skin or pressure sores), and spread to others is rarely associated with a clinical problem. The potential hazard is later transfer to a susceptible patient if the colonized resident is admitted to a surgical ward of a hospital.

Although eradication would be desirable from the public health viewpoint, this is rarely practicable or cost-effective, and could be unnecessarily disturbing to elderly, otherwise healthy people. However, screening may sometimes be desirable if the individual is to be admitted to a high-risk hospital ward, although this is usually carried out on admission. These community establishments are often not equipped for acute nursing care, and range from high-dependency units to those used for residence only. Establishments or wards that provide nursing care with associated medical procedures (e.g. urinary catheterization or intravenous lines) may need to be considered as low- to moderate-risk units (British Society for Antimicrobial Chemotherapy and Hospital Infection Society Working Party, 1995; British Society for Antimicrobial Chemotherapy, Hospital Infection Society and Infection Control Nurses Association Working Party, 1998).

Colonized patients can be admitted to long-term care establishments, or sent home, with minimal risk to other residents, staff or families. It is normal for 20–30% of healthy individuals to be nasal carriers of *Staphylococcus aureus* without harm to themselves or others, irrespective of whether or not the strain is resistant to methicillin. Nasal and skin treatment will not usually be used, although in some cases a course of treatment started in hospital will require completion. Instructions should be given by the hospital. Colonized residents should be given an explanatory leaflet for themselves and their family, but in most instances if the residents have not been in a hospital with an endemic situation, they will be unaware of whether or not they are colonized. However, a member of the staff of the residential establishment should be responsible for control of infection and receive at least some basic training (Public Health Medicine Group, 1996). A simple code of practice should be written, depending on the type of establishment. Colonized individuals with lesions (e.g. pressure sores) should be treated with care, staff should wear gloves and a plastic apron when performing dressing techniques, discarded dressings and aprons should be sealed in plastic bags, and bed linen should be carefully handled and washed at high temperatures. The hands should be washed after handling residents with lesions, whether colonized with MRSA or not.

Antibiotic policies are not commonly used in domiciliary practice, but should be introduced. Particular care is required in the use of topical agents (e.g. gentamicin, mupirocin, fusidic acid), which should not be used except in very special circumstances in hospital. Varicose ulcers and pressure sores are particularly likely to be colonized with antibiotic-resistant *Staphylococcus aureus* and Gram-negative bacilli. If it is thought necessary to use a topical antibiotic, the length of treatment should be no more than 7–10 days. The widespread use of expensive oral agents such as ciprofloxacin will encourage the emergence of resistant strains and restrict the use of a valuable agent for severe infections.

Care is necessary in the collection of specimens (see Chapter 7), and transport to the laboratory should be as rapid as possible. Urine specimens kept at room temperature for more than 3 hours may be useless due to growth of contaminants, haemolytic streptococci may die on dry swabs, and sputa are also rapidly overgrown with contaminating Gram-negative bacilli or yeasts.

Further guidance on aseptic and hygienic methods can be obtained from the CCDC or the infection control nurse or infection control doctor at the nearest district general hospital.

DISINFECTION OF LOANED EQUIPMENT

A variety of equipment is available on loan, including hospital beds. Contamination during the period of loan appears to present few practical difficulties.

Generally a deodorant/disinfectant is used, as unpleasant smells are the worst problem.

Decontamination should be carried out in the home before returning equipment to the central stores. Careful washing using a detergent such as washing-up liquid, followed by thorough drying, is usually adequate even if the patient was infected. If water cannot be used, 70% alcohol or methylated spirits is effective.

Fabric-covered commodes are widely used and are difficult to disinfect adequately. If the fabric is soiled although not contaminated with known pathogens, a carpet-cleaning solution, used in accordance with the manufacturer's instructions, may be effective in improving the appearance of the fabric. If it is contaminated with pathogens, then it should be replaced by the central stores.

Some warning about specific infection risks (e.g. enteric infections) should be given so that equipment can be collected and decontaminated by the hospital. Whenever possible, equipment supplied for home use should be as easy to decontaminate as that used in the hospital.

An area within the central stores of the hospital should be set aside for decontamination of loaned equipment. Adequate sinks and drainage should be available, and a member of staff should be thoroughly trained in equipment decontamination techniques.

REFERENCES

Begg, N.T., Gill, O.N. and White, J.M. (1989) COVER (Cover of Vaccination Evaluated Rapidly): description of the England and Wales scheme. *Public Health* 103, 81.

Benenson, A.S. (1995) *Control of communicable diseases manual*. Washington, DC: American Public Health Association.

British Medical Association (1989) *Code of practice for sterilization of instruments and control of cross-infection*. London: British Medical Association.

British Medical Association (1990) *A code of practice for the safe use and disposal of sharps*. London: British Medical Association.

British Society for Antimicrobial Chemotherapy and Hospital Infection Society Working Party (1995) Guidelines on the control of methicillin-resistant *Staphylococcus aureus* in the community. *Journal of Hospital Infection* 31, 1.

British Society for Antimicrobial Chemotherapy, Hospital Infection Society and Infection Control Nurses Association Working Party (1998) Revised guidelines for the control of methicillin-resistant *Staphylococcus aureus* in hospitals. *Journal of Hospital Infection* 39, 253.

Chief Medical Officer (1992) *Definition of food poisoning*. London: Department of Health.

Dean, A.G., Dean, J.A., Coulombier, D. *et al.* (1994) *Epi Info, Version 6: a word processing, database and statistics programme for epidemiology on microcomputers*. Atlanta, GA: Centers for Disease Control and Prevention.

Department of Health Expert Working Party (1995) *Food handlers' fitness to work. Guidance for food businesses, enforcement officers and health professionals*. London: Department of Health.

Department of Health Working Group (1994) *Management of outbreaks of foodborne illness*. London: Department of Health.

Fraise, A.P., Mitchell, K., O'Brien, S.J., Oldfield, K. and Wise, R. (1997) Methicillin-resistant *Staphylococcus aureus* (MRSA) in nursing homes in a major UK city: an anonymised point prevalence survey. *Epidemiology and Infection* 118, 1.

Guy, M. and Lynn, R. (eds) (1996) *Surveillance unit – 1995–96*. London: Surveillance Unit of the College of Paediatrics and Child Health.

Healing, T.D. (1992) The surveillance of communicable disease in the European community. *Communicable Disease Report* 2, R73.

Hoffman, P.N., Cooke, E.M., Larkin, D.P. *et al.* (1988) Control of infection in general practice: a survey and recommendations. *British Medical Journal* 297, 34.

Leigh, D.A. (1979) Treatment of familial staphylococcal infection. *Journal of Antimicrobial Chemotherapy* 5, 497.

Mandell, G.L., Bennett, J.E. and Dolin, R. (eds) (1995) *Mandell, Douglas and Bennett's principles and practice of infectious diseases*, 4th edn. New York: Churchill Livingstone.

Medical Devices Agency (1996) *The purchase, operation and maintenance of benchtop steam sterilizers*. London: Medical Devices Agency.

Medical Devices Agency (1998) *The validation and periodic testing of benchtop vacuum steam sterilizers*. London: Medical Devices Agency.

PHLS Meningococcal Infections Working Group (1995) Control of meningococcal disease: guidance for consultants for communicable disease control. *Communicable Disease Report* 5, R189.

PHLS Working Group (1993) Revised guidelines for the control of *Shigella sonnei* infection and other infective diarhoeas. *Communicable Disease Report* 3, R69.

Public Health Medicine Group (1996) *Guidelines on the control of infection in residential and nursing homes.* London: Deaprtment of Health.

Public Health Medicine Environmental Group (1996) *Guidelines on the control of infection in residential and nursing homes.* London: Department of Health.

Working Party of the PHLS Salmonella Committee (1995) The prevention of human transmission of gastrointestinal infections, infestations and bacterial intoxications: a guide for public health physicians and environmental health officers in England and Wales. *Communicable Disease Report* 5, R158.

Working Party of the Royal College of Obstetricians and Gynaecologists (1997) *HIV infections in maternity care and gynaecology.* London: Royal College of Obstetricians and Gynaecologists.

FURTHER READING

Advisory Committee on Dangerous Pathogens (1996) *Management and control of viral haemorrhagic fevers.* London: HMSO.

Bradley, D. and Warhurst, D.C. (1995) Malaria prophylaxis: guidelines for travellers from Britain. *British Medical Journal* 310, 709.

Button, J.T.H. (1994) *Communicable disease control: a practical guide to the law for health and local authorities.* London: Public Health Legal Information Unit in association with the Department of Health and the Welsh Office.

Cartwright, K.A.V., Begg, N.T. and Rudd, P. (1994) Use of vaccines and antibiotic prophylaxis in contacts and cases of *Haemophilus influenzae* type b (Hib) disease. *Communicable Disease Report* 4, R16.

Department of Health (1988) *Public health in England: the Report of the Committee of Inquiry into the future development of the Public Health Function.* London: Department of Health.

Department of Health (1991) *The health of the nation.* London: HMSO.

Healing, T.D., Hoffman, P.N. and Young, S.E.J. (1995) The infection hazards of human cadavers. *Communicable Disease Report* 5, R61.

Interdepartmental Working Group on Tuberculosis (1996) *Recommendations for the prevention and control of tuberculosis at local level.* London: Department of Health and Welsh Office.

NHS Management Executive (1993) *Public health: responsibilities of the NHS and the role of others.* Leeds: NHS Management Executive.

Newman, C.P.S. (1993) Surveillance and control of *Shigella sonnei* infection. *Communicable Disease Report* 3, R63.

Saunders, C.J.P., Joseph, C.A. and Watson, J.M. (1994) Investigating a single case of Legionnaires' disease: guidance for consultants in communicable disease control. *Communicable Disease Report*, 4, R112.

Subcommittee of the Joint Tuberculosis Committee of the British Thoracic Society (1994) Control and prevention of tuberculosis in the United Kingdom: code of Practice. *Thorax* 49, 1193.

Subcommittee of the PHLS Working Group on Vero cytotoxin-producing *Escherichia coli* (VTEC) (1995) Interim guidelines for the control of infections with Vero cytotoxin-producing *Escherichia coli*. *Communicable Disease Report* 5, R77.

UK Departments of Health (1998) *Guidance for clinical health care workers: protection against infection with blood-borne viruses*. London: Department of Health.

UK Health Departments (1992) *Immunisation against infectious disease*. London: HMSO.

UK Health Departments and the PHLS Communicable Disease Surveillance Centre (1995) *Health information for overseas travel*. London: HMSO.

Viral Gastroenteritis Subcommittee of the PHLS Virology Committee (1993) Outbreaks of gastroenteritis associated with SRSVs. *PHLS Microbiology Digest* 10, 2.

Wall, P.G., de Louvois, J., Gilbert, R.J. and Rowe, B. (1996) Food poisoning: notifications, laboratory reports and outbreaks – where do the statistics come from and what do they mean? *Communicable Disease Report* 6, R93.

BIBLIOGRAPHY

Altemeier, W.A., Burke, J.F., Pruitt, B.A. and Sandusky, W.R. (ed. Committee) (1984) *Manual on control of infection in surgical patients.* Philadelphia, PA: Lippincott.

Ayliffe, G.A.J., Coates, D. and Hoffman, P.N. (1993) *Chemical disinfection in hospitals,* 2nd edn. London: Public Health Laboratory Service.

Ayliffe, G.A.J., Babb, J.R. and Taylor, L.J. (1999) *Hospital-acquired infection. Principles and prevention,* 3rd edn. London: John Wright.

Bartlett, C.L.R., Macrae, A.D. and MacFarlane, J.D. (1986) *Legionella infections.* London: Edward Arnold.

Benenson, A.S. (1995) *Control of communicable disease in man,* 16th edn. New York: American Public Health Association.

Bennett, J.V. and Brachman, P.S. (1998) *Hospital infections,* 4th edn. Boston, MA: Little Brown.

Block, S.S. (2000) *Disinfection, sterilization and preservation.* 5th edn. Philadelphia, PA: Lea & Febiger.

Collins, C.H. and Kennedy, D.A. (1999) *Laboratory-acquired infections. History, incidence and preventions,* 4th edn. Oxford: Butterworth-Heinemann.

Crow, S. (1989) *Asepsis, the right touch.* Louisiana: Everett Co.

Damani, N.N. (1997) *Manual of infection control procedures.* London: Medical Media.

Emmerson, A.M. and Ayliffe, G.A.J. (eds) (1996) *Surveillance of nosocomial infections. Baillière's clinical infectious diseases.* Vol. 3. London: Baillière Tindall.

Gardner, J.F. and Peel, M.M. (1998) *Sterilization, disinfection and infection control,* 2nd edn. Edinburgh: Churchill Livingstone.

Greenwood, D., Slack, R. and Petherer, J. (eds) (1992) *Medical microbiology: a guide to microbial infections, pathogenesis, immunity, laboratory diagnosis and control,* 14th edn. Edinburgh: Churchill Livingstone.

Hobbs, B.C. and Roberts, D. (1993) *Food poisoning and food hygiene,* 6th edn. London: Edward Arnold.

Infection Control Nurses Association, London Regional Group (1995) *Infection control information resources.* Harpenden: Mediaprint.

International Federation of Infection Control (1995) *Education programme for infection control, basic concepts and training.* London: International Federation of Infection Control.

Johnston, I.D.A. and Hunter, A.R. (eds) (1984) *The design and utilization of operating-theatres.* London: Edward Arnold.

Kucers, A., Crowe, S.M., Grayson, M.L. and Hoy, J.F. (1997) *The use of antibiotics: a clinical review of antibacterial, antifungal and antiviral drugs,* 5th edn. Oxford: Butterworth-Heinemann.

Mandell, G.L., Bennett, J.E. and Dolin, R. (2000) *Principles and practice of infectious disease.* 5th edn. Edinburgh: Churchill Livingstone.

Maurer, I.M. (1985) *Hospital hygiene.* 3rd edn. London: Edward Arnold.

Mayhall, C.G. (ed.) (1999) *Hospital epidemiology and infection control.* Baltimore, MD: Williams and Wilkins.

Meers, P., McPherson, M. and Sedgwick, J. (1997) *Infection control in healthcare.* Cheltenham: Stanley Thornes.

Mehtar, S. (1992) *Hospital infection control. Setting up a cost-effective programme with minimal resources.* Oxford: Oxford Medical Publications.

Moi Lin, L., Ching Tai Yin, P. and Wing Hong, S. (1999) *A handbook of infection control for the Asian healthcare worker.* Hong Kong: Excerpta Medica Asia Ltd.

O'Grady, F.W., Lambert, H.P., Finch, R.G. and Greenwood, D. (1997) *Antibiotic and chemotherapy. Anti-infective agents and their use in therapy,* 7th edn. Edinburgh: Churchill Livingstone.

Philpott-Howard, J. and Casewell, M. (1994) *Hospital infection control: policies and practical procedures.* London: Saunders.

Russell, A.D., Hugo, W.B. and Ayliffe, G.A.J. (eds) (1999) *Principles and practice of disinfection, preservation and sterilization.* 3rd edn. Oxford: Blackwell Science.

Shanson, D. (1999) *Microbiology in clinical medicine,* 3rd edn. Oxford: Butterworth-Heinemann.

Slade, N. and Gillespie, W.A. (1985) *The urinary tract and the catheter: infection and other problems.* Chichester: John Wiley.

Taylor, E.W. (ed.) (1992) *Infection and surgical practice.* Oxford: Oxford Medical Publications.

Wenzel, R.P. (ed.) (1997) *Prevention and control of nosocomial infections.* 3rd edn. Baltimore, MD: Williams & Wilkins.

Wilson, J. (1995) *Infection control in clinical practice.* London: Baillière Tindall.

World Health Organization (1996) *Guidelines for preventing HIV, HBV and other infections in the health care setting.* New Delhi: Regional Office for South East Asia.

Worsley, M.A., Ward, K.A., Parker, L., Ayliffe, G.A.J. and Sedgwick, J.A. (1990) *Infection control: guidelines for nursing care.* London: Infection Control Nurses Association.

INDEX

Page references in *italics* refer to figures; those in **bold** refer to tables